Comparative Cardiac Imaging
A Case-based Guide

Comparative Cardiac Imaging
A Case-based Guide

Chief Editor
Jing Ping Sun, MD, FACC, FAHA
Visiting Professor
Division of Cardiology
Department of Medicine and Therapeutics
Prince of Wales Hospital
The Chinese University of Hong Kong
Hong Kong SAR

Associate Editor
Xing Sheng Yang, MD, PhD, FACC, FAHA
Visiting Professor
Division of Cardiology
Department of Medicine and Therapeutics
Prince of Wales Hospital
The Chinese University of Hong Kong
Hong Kong SAR

Associate Editor
Bryan P. Yan, MD, FACC, FRACP, FESC, FRCPE
Associate Professor,
Division of Cardiology
Department of Medicine and Therapeutics
Prince of Wales Hospital
The Chinese University of Hong Kong
Hong Kong SAR

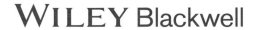

Registered Office(s)
John Wiley & Sons, Inc., 111 River Street, Hoboken, NJ 07030, USA
John Wiley & Sons Ltd, The Atrium, Southern Gate, Chichester, West Sussex, PO19 8SQ, UK

Editorial Office
9600 Garsington Road, Oxford, OX4 2DQ, UK

For details of our global editorial offices, customer services, and more information about Wiley products visit us at www.wiley.com.

Wiley also publishes its books in a variety of electronic formats and by print-on-demand. Some content that appears in standard print versions of this book may not be available in other formats.

Library of Congress Cataloging-in-Publication Data
Names: Sun, Jingping, editor. | Yang, Xingsheng, editor. | Yan, Bryan P., editor.
Title: Comparative cardiac imaging : a case-based guide / edited by Jing Ping Sun, Xing Sheng Yang, Bryan P. Yan.
Other titles: Comparative cardiac imaging (Sun)
Description: Hoboken, NJ : Wiley, 2018. | Includes bibliographical references and index. |
Identifiers: LCCN 2017050778 (print) | LCCN 2017051146 (ebook) | ISBN 9781119453178 (pdf) |
    ISBN 9781119453208 (epub) | ISBN 9781119453192 (oBook) | ISBN 9780470656372 (cloth)
Subjects: | MESH: Heart Diseases–diagnostic imaging | Heart–diagnostic imaging |
    Cardiac Imaging Techniques–methods | Case Reports
Classification: LCC RC670 (ebook) | LCC RC670 (print) | NLM WG 141 | DDC 616.1/2075–dc23
LC record available at https://lccn.loc.gov/2017050778

Cover Design: Wiley
Cover Image: © temet/Gettyimages

Set in 9.5/12pt Minion by SPi Global, Pondicherry, India

Printed in Singapore by C.O.S. Printers Pte Ltd

10 9 8 7 6 5 4 3 2 1

Contents

Part II Artery Disease

Part III Cardiac Mass

Part IV Cardiomyopathy and Myocarditis

Part V Diversification

Notes on Contributors

Yuanqing Cai

Department of Ultrasound, Xinqiao Hospital, Third Military Medical University, Chongqing, China
wctsai@seed.net.tw

Anna K. Y. Chan

Division of Cardiology, Department of Medicine and Therapeutics, Prince of Wales Hospital, The Chinese University of Hong Kong, Hong Kong
ccp639@ha.org.hk

Doris T. Chan

Division of Cardiology, Department of Medicine and Therapeutics, Prince of Wales Hospital, The Chinese University of Hong Kong, Hong Kong

Liu Chen

Department of Cardiology, West China Hospital of Sichuan University, Chengdu, Sichuan Province, China
297521926@qq.com

Ming Chen

Department of Ultrasound in Medicine, Shanghai East Hospital, Tongji University School of Medicine, Shanghai, China
mingchen1283@vip.163.com

Ligang Fang

Department of Cardiology, Affiliated Hospital of Peking Union Medical College, Beijing, China
fanglgpumch@sina.com

Yuan Feng

Department of Cardiology, West China Hospital of Sichuan University, Chengdu, Sichuan Province, China
fynotebook@hotmail.com

Ran Guo

Department of Cardiology, First Affiliated Hospital of Dalian Medical University, Dalian, China
guo2652402@163.com

Changchun Hao

Qinglong Country Hospital, Hebei Province, China
1058899098@qq.com

Ben He

Department of Cardiology, Renji Hospital, Tongji University School of Medicine Shanghai, China
drheben@126.com

Junli Hu

Department of Ultrasonography, Affiliated Hospital of Jining Medical University, Jining, Shandong Province, China
hujunli517@126.com

Shuran Huang

Department of Intensive Care Unit, Affiliated Hospital of Jining Medical University, Jining, Shandong Province, China
isabeir@163.com

Yong Huo

Department of Cardiology, Peking University First Hospital, Beijing Medical School Beijing, China
drhuoyong@163.com

Yong Jiang

Department of Ultrasound, Fuwai Hospital, Beijing, China
yangjian1212@hotmail.com

Kevin Ka-Ho Kam

Division of Cardiology, Department of Medicine and Therapeutics
Prince of Wales Hospital, The Chinese University of Hong Kong, Hong Kong
Kk381@ha.org.hk

Alex Pui-Wai Lee

Division of Cardiology, Department of Medicine and Therapeutics
Prince of Wales Hospital, The Chinese University of Hong Kong, Hong Kong
alexpwlee@cuhk.edu.hk

Cheng-Han Lee

Divisions of Cardiology, Department of Internal Medicine, School of Medicine, National Cheng Kung University, Taiwan
appollolee@hotmail.com

Yi Liang

Department of Cardiology, Affiliated Hospital of Zhenjiang Medical College, Zhenjiang, Jiangsu Province, China
13918196530@139.com

Ping-Yen Liu

Divisions of Cardiology, Department of Internal Medicine, School of Medicine, National Cheng Kung University, Taiwan
larry@mail.ncku.edu.tw

Yi Liu

Department of Ultrasound in Medicine, Shanghai East Hospital, Tongji University School of Medicine, Shanghai, China
13918196530@139.com

Jen-Li Looi

Division of Cardiology, Department of Medicine and Therapeutics, Prince of Wales Hospital, The Chinese University of Hong Kong, Hong Kong
Jenli.Looi@middlemore.co.nz

Lan Ma

Echocardiographic Department, Shanghai Chest Hospital, Jiaotong University, Shanghai, China
majing0709@163.com

Fanxia Meng

Department of Ultrasound in Medicine, Shanghai East Hospital, Tongji University School of Medicine, Shanghai, China
mengmeng8219@hotmail.com

Xianda Ni

Department of Ultrasonography, The First Affiliated Hospital of Wenzhou Medical University, Wenzhou, Zhejiang Province, China
xianda.ni@gmail.com

Litong Qi

Department of Cardiology, Peking University First Hospital, Beijing Medical School, Beijing, China
qilitong2013@outlook.com

Zhiqing Qiao

Department of Cardiology, Renji Hospital, School of Medicine, Shanghai Jiaotong University Shanghai, China
oq1z2q3@yeah.net

Xuedong Shen

Department of Cardiology, Renji Hospital, School of Medicine, Shanghai Jiaotong University, Shanghai, China
shenxd@hotmail.com

Ming-Ming Sim

Department of Cardiology, Landseed Hospital, Taiwan

Guiling Sui

Department of Ultrasonography, Affiliated Hospital of Jining Medical University, Jining, Shandong Province, China
sgl671231@163.com

Jing Ping Sun

Division of Cardiology, Department of Medicine and Therapeutics
Prince of Wales Hospital, The Chinese University of Hong Kong, Hong Kong
Jingpingsun6@gmail.com, Jingpingsun6@yahoo.com

Zhanguo Sun

Shandong Provincial Key Laboratory of Cardiac Disease Diagnosis and Treatment, Affiliated Hospital of Jining Medical University, Jining, Shandong Province, China
yingxiangszg@163.com

Hong Tang

Department of Cardiology, West China Hospital of Sichuan University, Chengdu, Sichuan Province, China
hxyyth@qq.com

Wei-Chuan Tsai

Divisions of Cardiology, Department of Internal Medicine, School of Medicine, National Cheng Kung University, Taiwan
wctsai@seed.net.tw

Hao Wang

Department of Ultrasound, Fuwai Hospital, Beijing, China
hal6112@gmail.com

Hongjun Wang
Department of Ultrasonography, Affiliated
Hospital of Jining Medical University,
Jining, Shandong Province, China
wanghongjunjyfy@163.com

Jingjin Wang
Department of Ultrasound, Fuwai Hospital,
Beijing, China
jingjin0305@yahoo.com

Shaochun Wang
Department of Ultrasonography, Affiliated
Hospital of Jining Medical University,
Jining, Shandong Province, China
jn_usm@163.com

Yining Wang
Department of Cardiology, Affiliated
Hospital of Peking Union Medical College,
Beijing, China
liu987@vip.sina.com

Ka-Tak Wong
Division of Radiology, Prince of Wales Hospital,
The Chinese University of Hong Kong,
Hong Kong
wongkatak@gmail.com

Weihua Wu
Echocardiographic Department, Shanghai Chest
Hospital, Jiaotong University, Shanghai, China
liu987@vip.sina.com

Hongmei Xia
Department of Ultrasound, Xinqiao Hospital,
Third Military Medical University, Chongqing,
China
xiahm985206@126.com

Lianghua Xia
Department of Ultrasound in Medicine,
Shanghai East Hospital, Tongji
University School of Medicine,
Shanghai, China
huaoo4@163.com

Min Xu
Department of Ultrasound in Medicine,
Shanghai East Hospital, Tongji
University School of Medicine,
Shanghai, China
autumnsky_1204@163.com

Nan Xu
Department of Ultrasound in Medicine, Shanghai
East Hospital,
Tongji University School of Medicine, Shanghai,
China
southmuch@hotmail.com

Yali Xu
Department of Ultrosound, Xinqiao Hospital,
The Military Medical University, Chonqging,
China
xuyali1976@163.com

Bryan P. Yan
Division of Cardiology, Department of Medicine
and Therapeutics
Prince of Wales Hospital, The Chinese University
of Hong Kong, Hong Kong
bryan.yan@cuhk.edu.hk

Jinchuan Yan
Department of Cardiology, Affiliated Hospital of
Zhenjiang Medical College, Zhenjiang, Jiangsu
Province, China
yanjinchuan@hotmail.com

Li-Tan Yang
Divisions of Cardiology, Department of Internal
Medicine, School of Medicine, National Cheng
Kung University, Taiwan
litanyang@yahool.com.tw

Xing Sheng Yang
Division of Cardiology, Department of Medicine
and Therapeutics
Prince of Wales Hospital, The Chinese
University of Hong Kong, Hong Kong
Xingshengyang0018@gmail.com

Ying Yang
Department of Cardiology, Peking
University First Hospital, Beijing
Medical School
Beijing, China
yangying1527@163.com

Guozhen Yuan
Department of Ultrasonography,
Affiliated Hospital of Jining
Medical University,
Jining, Shandong Province, China
yuanguozhen@126.com

Bo Zhang

Department of Ultrasound in Medicine, Shanghai
East Hospital, Tongji University School of
Medicine, Shanghai, China
zhangbodongfang@qq.com

Chengzheng Zhang

Department of Ultrasonography, Affiliated
Hospital of Jining Medical University,
Jining, Shandong Province, China
120098555@qq.com

Fen Zhang

Department of Cardiology, Affiliated Hospital of
Zhenjiang Medical College, Zhenjiang, Jiangsu
Province, China
987971534@qq.com

Haiping Zhang

Department of Ultrasonography, The Second
Affiliated Hospital of Wenzhou Medical
University, Wenzhou, Zhejiang Province, China

Lei Zhang

Department of Radiology, Shanghai East
Hospital, Tongji University School of Medicine,
Shanghai, China
zhanglei4302@hotmail.com

Ying Zheng

Department of Cardiology, Renji Hospital,
Shanghai Jiaotong University School of Medicine,
Shanghai, China
drzhengying@163.com

Foreword

Advances in cardiac imaging have been spectacular over the past several decades. The anatomic and functional detail offered by echocardiography, cardiac magnetic resonance, and computed tomographic angiography allows precise delineation of the pathophysiology of both congenital and acquired cardiac diseases. However, each imaging specialist tends to be highly skilled in only one imaging technique, yet the practicing cardiologist needs to be able to interpret and integrate data correctly from all the modalities. Over the past decade a number of advanced training programs in cardiac imaging have striven to train cardiovascular specialists broadly in the use of these imaging methods and this has resulted in a modest number of recently trained physicians being skilled in all modalities. Yet there is a need for all cardiologists to become better informed about the advantages of each technique as well as their similarities and differences.

Dr. Sun with this publication *Cardiac Imaging – A Case-based Guide*, has greatly assisted cardiologists in acquiring this knowledge. She has collected a series of cases that present rather rare and challenging congenital cardiac disorders as well as complex acquired cardiac diseases where precise cardiac imaging is essential. She shows all the imaging modalities for each cardiac lesion, compares the contributions of each imaging modality, and discusses the history and pathophysiology of each specific defect. Key references are provided for each of the often unusual diseases. The reader will quickly gain an overview of the exquisite details provided by contemporary cardiac imaging, which is of great value. Using the format of standard case presentations with static images plus the technological advance of imbedded cine loops from each imaging technique, Dr. Sun has provided a readily accessible approach to a better appreciation of normal cardiac anatomy, the complex anatomic alterations of cardiac malformations, and the structural changes associated with acquired cardiac diseases. Reading and studying this collation of clinical cases will be an enjoyable learning experience for cardiac imaging specialists as well as pediatric and adult cardiologists.

Robert C Bahler, M.D.
Emeritus Professor of Medicine
Case Western Reserve University School of Medicine
at MetroHealth Medical Center
Cleveland, OH, United States

Preface

Noninvasive cardiac imaging includes a combination of different modalities that can be used to evaluate both cardiac structure and function. As a result of technological advances, the number of available noninvasive cardiac tests in the physician's armamentarium has increased substantially over the last decade. Anatomic and functional information obtained from echocardiography, cardiac magnetic resonance and computed tomographic angiography allows precise delineation of pathophysiology of both congenital and acquired cardiac diseases. However, each imaging specialist tends to be highly skilled in only one imaging technique, yet the practicing cardiologist needs to be able to correctly interpret and integrate data from all the modalities.

Case-based learning is a time-honored tradition in cardiac imaging training. Students or fellows often spend many years in the echocardiography laboratory or radiology department to chance encounter the wealth and breadth of cardiac pathologies that are referred for noninvasive assessment. However, there can be inconsistency and variability in this method of learning between individual experiences. We have collected a spectrum of interesting and rare cases in this book to provide physicians a readily accessible resource or reference to enable them to appreciate better the normal cardiac anatomy, complex cardiac malformations, congenital, and acquired cardiac diseases. These cases mainly come from China which is a large country covering approximately one-fifteenth of the world's total land mass and 20% of the world's population. Each case is presented with a short vignette, key imaging findings (both still frame and videos), with expert interpretation, differential diagnosis, discussion of pathology and disease management, and comparison between imaging modalities used.

With rapidly improving healthcare access for both the urban and rural Chinese population and physician experience in noninvasive cardiac imaging, we have been overwhelmed by the range of cardiac pathologies that are educational, some rarely seen or published in Western literature. We hope our selection of cases will offer a window of opportunity for both students and experts to discover some hidden treasures and mysteries from the orient.

Jing Ping Sun, MD, FACC, FAHA

Xing Sheng Yang, MD, PhD, FACC, FAHA

Bryan P. Yan, MD, FACC

Abbreviations

2D	Two dimensional
3D	Three-dimensional
A2C	Apical two chamber
A3C	Apical three chamber
A4C	Apical four chamber
A5C	Apical five chamber
AAO	Ascending aorta
ABD	Abdomen aorta
AO	Aorta
AV	Aortic valve
CS	Coronary sinus
DAO	Descending aorta
LA	Left atrium
LA	Left atrium
LV	Left ventricle
LV	Left ventricle
M-mode	Time motion mode
MV	Mitral valve
PA	Pulmonary artery (right = RPA; left = LPA)
PEff	Pericardial effusion
PLAx	Parasternal long axis
PlEff	Pleural effusion
PSAx	Parasternal short axis
PV	Pulmonic valve
PVn	Pulmonary vein (left upper pulmonary vein = LUPV; right upper = RUPV)
RA	Right atrium
RV	Right ventricle
SC	Subcostal
SSN	Suprasternal notch
TEE	Transesophageal echocardiography or transoesophageal echocardiogram
TTE	Transthoracic echocardiography
TV	Tricuspid valve

About the Companion Website

This book is accompanied by a companion website:

www.wiley.com/sun/comparative_cardiac_imaging

The Web site includes:
• Videos showing cardiac images described in the book.

The videos are clearly signposted throughout the book. Look out for .

Part I
Congenital Heart Disease in the Adult

1 Aneurysmal Aorto–Left Ventricular Tunnel and Bicuspid Aortic Valve with Severe Stenosis

Fanxia Meng[1], Bo Zhang[1], Nan Xu[1], and Jing Ping Sun[2]

[1] Tongji University, Shanghai, China
[2] The Chinese University of Hong Kong, Hong Kong

History

A 60-year-old male presented with increasing shortness of breath over 2 years.

Physical Examination

The heart rate was 80 bpm, with frequent premature beats. On auscultation, there were 3/6 systolic and diastolic murmurs at the left parasternal edge in the third intercostal space.

Transthoracic Echocardiogram

A transthoracic echocardiogram showed that the aortic valves were severely calcified (Figure 1-1*) with stenosis (peak velocity was 6 m/s) and mild regurgitation. An aorto–left-ventricular tunnel (ALVT) (T) with entry from the aorta (thick arrow) and exit (thin arrow) into the left ventricle (LV) was seen (Figure 1). Blood flows from the aorta into the ALVT (T), and then into the LV cavity which can be seen by the color Doppler (Figure 1-1B). Left ventricle hypertrophy with normal systolic function was noted (Video 1-1). Nonvalvular regurgitation (thick arrow) and a shunt from aorta into ALVT (thin arrow) was seen by color Doppler (Figure 1-1D, Video 1.2).

A computer angiogram showed that the ascending aorta was dilated, with an aneurysmal ALVT (T) arising from the aortic root and connected with the LV (*) (Figure 1-2A). The aortic annulus, aortic valves, and tunnel (T) were severely calcified (arrow), (Figure 1-2B). The connection (*) between the aortic root and ALVT (T) could be seen (Figure 1-2C). Three-dimensional reconstruction computed tomography imaging showed aneurysmal ALVT (arrow), left coronary artery (LCA) arising from aortic root (arrow) behind the aneurysmal ALVT, and significantly dilated ascending AO (Figure 1-2D).

Management

The patient underwent open heart surgery. Surgical inspection revealed a 3 cm aneurysmal tunnel with smooth surface, it was (white arrow) arising from the left Valsalva sinus, located at below the LCA orifice (Figure 1-3). The aortic valve was bicuspid and severely

Comparative Cardiac Imaging: A Case-based Guide, First Edition.
Edited by Jing Ping Sun, Xing Sheng Yang, and Bryan P. Yan.
© 2018 John Wiley & Sons Ltd. Published 2018 by John Wiley & Sons Ltd.
Companion website: www.wiley.com/sun/comparative_cardiac_imaging

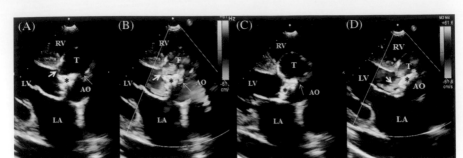

Figure 1-1 Transthoracic echocardiogram showed: A. Aortic valves displayed severe calcification (Figure 1-1.*). An aorto-left ventricular tunnel (ALVT) (T) was seen with entry from the aorta (thin arrow) and exit (thick arrow) into the left ventricle (LV). B. The blood flow from the aorta into the ALVT (T) and out of the tunnel into the LV were seen with color Doppler. C. The outline of the tunnel (T) with the entrance from the aorta was clearly seen. D. A nonvalvular regurgitation (thick arrow) and a shunt from the aorta into the ALVT (thin arrow) were seen with color Doppler.

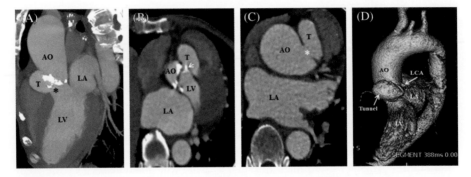

Figure 1-2 Computer angiogram showed: A. Computed tomography scan, long-axis view, showed the dilated ascending aorta, an aneurysmal ALVT (T) arising from aortic root and connected with the LV (*). B. The short-axis view showed the aortic annulus with calcification, and calcificatiive connection (arrow) between the LV and tunnel (T). C. The short-axis view showed the connection (*) between the aortic root and ALVT (T). D. Computed tomography three-dimensional reconstruction imaging showed aneurysmal ALVT (arrow), left coronary artery (LCA) arising from the aortic root (arrow) behind the aneurysmal ALVT, and significantly dilated ascending AO.

calcified. The aortic and LV orifices of the ALVT were repaired, and the aortic valve was replaced. The patient recovered well after the operation. A follow-up echocardiogram showed a well-seated and functioning prosthetic aortic valve.

Discussion

An aorto–left-ventricular tunnel (ALVT) is a congenital extracardiac channel connecting the ascending aorta to either left or right ventricular cavity. It is extremely rare with incidence as low as 0.001% of all congenital heart diseases [1]. Hovaguimian and colleagues [2] classified the ALVT into four types (I, II, III, and IV) that have a bearing on the appropriate surgical techniques of repair: A slitlike opening at the aortic end with no valve distortion in type I (prevalence, 24%), a large extracardiac aneurysm in type II (44%), an intracardiac aneurysm of the septal portion of the tunnel with or without right

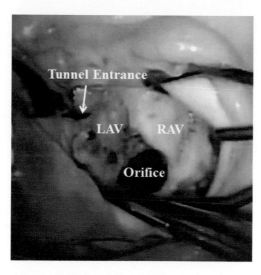

Figure 1-3   Intraoperative picture showed the entrance of tunnel (white arrow) arising from the left Valsalva sinus, located at below and in front of the LCA orifice in the ascending aorta.

ventricular outflow tract obstruction in type III (24%), and a combination of types II and III in type IV (8%). In most cases, the aortic orifice of the tunnel arises from the right coronary sinus and is on the anterolateral side of the ascending aorta [2].The ALVT rarely arises from the left coronary sinus, and there are only a few reports of this presentation [3, 4].

In our patient the aortic orifice of the aneurysmal tunnel arises from the left coronary sinus below the orifice of the left coronary artery.The exit of the tunnel into the left ventricle appears narrow and has severe calcification. This patient had congenital ALVT associated with a bicuspid aortic valve with severe calcification and stenosis. To the best of our knowledge, this is very rare in the literature.

Associated Anomalies

Aortic valve abnormalities like dysplastic or bicuspid valve with stenosis are frequent [5], but aortic atresia has rarely been reported [6]. Stenosis of the pulmonary valve [7] and subvalvular pulmonary obstruction due to a tunnel have been reported [8]. Proximal coronary anomalies like coronary ostium lying within the tunnel or atresia of coronary ostium have been documented [9].

Clinical Presentation

The clinical presentation of ALVT varies depending upon the compression of the coronary arteries, the presence of right or left ventricular outflow obstruction, and the diameter of the tunnel [10–12]. Congestive heart failure frequently develops during the first year of life [10]. The onset, severity, and progression of heart failure vary and range from *in utero* fetal death [13] to asymptomatic adulthood [14], and this depends on the cross-sectional area of tunnel and the amount of aortic regurgitation [15]. Chronic preload due to regurgitation leading to LV dilatation is seen in asymptomatic grown-up patients. Early diagnosis and surgical correction are essential to prevent irreversible myocardial dysfunction and heart failure. Untreated cases may progress to the development of native aortic valve regurgitation. The development of symptoms may be delayed if the tunnel terminates in the right ventricle and has a significant right ventricular outflow tract obstruction, thereby limiting the magnitude of the shunt [16].

In our case, the tunnel terminus was narrow, which limited the regurgitation from the aorta and resulted in the ALVT becoming aneurysmal. Due to a small amount of regurgitation, there was no left ventricular dilatation and heart failure until the patient was 60 years old. Shortness of breath is caused by bicuspid aortic valve stenosis.

Diagnosis

Echocardiography is the most important test for the diagnosis of ALVT; cardiac catheterization is required only in those cases with inadequate information about coronary artery anatomy [17]. Parasternal views are particularly useful in understanding the origin of the tunnel and its relation with the coronary ostium, its length and opening into one of the ventricles. An ALVT never passes through myocardium to reach the cavity of the ventricle, a feature that differentiates it from a coronary-cameral fistula. Fistulous connections of the coronary arteries, however, always pass through the myocardium to reach the lumen of a cardiac chamber, and do not involve the hingepoint of an aortic valvar leaflet. As we will see, these features do not always serve to distinguish a fistula from a tunnel extending to open within the right ventricle but they do contrast with most tunnels that open within the left ventricle [18]. Another close differential diagnosis is a ruptured sinus of Valsalva aneurysm, which has its orifice in the sinus of the aortic valve.

The computer tomogram has the advantage of providing three-dimensional information, which helps in understanding the close relation around ALVT. In our case, the CT images clearly indicate the anatomic arrangement underscoring the malformations.

Treatment

Without surgical treatment, most patients die early in life due to congestive heart failure. Therefore, medical management should only be to prepare the patient for surgery.

Transcatheter closure. Although, aorto-left ventricular tunnel could be treated by transcatheter closure using amplatzer duct occluder in literatures [19, 20], it is not the established method of tunnel closure due to the complex anatomy of the tunnel, such as its proximity to the aortic cusp and right coronary ostium, or the coronary ostium inside the tunnel wall, or already distorted cusp anatomy with valvular regurgitation. The tunnel itself is a significantly distensible structure. Hence, careful selection is needed for transcatheter closure.

Surgical Management

Volume overload due to severe regurgitation is a feature of ALVT; hence, it warrants correction as soon as the diagnosis is made. Survival following surgical repair has improved from around 20% to nearly 100% [21].

Even if the patients are treated, they should be followed up in case the tunnel persists, and also for aortic aneurysm because of the occurrence of aortic insufficiency in the long term and worsening heart failure. The incidence of aortic insufficiency in patients with ALVT following surgery ranges from 16–60%, and the requirement for aortic valve replacement ranges from 0–50% [22, 23].

Key Points

1. Aorto-left ventricular tunnel is a rare congenital extracardiac channel with progressive left ventricular dilatation, which needs early correction.
2. After the treatment, all patients should be followed up for tunnel recurrence, aortic valve incompetence, left ventricular dysfunction, and aortic aneurysm throughout their lives.
3. In ALVT, coronary artery abnormalities and other associated abnormalities should be observed.

References

1. Okoroma, E.O., Perry, L.W., Scott, L.P. et al. (1976). Aortico-left ventricular tunnel: Clinical profile, diagnostic features and surgical considerations. *J Thorac Cardiovasc Surg* 71: 238–244.
2. Hovaguimian, H., Cobanoglu, A. and Starr, A. (1988). Aortico-left ventricular tunnel: A clinical review and new surgical classification. *Ann Thorac Surg* 45: 106–112.
3. Ono, M., Goerler, H., Boethig, D. et al. (2008). Surgical repair of aortico-left ventricular tunnel arising from the left aortic sinus. *Interact Cardiovasc Thorac Surg* 7 (3): 510–511.
4. Nezafati, M.H., Maleki, M.H., Javan, H. et al. (2010). Repair of aorto-left ventricular tunnel arising from the left sinus of Valsalva. *J Card Surg* 25 (3): 345–346.
5. Martins, J.D., Sherwood, M.C., Mayer, J.E., Jr et al. (2004). Aortico-left ventricular tunnel: 35-year experience. *J Am Coll Cardiol* 44: 446–450.
6. Bitar, F.F., Smith, F.C., Kavey, R.E. et al. (1993). Aortico-left ventricular tunnel with aortic atresia in the newborn. *Am Heart J* 126: 1480–1482.
7. Martin Jimenez, J., Gonzales Diegues, C.C., Quero Jimenez, C. et al. (1996). Aortico-left ventricular tunnel associated with pulmonary valve stenosis. *Rev Esp Cardiol* 49: 921–924.
8. Knott-Craig, C.J., van der Merwe, P.L., Kalis, N.N. et al. (1992). Repair of aortico-left ventricular tunnel associated with subpulmonary obstruction. *Ann Thorac Surg* 54: 557–559.
9. Bonnet, D., Bonhoeffer, P., Sidi, D. et al. (1999). Surgical angioplasty of the main coronary arteries in children. *J Thorac Cardiovasc Surg* 117: 352–357.
10. McKay, R. (2007). Aorto-ventricular tunnel. *Orphanet J Rare Dis* 2: 41.
11. Martins, J.D., Sherwood, M.C., Mayer, J.E. Jr et al. (2004). Aortico-left ventricular tunnel: 35-year experience. *J Am Coll Cardiol* 44 (2). 446– 50.
12. Norman, R. and Kafka, H. (2009). Aortico left ventricular tunnel in adulthood: Twenty-two year follow up. *Int J Cardiol* 134 (1): e20–2.
13. Sousa-Uva, M., Touchot, A., Fermont, L. et al. (1996). Aortico-left ventricular tunnel in fetuses and infants. *Ann Thorac Surg* 61: 1805–1810.
14. Kafka, H., Chan, K.L. and Leach, A.J. (1989). Asymptomatic aortico-left ventricular tunnel in adulthood. *Am J Cardiol.* 63: 1021–1022.
15. Kouchoukos, N.T., Blackstone, E.H., Hanley, F.L., and Kirklin, J.K. (2013). Congenital sinus of valsalva aneurysm and aortic left ventricular tunnel. *Kirklin/Barratt-Boyes Cardiac Surgery*, 4th edn, 1326–1341. Philadelphia, PA: Elsevier.
16. Mueller, C., Dave, H., and Prêtre, R. (2012). Surgical repair of aorto-ventricular tunnel. *Multimed Man Cardiothorac Surg.* doi:10.1093/mmcts/mms006
17. Sadeghpour, A., Peighambari, M., Dalirrooyfard, M. et al. (2006). Aorta-to-left ventricle tunnel associated with noncompaction left ventricle. *J Am Soc Echocardiogr* 19: 1073.
18. McKay, R., Anderson, R.H., and Cook, A.C. (2002). The aorto-ventricular tunnels. *Cardiol Young* 12: 563–580.
19. Vida, V.L., Bottio, T., and Stellin, G. (2004). An unusual case of aorto-left ventricular tunnel. *Cardiol Young* 14: 203–205.
20. Chessa, M., Chaudhani, M., and De Giovanni, J.V. (2000). Aorto-left ventricular tunnel: Transcatheter closure using amplatzer duct occluder device. *Am J Cardiol* 86: 253–254.

21. McKay, R., Anderson, R.H., and Cook, A.C. (2002). The aorto-ventricular tunnels. *Cardiol Young* 12: 563–580.

22. Myers, J.L. and Mehta, S.M. (2000). Congenital heart surgery nomenclature and database project: Aortico-left ventricular tunnel. *Ann Thorac Surg* 69: 164–169.

23. Honjo, O., Ishino, K., Kawada M., et al. (2006). Late outcome after repair of aortico-left ventricular tunnel: 10-year follow-up. *Circ J* 70: 939–941.

2 Anomalous Origin of the Left Coronary Artery from the Pulmonary Trunk

Weihua Wu[1] and Jing Ping Sun[2]

[1] Jiaotong University, Shanghai, China
[2] The Chinese University of Hong Kong, Hong Kong

History

A 59-year-old female presented with a 5-year history of chest discomfort and two episodes of syncope.

Physical Examination

Heart rate was 70 bpm. Blood pressure was 120/80 mm Hg. There was a 3/6 grade systolic murmur at the apical area.

Laboratory

A 24-hour Holter monitor showed multiple atrial and ventricular premature beats with short runs of ventricular tachycardia.

Chest X-ray

This revealed cardiomegaly and pulmonary congestion.

Echocardiography

An apical four-chamber view showed the left atrium and ventricle were significantly enlarged with borderline systolic function (LVEF = 50%). Continuous color Doppler flow was seen within the ventricular septum; the direction of blood flow was towards the LV cavity during diastole. A parasternal short axis view also showed intraseptum blood flow (Figure 2-1, Figure 2-2; Video 2-1, and Video 2-2). There was retrograde blood flow into the main pulmonary artery. The left coronary artery orifice could not be visualized in the aortic root, which suggested an anomalous origin left coronary artery.

Coronary Angiography

Angiography showed an anomalous left coronary artery arising from the pulmonary artery (Figure 2-3; Video 2-3) and a dilated right coronary artery originating from the aortic root. There were many collateral arteries with retrograde flow from the right to the anomalous left coronary artery.

Comparative Cardiac Imaging: A Case-based Guide, First Edition.
Edited by Jing Ping Sun, Xing Sheng Yang, and Bryan P. Yan.
© 2018 John Wiley & Sons Ltd. Published 2018 by John Wiley & Sons Ltd.
Companion website: www.wiley.com/sun/comparative_cardiac_imaging

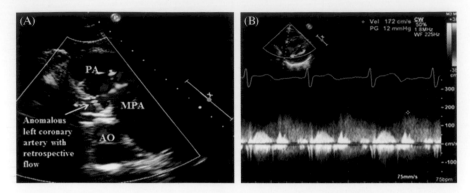

Figure 2-1   A. Atypical parasternal short-axis view showed anomalous left coronary artery with retrospective flow arrow (arrow). B. Continuous wave Doppler recorded from a short-axis view showed coronary flow into septum during cardiac cycle, predominately in diastole.

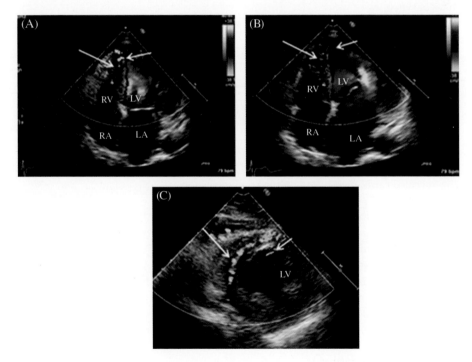

Figure 2-2   A. Apical four-chamber view showed left atria and ventricle were significantly enlarged with a color Doppler flow in the ventricular septum (long arrow) communicating with the left ventricular cavity continuously. The blood flowed back to septum during systole (short arrow) and B. into the LV cavity during diastole (short arrow). C. A parasternal short-axis view showed the intraseptal blood flow (long arrow) and the flow from the interventricular septal into the LV (short arrow).

Computed Tomography

Cardiac 64-slice multidetector computed tomography (MDCT) was performed to better define the origin and course of the anomalous left coronary artery. This confirmed the

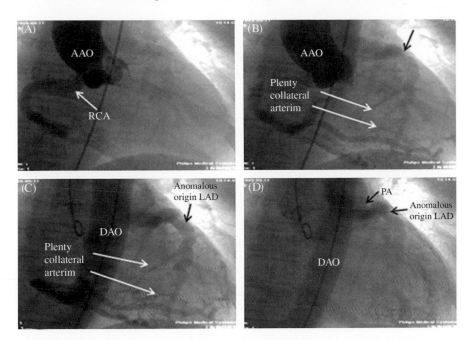

Figure 2-3   A series of angiograms showed that: A. The right coronary artery was original from aorta, B. plenty collateral arteries between right and left coronary, and C. anomalous origin of left coronary artery was from pulmonary artery, and plenty collateral arteries between right and left coronary, D. anomalous LAD with retrospective flow (arrow) from collateral arteries.

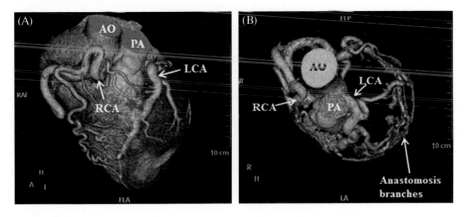

Figure 2-4   Computed tomography reconstructive imaging: A. A three-dimensional CT reconstruction image showed the RCA originating from the aorta, but the LCA originating from the pulmonary artery. B. A three-dimensional CT reconstruction image showed numerous anastomosis branches between right and left coronary arteries, and the RCA originating from the aorta, but the LCA originating from the pulmonary artery.

right coronary artery (RCA) originating from the aorta and the left coronary artery (LCA) originating from the pulmonary artery. There were many branches of anastomosis between the right and left coronary arteries (Figure 2-4).

Operation Findings

Bypass surgery was successfully performed without any complications. The surgeon found that the LCA originated from the main pulmonary artery, and the orifice of the LCA was located above the pulmonary valve about 10 mm; the LCA was ligated close to its connection with the main pulmonary artery, and an internal mammary artery bypass to the LCA was performed.

The patient improved quickly after operation and is still being followed up with normal left ventricular systolic function.

Discussion

An anomalous origin of the left coronary artery from the pulmonary artery (ALCAPA) is a rare congenital coronary abnormality associated with early infant mortality and adult sudden death. The incidence of ALCAPA is estimated at 1/300 000 live births comprising between 0.24% and 0.46% of all congenital heart defects. Left untreated, about 90% of infants die in the first year of life as a result of intractable left ventricular failure [1]. In a review of 25 infant and adult cases, Kaunitz [2] noted RCA dilation and significant development of collateralization from the RCA to the LCA in the adult cases. This became the first distinction proposed between infants who die in the first year and those who survive to adulthood. Several pathophysiologic mechanisms have been invoked to explain why ALCAPA is well tolerated in the early neonatal period and why some patients survive until adulthood.

During fetal and early neonatal life, the pulmonary pressure equals systemic pressure. This leads to antegrade flow in the anomalous left coronary artery and the normal RCA. A gradual decline in the pulmonary pressure after birth results in low perfusion pressure, hypoxic blood, and reversal of flow in the LCA [3]. In the infant type of ALCAPA, there is little or no collateral flow between the RCA and the LCA. When reversal of flow in the LCA is established, reduced blood supply to the myocardium leads to myocardial infarction [3].

In the adult type, reversal of flow in the LCA triggers formation of interarterial collaterals. With time, marked dilatation of the RCA and LCA causes preferential blood flow into the low-pressure pulmonary system rather than into the high- resistance myocardium. This results in a coronary steal phenomenon [3].

Since the late 1990s, the number of reported patients with ALCAPA aged over 50 years has increased.

Imaging Diagnosis

This diagnosis in an older cohort correlates with advances in echocardiography and the introduction of cardiac CT and MRI as new noninvasive techniques for evaluation of coronary anatomy. Cardiac CT and MRI are not only useful in diagnosis but may also offer prognostic information, allowing risk stratification, and may be utilized for long-term follow-up imaging.

Echocardiography and MRI

Echocardiography and MRI also can evaluate myocardial function, ischemia, and viability. Imaging has reached such an advanced stage of sophistication and precision that these techniques may eventually allow for the establishment of definite clinical guidelines for managing this congenital condition.

Transthoracic echocardiography is an essential tool for the diagnosis of ALCAPA. In pediatric patients, the echocardiographic diagnosis of this anomaly has improved.

However, in the adult group, the location of the RCA ostiumis is always difficult to detect by transthoracic two-dimensional imaging because of a low spatial resolution with poor penetration through the chest wall [4]. In our case, we found several characteristics: (i) There is a color Doppler flow in ventricular septum that communicated with left ventricular cavity continuously; the blood flow was back to septum during systole and into LV cavity during diastole; this phenomenon suggest that there is abnormal communication with coronary circulation. (ii) There is an abnormal blood flow retrospectively into the main pulmonary artery. (iii) The orifice of LCA could not be found from the aortic root, which leads to suspicion of an anomalous origin of the LCA.

Angiography

The complete coronary angiography provided detailed anatomic information of origin, course, and relationships of the anomalous coronary artery.

An anomalous origin of the left coronary artery from the pulmonary artery was diagnosed by the echocardiography initially, and confirmed by the CT and angiogram. Imaging information helps surgeons to perform surgery successfully.

Cardiac Computed Tomography

Coronary angiogram and cardiovascular magnetic resonance provide excellent visualization of coronary artery anomalies. In our case, CT showed that the RCA originated from the aorta, but the LCA originated from the pulmonary artery; there are plenty of anastomosis branches between the right and left coronary arteries. An accurate diagnosis was made by these findings.

Treatment

Surgical repair outcomes are quite excellent in most patients. Most of the patients with ALCAPA present with findings of decreased left ventricular function and mitral regurgitation secondary to myocardial ischemia and papillary muscle damage, respectively [4]. Immediate coronary reimplantation and early improvement of left ventricular function are essential for recovery. After successful repair, ventricular function, dilatation, and mitral regurgitation improve gradually [5]. The patient reported here underwent successful surgical treatment. At the time of this writing, she remains asymptomatic more than 2.5 years post operation.

Conclusion

An anomalous origin of the left coronary artery from the pulmonary artery is a rare and life-threatening condition. The availability of newer diagnostic modalities correlates with an increasing incidence in an older cohort. A comprehensive review of adult ALCAPA suggests that older patients experience less frequent life-threatening presentations and sudden death. Nevertheless, surgical correction should be considered for all patients. Finally, the lack of adequate comparative surgical and follow-up data in adults indicate the need for this information in future studies [6].

Key Points

1. Anomalous origin of the left coronary artery from the pulmonary artery is a rare but serious congenital cardiac anomaly.
2. Early diagnosis using echocardiography with color flow mapping and improvements in surgical techniques (e.g., myocardial preservation) dramatically improve prognosis.

References

1. Keith, J.D. (1959). The anomalous origin of the left coronary artery from the pulmonary artery *Br. Heart J.* 21: 149–161.
2. Kaunitz, P.E. (1947). Origin of left coronary artery from the pulmonary artery: review of the literature and report of two cases. *Am. Heart J.* 33: 182–206.
3. Driscoll, D.J., Nihill, M.R., Mullins, C.E. et al. (1981). Management of symptomatic infants with anomalous origin of the left coronary artery from the pulmonary artery. *Am. J. Cardiol.* 147: 642–648.
4. Dodge-Khatami, A., Mavroudis, C. and Backer, C.L. (2002). Anomalous origin of the left coronary artery from the pulmonary artery: collective review of surgical therapy. *Ann. Thorac. Surg.* 74: 946–955.
5. Case, R.B., Morrow, A.G., Stainsby, W. et al. (1958). Anomalous origin of the left coronary artery: Physiologic defect and suggested surgical treatment. *Circulation* 17 (6): 1062–1068.
6. Yau, J.M., Singh, R., Halpern, E.J. et al. (2011). Anomalous origin of the left coronary artery from the pulmonary artery in adults: a comprehensive review of 151 adult cases and a new diagnosis in a 53-year-old woman. *Clin. Cardiol.* 34 (4): 204–210.

3 Anomalous Origin of Right Coronary Artery

Kevin Ka-Ho Kam, Jing Ping Sun, and Xing Sheng Yang

The Chinese University of Hong Kong, Hong Kong

History

A 26-year-old gentleman with situs inversus and detrocardia presented with worsening atypical chest pain for more than 10 years. Chest pain was not related to exertion.

Physical Examination

Situs inversus was diagnosed at the age of 2 years. Jaundice developed at the age of 3 years due to congenital biliary atresia. Corrective surgery was performed at the time and there have been no major health issues until this presentation. Cardiovascular examination demonstrated dextrocardia and a soft pansystolic murmur at the apex.

Exercise Stress Electrocardiogram

The exercise stress electrocardiogram showed ST segment depression in the inferior leads during the Bruce stage 4 exercise up to 13.2 METS but no chest pain during or after the test.

Echocardiogram

The left ventricle (LV) ejection fraction was normal. There was no resting LV regional wall motion abnormality. Bicycle ergometer exercise stress echocardiogram was performed. Target heart rate was achieved with maximum workload of 125 W and total exercise time of 19 min. There was no stress-induced regional wall motion abnormality.

Computed Tomography

The left main stem (LMS) arose from the left coronary cusp, which then gave rise to left anterior descending artery (LAD) and left circumflex artery (LCX) with normal caliber. The origin of the right coronary artery (RCA) was anomalous arising from the LMS (Figure 3-1). The RCA ran in an epicardial interarterial course between the aortic root and right ventricular outflow (RVOT) (Figure 3-2). The proximal RCA segment was compressed by the two great vessels into a smooth slit (Figure 3-2).

Comparative Cardiac Imaging: A Case-based Guide, First Edition.
Edited by Jing Ping Sun, Xing Sheng Yang, and Bryan P. Yan.
© 2018 John Wiley & Sons Ltd. Published 2018 by John Wiley & Sons Ltd.
Companion website: www.wiley.com/sun/comparative_cardiac_imaging

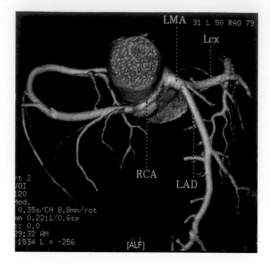

Figure 3-1 The left main stem arose from the left coronary cusp, which then gave rise to the left anterior descending artery and left circumflex artery with normal caliber. The right coronary artery shared the common origin of the LMS, originating from the left coronary cusp.
Notes: LMS, left main stem coronary; LAD, left anterior descending artery; LCX, left circumflex artery; RCA, right coronary artery.

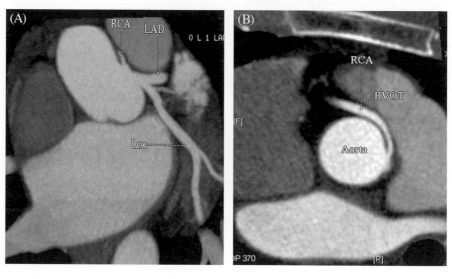

Figure 3-2 A. The right coronary artery shared the common origin of LMS, originating from the left coronary cusp. B. The proximal RCA run in an epicardial interarterial course between the aortic root and the right ventricular outflow tract, in which the sandwiched proximal segment is smoothly narrowed.
Note: RVOT, right ventricular outflow tract.

Management

The patient was warned of the risk of sudden cardiac death and advised to avoid vigorous exercise. Conservative management was adopted in view of the absence of myocardial ischemia during stress echo.

Discussion

Anomalies of coronary arteries are common, accounting for nearly 1% of patients undergoing cardiac catherization [1]. Most of them are asymptomatic and majority are discovered incidentally [2]. About a quarter of sudden cardiac deaths of young adults are due to coronary anomalies. In a study done by the Minneapolis Heart Institute Foundation Registry from 1980 to 2005, anomalous coronary arteries were the second commonest causes of sudden cardiac death in young competitive athletes, accounting for 17% of cases [3].

Transthoracic echocardiography is the recommended primary noninvasive modality. In most patients it can delineate both coronary ostia; however, color Doppler provides good anatomic definition of the proximal intramural course of the anomalous vessel. In cases of diagnostic doubt, transesophageal echocardiography can identify the origin of the coronary arteries.

Multidetector Computed Tomography (MDCT) Angiography

The definitive diagnosis was achieved by MDCT in our patient. Magnetic resonance imaging can clearly delineate the anatomy and has recently replaced angiography as a definitive diagnostic tool. Currently ECG-gated MDCT coronary angiograms are the gold standard for diagnosing anomalous coronaries [4].

The pathophysiology of coronary anomaly is complex and reasons for morbidity and mortality can be multifactorial. Vigorous physical activity plays an important role, as exercise promotes sympathetic drive, increasing myocardial oxygen consumption. The expansion of the proximal aorta and pulmonary artery is a contributing factor in the sudden collapse of the proximal anomalous coronary artery [5].

Possible mechanisms of the coronary flow restriction are below:

- Acute angulation at the takeoff of the coronary artery [6].
- A slitlike orifice and the presence of an ostial ridge [6].
- Variable lateral luminal compression of the intramural trunk during systole as the proximal anomalous coronary artery run intramural course [7].
- Impingement of the proximal anomalous coronary artery between the aorta and the pulmonary artery during vigorous exercise, causing kinking of the artery [8].

Anomalous origin of right coronary artery (RCA) from the left coronary sinus with a course between the aorta and the RVOT is very rare. However, sudden cardiac death as a result of an anomalous RCA is far less common than an anomalous LCA [5]. One study showed that a slitlike ostium and an acute angle takeoff of the coronary artery are more frequent in sudden cardiac death [9]. Thus those patients may be suitable candidates for surgical treatment [9].

Regarding the management plan, there has so far been no randomized controlled trial to compare aggressive versus conservative approaches. Pelliccia [10] suggested the treatment policy as follows:

- Young patients (<35 years) with symptoms and / or myocardial ischemia should be operated on.
- The best therapy method is uncertain for young patients (<35 years) without symptoms and / or myocardial ischemia.
- Older patients (>35 years) without symptom or ischemia need no surgical therapy.

The physician should advise the patient to avoid severe physical activity [5, 10] as it may induce myocardial ischemia as a result of coronary flow restriction. If there is clinical evidence of myocardial ischemia, surgical treatment should be recommended.

These comprise unroofing procedure, percutaneous coronary intervention, coronary artery bypass graft, pulmonary artery translocation, and direct coronary reimplantation [10].

Key Points

1. Anomalies of coronary arteries are common, accounting for nearly 1% of patients undergoing cardiac catheterization. About a quarter of sudden cardiac deaths of young adults are due to coronary anomaly.
2. A definitive diagnosis could be achieved by MDCT.
3. A young patient (<35 years) with symptoms and/or myocardial ischemia should be operated on.
4. The best therapy for a young patient (<35 years) without symptoms and/or myocardial ischemia is uncertain.
5. An older patient (>35 years) without symptoms or ischemia do not need surgical therapy.

References

1. Yamanaka, O. and Hobbs, R.E. (1990) Coronary artery anomalies in 126 595 patients undergoing coronary arteriography. *Cathet Cardiovasc Diagn* 21: 28–40.
2. Kardos, A., Babai, L., Rudas, L. et al. (1997). Epidemiology of congenital coronary artery anomalies: a coronary arteriography study on a central European population. *Cathet Cardiovasc Diagn* 42: 270–275.
3. Maroon, B.J., Shirani, J., Poliac, L.C. et al. (1996). Sudden death in young competitive athletes. Clinical, demographic, and pathological profiles. *JAMA* 276: 199–204.
4. Datta, J., White, C.S., Gilkeson, R.C. et al. (2005). Anomalous coronary arteries in adults: Depiction at multi-detector row CT angiography. *Radiology* 235: 812–818.
5. Cheitlin, M.D. and MacGregor, J. (2009). Congenital anomalies of coronary arteries: Role in the pathogenesis of sudden cardiac death. *Herz* 34: 268–279.
6. Virmani, R., Chun, P.K., Goldstein, R.E. et al. (1984). Acute takeoffs of the coronary arteries along the aortic wall and congenital coronary ostial valve-like ridges: Association with sudden death. *J Am Coll Cardiol* 3: 766–771.
7. Angelini, P. (2002) Coronary artery anomalies – current clinical issues, definitions, classification, incidence, clinical relevance, and treatment guidelines. *Tex Heart Inst J* 29: 271–278.
8. Taylor, A.J., Byers, J.P., Cheitlin, M.D. et al. (1997) Anomalous right or left coronary artery from the contralateral coronary sinus: "High-risk" abnormalities in the initial coronary artery course and heterogeneous clinical outcomes. *Am Heart J* 133: 428–435.
9. Lee, B.Y., Song, K.S., Jung, S.E. et al. (2009). Anomalous right coronary artery originated from left coronary sinus with interarterial course: Evaluation of the proximal segment on multidetector row computed tomography with clinical correlation. *J Comput Assist Tomogr* 33: 755–762.
10. Pelliccia, A. (2001). Congenital coronary artery anomalies in young patients: New perspectives for timely identification. *J Am Coll Cardiol* 37: 598–600.

4 Interrupted Aortic Arch associated with Aortopulmonary Window

Yali Xu[1] and Jing Ping Sun[2]

[1] The Military Medical University, Chonqging, China
[2] The Chinese University of Hong Kong, Hong Kong

History

A 6-year-old boy was referred due to dyspnea on exertion and cyanosis for 3 years.

Physical Examination

The child had clubbing of his fingers. Blood pressure in the upper extremity was 100/60 mmHg on the right and 95/61 mmHg on the left and in the lower extremity, 106/57 mmHg on the right and 115/52 mmHg on the left. There was no heart murmur on auscultation.

Laboratory

Peripheral pulse oximetry was 92%, 92%, 89% and 86% in the left arm, right arm, left leg, and right leg, respectively.

Transthoracic Echocardiogram

A parasternal short axis view showed a large aortopulmonary window with a large defect about 28 mm between the ascending aorta (AAO) and pulmonary artery (PA) (Figure 4-1A; Video 4-1). A suprasternal notch view showed an aortic arch (ARCH) interrupted distal to the origin of the left subclavian artery (arrow), and the right pulmonary artery was arising from the ascending aorta (Figure 4-1B). A parasternal short axis view showed a large patent ductus arteriosus (PDA) connected to the descending thoracic aorta (DAO) (Figure 4-1C). There was severe pulmonary hypertension with peak systolic pulmonary pressure of 95 mmHg estimated by the velocity of tricuspid regurgitation.

Computed Tomography

Multidetector computed tomography angiography showed a large aortopulmonary window (arrow) between the AAO and the main pulmonary artery (MPA) (Figure 4-2A). The right pulmonary artery was arising from the AAO and the left pulmonary artery from main pulmonary artery (Figure 4-2A). A lateral view showed a patent ductus arteriosus (PDA) continuing into the descending thoracic aorta (DAO) (Figure 4-2B). A posterior view with a three-dimensional volume rendering image showed the MPA with

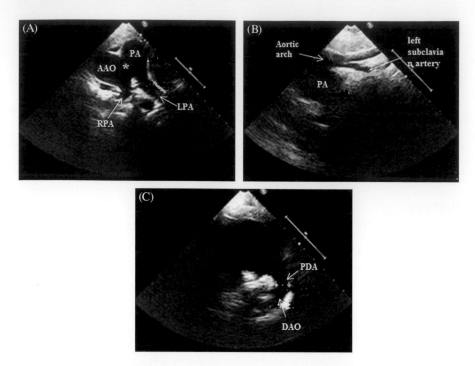

Figure 4-1   Echocardiography: A. A parasternal short axis view showed a large aortopulmonary window (*) between the ascending aorta (AAO) and the pulmonary artery (PA), the right pulmonary artery was arising from ascending aorta. B. A suprasternal notch view showed an aortic arch (ARCH) interrupted at distal to the origin of the left subclavian artery (arrow). C. The parasternal short axis view showed a large patent ductus arteriosus (PDA) extending into the thoracic aorta (DAO).

a PDA continuing into the thoracic aorta, and aortic arch interruption occurred distal to the origin of the left subclavian artery (Figure 4-2C). An anterior view with a three-dimensional volume rendering image showed a large aortopulmonary window (about 27.2 mm, arrow) between the ascending aorta and the main pulmonary artery and a type A interrupted aortic arch (Figure 4-2D).

Surgery was contraindicated for this case due to severe pulmonary hypertension.

Discussion

An interrupted aortic arch (IAA) associated with an aortopulmonary window (APW) is a rare congenital cardiac anomaly. Isolated APW occurs in 0.2% cases of congenital heart disease and about 52% of cases with APW coexist with other cardiac anomalies like patent ductus arteriosus (PDA), ventricular septum defect (VSD), IAA,or aortic coarctation [1]. In IAA cases, the occurrence of the coexistence of APW and IAA was 3.5%–4.2%, or 5.3% [1, 2]. Early diagnosis, classification, and surgical correction are particularly important because the high mortality in newborns and infants results from pulmonary hypertension and heart failure.

Richardson's anatomic classification [3] describes three types of APW. In type I, the defect is located between the AAO and the MPA proximal to the sinuses of Valsalva due to incomplete separation of the aortopulmonary trunk; type II, a more distal defectwas

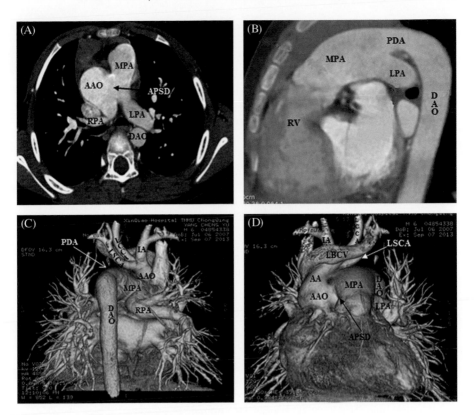

Figure 4-2 Computed tomography images: A. Axial maximum intensity projection image showed a large aortopulmonary window (arrow) between the ascending aorta (AAO) and the pulmonary artery (MPA), right and left pulmonary arteries and descending aorta (DAO). B. Lateral view showed right ventricle (RV), main pulmonary artery (MPA) with left pulmonary artery (LPA), and a patent ductus arteriosus (PDA) extending into the thoracic aorta (DAO). C. A posterior view with a three-dimensional volume rendering image showed the main pulmonary artery with a patent ductus arteriosus extending in the thoracic aorta and aortic arch interruption distal to the origin of the left subclavian artery. D. Anterior view with three-dimensional volume rendering showing a large aortopulmonary window (arrow) between the ascending aorta and the main pulmonary artery, and a type A interrupted aortic arch.
Notes: APSD, aortopulmonary window; RPA, right pulmonary artery; LSCA, left subclavian artery; LCCA, left common carotid artery; IA, Innominate artery; RPA, right pulmonary artery; LPA, left pulmonary artery; LBCV, left brachiocephalic vein; AAO, ascending aorta; AA, aortic arch.

demonstrated between the AAO and the origin of the RPA from the MPA due to abnormal migration of sixth aortic arch; type III presents with a complete separation between aorta and MPA, and the RPA usually originates from the AAO.

Interrupted aortic arch has been classified into three types (A, B, and C) based on the site of aortic interruption. In type A interrupted left aortic arch, the arch interruption occurs distal to the origin of the left subclavian artery. In type B interrupted left aortic arch, the interruption occurs distal to the origin of the left common carotid artery. In type C interrupted left aortic arch, the interruption occurs between the innominate artery and the left common carotid artery [4].

According to the classification above, our case should belong to a type A IAA (with an interruption located distal to the left subclavian artery) and type III APW (presented with a complete separation of the lumen between AAO and MPA) and coexisted with PDA as well as PFO.

An echocardiogram is always the first image technique to detect the abnormalities; CT or MRI angiography can provide the anatomy in detail.

Most of these patients died in childhood due to congestive heart failure and severe pulmonary hypertension. A report of five cases of IAA and APW showed that the median age was 1.6 years with the maximum age of 13 [5]. Ucak reported a case of IAA associated with APW in a 20-year-old man [6].

Pulmonary hypertension is an early complication in patients with IAA and APW due to the direct shunt between the AA and MPA. Surgical correction is the only way to save the life of the patients. Unfortunately, some patients lost this chance due to the severe pulmonary hypertension. This happened in our case. It is therefore extremely important to detect the cardiac anomaly as early as possible.

In conclusion, we have presented a case of IAA associated with APW. These congenital malformations were detected by echocardiography and the anatomical features were provided in detail by MSCT.

Key Points

1. Isolated APW occurs in 0.2% cases of congenital heart disease and about 52% of cases with APW coexist with other cardiac anomalies like PDA, VSD, IAA or aortic coarctation.
2. Surgical correction is the only way to save the life of the patient. Unfortunately, some patients lost this chance due to severe pulmonary hypertension. It is therefore extremely important to detect the cardiac anomaly as early as possible.

References

1. Konstantinov, I.E., Karamlou, T., Williams, W.G. et al. (2006). Surgical management of aortopulmonary window associated with interrupted aortic arch:a congenital heart surgeons society study. *J Thorac Cardiovasc Surg* 131: 1136–1141.
2. Yildirim, N., Dogan, S.M., Aydin, M. et al. (2008). Isolated interrupted aortic arch, a rare cause of hypertension in adults. *Int J Cardiol* 127: e52–e53.
3. Richardson, J.V., Doty, D.B., Rossi, N.P. et al. (1979). The spectrum of anomalies of aortopulmonary septation. *J Thorac Cardiovasc Surg* 78: 21–27.
4. Mishra, P.K. (2009) Management strategies for interrupted aortic arch with associated anomalies. *Eur J Cardiothorac Surg* 35: 569–576.
5. Wang, D., Liu, Y., Su, J. et al. (2012). Surgical treatment of five patients with interrupted aortic arch and aortopulmonary window. *J Cardiovasc Pulmonary Dis* 5: 537–539.
6. Ucaka, A., Inan, K., Onan, B. et al. (2011). Interrupted aortic arch associated with aortopulmonary window in a 20 year-old young adult. *Int J Cardiology* 149: e120–e122.

5 Congenitally Corrected Transposition of the Great Arteries

Ming-Ming Sim[1] and Jing Ping Sun[2]

[1] Landseed Hospital, Taiwan
[2] The Chinese University of Hong Kong, Hong Kong

History

A 50-year-old woman with mild exertional dyspnea for years was seen for a preoperative cardiac risk evaluation due to an abnormal ECG. Her medical history was unremarkable.

Physical Examination

Blood pressure: 154/90 mm Hg; pulse rate: 84 bpm.
Heart: Grade 2/6 systolic murmur. Edema (−). Cyanosis (−). Clubbing (−).
No jugular venous distension.

Electrocardiogram

Electrocardiogram showed normal sinus rhythm with a left-axis deviation, QS waves in II, III, AVF and absence of Q waves in leads V4–V6 (Figure 5-1).

Chest X-ray

A posteroanterior chest X ray showed a normal cardiac silhouette. The ascending aortic shadow and the main pulmonary artery segment are absent (Figure 5-2).

Echocardiography

Major ultrasound features in congenitally corrected transposition of the great arteries were demonstrated by echocardiography. In the apical four-chamber view, Reversed off-setting of the septal attachments of the atrioventricular valves, with the mitral valve on the right side attached appreciably higher than the tricuspid valve (TV) on the left side of the heart. The left atrium (LA) is connected to a morphological right ventricle, which is characterized by myocardial trabeculations; in addition, the morphological left ventricle (LV) is connected with the right atrium, positioned on the right side (Figure 5-3).

Computed Tomography

Note the main pulmonary artery arising from the morphology left ventricle (MLV). The aorta arises from the anterior position of the morphology right ventricle (MRV), the pulmonary veins return to left atrium (Figure 5-4).

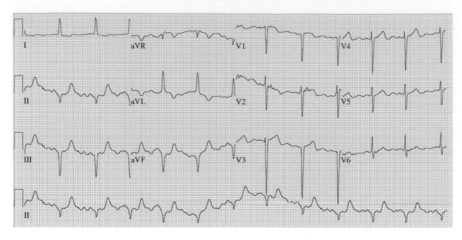

Figure 5-1 Electrocardiogram showing normal sinus rhythm with a left-axis deviation, QS waves in II, III, AVF and absence of Q waves in leads V4–V6.

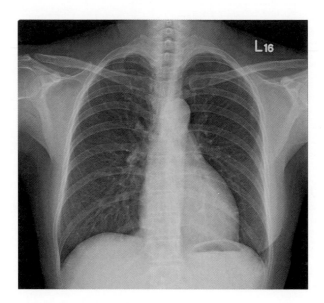

Figure 5-2 Chest X ray. Posteroanterior chest X-ray showing a cardiac silhouette. The ascending aortic shadow and the main pulmonary artery segment are absent.

A three-dimensional volume-rendered image showed the spatial relationship of great arteries, ascending aorta was anterior to left of-the main pulmonary artery. Anterior descending and circumflex coronary artery arise from left common coronary artery (LMA); LMA arises from anterior aortic sinus. Right coronary artery arises from posterior aortic sinus (Figure 5-5).

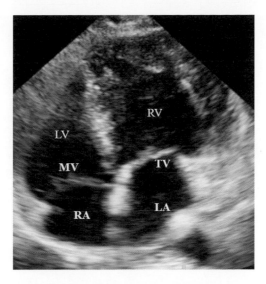

Figure 5-3 Echocardiography. In the apical four-chamber view, there is reversed offsetting of the attachments of the atrioventricular valves to the septum, with the mitral valve on the right side attached appreciably higher than the tricuspid valve (TV) on the left side of the heart. The left atrium (LA) is connected to a morphological right ventricle, which is characterized by myocardial trabeculations; in addition, the morphological left ventricle (LV) is connected with the right atrium (RA), positioned on the right side.

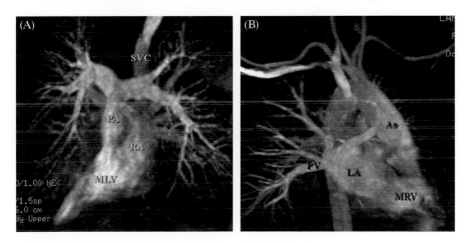

Figure 5-4 Computed tomography. A. Note the main pulmonary artery arising from the morphology left ventricle (MLV). B. The aorta arises from the anterior position of the morphology right ventricle (MRV), the pulmonary veins return to left atrium.

Discussion

Congenitally corrected transposition of the great arteries is rare, occurring in less than 1% of all forms of congenital heart disease [1]. The ventricular septal defect and pulmonic stenosis are seen in 98% of cases [2]. Other associated lesions include pulmonary

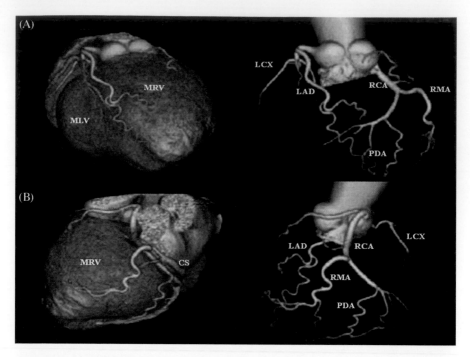

Figure 5-5 Three-dimensional volume-rendered image shows spatial relationship of great arteries with ascending aorta locating at anterior and to left of main pulmonary artery. Anterior descending artery and circumflex artery arise from common left ventricular coronary artery off of anterior aortic sinus. Right coronary artery arises from posterior aortic sinus.

atresia, and tricuspid valve regurgitation, Ebsteinlike anomaly of the tricuspid valve, atrial septal defect, and coarctation of the aorta [3].

Late complications include systemic ventricular dysfunction, progressive systemic atrioventricular valvular regurgitation, congestive heart failure, infective endocarditis, and conduction abnormalities such as complete heart block, Wolff–Parkinson–White syndrome, and supraventricular tachyarrhythmias such as atrial fibrillation and atrial flutter [1, 2, 4]. Only 1–10% of individuals with congenitally corrected transposition of the great vessels have no associated defects [5].

Because of the abnormal direction of the initial depolarization of the septum from right to left leads, the Q waves appear in the right precordial leads but are absent from the left precordial leads. The greater distance between the atrioventricular node and the base of the interventricular septum also results in a longer bundle of His. This explains the atrioventricular conduction delay that is frequently seen [6]. First-degree atrioventricular block is found in around 50% of cases, while its progression to complete heart block occurs at a rate of 2% per year [7]. In some patients there is also an accessory pathway that provides the anatomical substrate for pre-excitation [6]. Because of the characteristics of the systemic conduction, ECG contributes significantly to the diagnosis. The abnormal ECG QS waves in II, III, AVF, and the absence of Q waves in leads V4–V6 were the important clues to diagnosis in our case.

In corrected transposition, the coronary arteries are distributed in a similar way to the ventricles. The anterior descending branch and the circumflex artery supply the morphological left ventricle while the right coronary artery supplies the morphological right ventricle [6]. The CT images demonstrate that the right coronary artery and its branches are larger than the left coronary artery system in the present case.

Because the right ventricle is subjected to systemic pressures, its muscle mass in a congenitally corrected transposition of the great arteries is significantly increased in comparison with the right ventricular muscle mass in the normal heart. This increased systemic pressure results in an increased right-ventricular workload, necessitating an increase in oxygen delivery. The large size of the right coronary artery in our case may be the mechanism to increase the oxygen supply in order to satisfy the increased demand.

The clinical course of corrected transposition of the great vessels depends on the presence and severity of the associated defects. Even in the absence of such anomalies, or after their surgical repair, the question remains of whether the anatomical right ventricle is capable of maintaining an adequate cardiac output over a long period [7].

Even though the right ventricle and the tricuspid valve are morphologically normal, they are inferior to the left ventricle and the mitral valve regarding the long-term maintenance of systemic circulation. The particular morphology of the tricuspid valve, the smaller papillary muscles, the conduction system and the single-vessel perfusion of the systemic ventricle by the right coronary artery, all tend to work against their functions [8].

Dysfunction of the morphology right ventricle is the cause of death in more than 50% of patients [9]. In most cases, it is accompanied by severe insufficiency of the systemic atrioventricular valve. It is not clear whether the latter is the cause of the ventricular dysfunction or the result [10].

A normal life span is possible with a totally "corrected transposition," but in most instances some impairment of cardiac function will occur. Heart block may occur suddenly after age 20 and lead to progressive heart failure and death [11]. Van Son JA et al. suggested that the results of systemic atrioventricular valve replacement in corrected transposition have improved significantly since the mid-2000s. To preserve systemic ventricular function, we suggest that operation be considered at the earliest sign of progressive ventricular dysfunction (ejection fraction >45%) as assessed by serial clinical evaluation and echocardiography [12]. When tricuspid insufficiency is combined with dysfunction of the systemic right ventricle, the double switch operation (arterial and atrial) is considered appropriate [13, 14].

Imaging in Adult Congenital Heart Disease

Echocardiography (both transthoracic and transesophageal) remains the technique of choice for the routine assessment and follow up of patients with congenital heart disease. It is also used extensively in regional centers but requires a level of expertise that is beyond many technician sonographers and general cardiologists. Again, both functional and anatomical data are available using this technique if local expertise allows.

With multiple direction computed tomography (MDCT) machines becoming more commonplace, cardiac MDCT is now also emerging as a complement to established techniques and a viable alternative to cardiac magnetic resonance (CMR) in those patients who are unable or unwilling to undergo it. Patient selection remains important as multiphase reformatting of MDCT data uses retrospective gating techniques and therefore requires a stable heart rhythm. Patients with atrial fibrillation and other rhythms with wide beat-to-beat variation may introduce significant artifacts to the dataset.

With CMR, the lack of ionizing radiation and the fast temporal resolution allow high-quality anatomical and functional data to be obtained at almost no risk to the patient. The functional data derived from CMR, in particular, include both ventriculography, importantly, blood-flow data and the quantitative assessment of stenotic and regurgitant valves. However, there are important limitations with CMR and these include the lack of availability of machines, time for cardiac studies (requiring at least 30–60 min per study), and local expertise required to interpret and reformat acquired data.

International publications contain very few cases of adult patients with congenitally corrected transposition of the great arteries without associated defects or surgical intervention. Our patient adds one more case to this short list.

Key Points

1. Congenitally corrected transposition of the great arteries is a rare, occurring in less than 1% of all forms of congenital heart disease.
2. A normal life span is possible with a totally "corrected transposition," but in most instances some impairment of cardiac function will occur.
3. Cardiac imaging is dedicated tool for diagnosis.

References

1. Connelly, M.S., Liu, P.P., Williams, W.G. et al. (1996). Congenitally corrected transposition of the great arteries in the adult: Functional status and complications. *J Am Coll Cardiol* 27: 1238–1243.
2. Graham, T.P. Jr, Bernard, Y.D., Mellen, B.G. et al. (2000). Longterm outcome in congenitally corrected transposition of the great arteries: Amulti-institutional study. *J Am Coll Cardiol* 36: 255–261.
3. Lundstrom, U., Bull, C., Wyse, R.K. et al. (1990). The natural and "unnatural" history of congenitally corrected transposition. *Am J Cardiol* 65: 1222–1229.
4. Beauchesne, L.M., Warnes, C.A., Connolly, H.M. et al. (2002). Outcome of the unoperated adult who presents with congenitally corrected transposition of the great arteries. *J Am Coll Cardiol* 40: 285–290.
5. Ikeda, U., Furuse, M., Suzuki, O. et al. (1992). Long-term survival in aged patients with corrected transposition of the great arteries. *Chest* 101: 1385.
6. Braunwald, E. (2001). *Heart Disease*, 6th edn, 1571–1572. W.B. Saunders.
7. Beauchesne, L.M., Warnes, C.A., Connolly, H.M. et al. (2002). Outcome of the unoperated adult who presents with congenitally transposition of the great arteries. *J Am Coll Cardiol* 40: 285–290.
8. Van Praagh, R., Papagiannis, J., Grunenfelder, J. et al. (1998). Pathologic anatomy of corrected transposition of the great arteries: Medical and surgical implications. *Am Heart J* 135: 772–785.
9. Connelly, M.S., Liu, P.P., Williams, W.G. et al. (1996). Congenitally corrected transposition of the great arteries in the adult: Functional status and complications. *J Am Coll Cardiol* 27: 1238–1243.
10. Graham, T.P. Jr, Parrish, M.D., Boucek, R.J. Jr et al. (1983). Assessment of ventricular size and function in congenitally corrected transposition of the great arteries. *Am J Cardiol* 51: 244–251.
11. Cumming, G.R. (1962). Congenital corrected transposition of the great vessels without associated intracardiac anomalies. *Am J Cardiol* 10: 605–614.
12. Van Son, J.A., Danielson, G.K., Huhta, J.C. et al. (1995). Late results of systemic atrioventricular valve replacement in corrected transposition. *J Thorac Cardiovasc Surg* 109: 642–652.
13. Imai, Y. (1997). Double-switch operation for congenitally corrected transposition. *Adv Cardiac Surg* 9: 65–86.
14. Karl, T.R., Weintraub, R.G., Brizard, C.P. et al. (1997). Senning plus arterial switch operation for discordant (congenitally corrected) transposition. *Ann Thorac Surg* 64: 495–502.

6 Coronary Fistula

Fanxia Meng[1], Jing Ping Sun[2], Ming Chen[1], and Lei Zhang[1]

[1] Tongji University School of Medicine, Shanghai, China
[2] The Chinese University of Hong Kong, Hong Kong

History

An 18-year-old girl complained of exertional dyspnea for 1 year.

Physical Examination

Blood pressure 110 / 80 mmHg. Breathing 28 times / min, heart rate: 98 bpm. A grade 2/6 systolic decrescendo murmur is heard best at the fourth right intercostal space.

Chest X-ray

There is vascular congestion with increased interstitial markings findings indicating mild pulmonary vascular congestion. There is mild cardiomegaly.

Transthoracic Echocardiography

The proximal segments of the left and right coronaries are dilated, filling with high-velocity color Doppler flow. Multiple color flows from ventricular septal, anterior, inferior and posterior wall drainage into left ventricular cavity were seen at parasternal short axis, atypical two-chamber views (Figure 6-1, Video 6-1, and Video 6-2). Multiple color flows from right ventricle (RV) free wall drainage into RV cavity at atypical four-chamber view and parasternal short axis views (Figure 6-1, Video 6-3, and Video 6-4).

Computed Tomography Angiography

Volume-rendered image from computed tomography (CT) (Figure 6-2) showed the right coronary artery expands over the entire length; and the left main coronary artery derived into three branches, which are dilated over the entire length along the anterior surface of the ventricle; the terminal of branches are communicating with the left ventricle cavity.

Coronary Angiography

The coronary system appeared to be the right-dominant type. The right coronary was significantly dilated; the left main coronary derived three branches in general expansion. The distal vessels of LAD branches formed a rich vascular network. Contrast agent diffused into the left ventricle myocardium and a cavity.

Comparative Cardiac Imaging: A Case-based Guide, First Edition.
Edited by Jing Ping Sun, Xing Sheng Yang, and Bryan P. Yan.
© 2018 John Wiley & Sons Ltd. Published 2018 by John Wiley & Sons Ltd.
Companion website: www.wiley.com/sun/comparative_cardiac_imaging

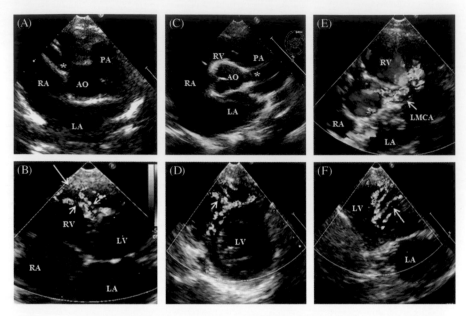

Figure 6-1 Two-D Echocardiography showed: A. Parasternal short-axis view at aortic level showed dilated RCA (*). B. Atypical apical four-chamber view showed multiple shunts from RV free wall (long arrow) into RV cavity (small arrows). C. Parasternal short axis view at aortic valve level showed dilated LCA (*). D. Parasternal short-axis view with color Doppler at papillary muscle level showed three fistula flows from ventricular septum into RV cavity. E. Parasternal short-axis view with color Doppler at aortic valve level showed dilated LCA filling with color flow (arrow). F. Atypical apical two-chamber view with color Doppler showed multiple fistula flows (arrow) from LV anterior wall into LV cavity.
Notes: RA, right ventricle; LA, left atrium; AO, aorta; PA, pulmonary artery; LV, left ventricle and LMCA, left main coronary artery.

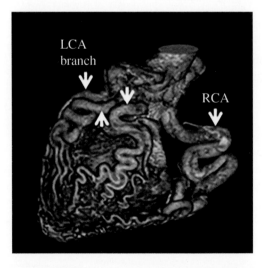

Figure 6-2 Volume-rendered image from computed tomography (CT) showed RCA dilated over the entire length (arrow); and the left main coronary artery derived into three branches (arrows), which are dilated over the entire length along the anterior surface of the ventricle.

Discussion

The coronary artery fistula (CAF) is defined as direct communication of a coronary artery with a cardiac chamber, great vessel, or other vascular structure, bypassing the myocardial capillary bed. The incidence, angiographic characteristics, and natural history of coronary artery fistulas in patients undergoing diagnostic cardiac catheterization have not been well defined. Coronary artery fistula is a rare condition. Of 33 600 patients who had diagnostic cardiac catheterization, 34 (0.1%) had coronary artery fistula. Nineteen (56%) fistulas originated from the right, 11 (32%) from the left anterior descending, and 4 (12%) from the circumflex coronary arteries, respectively [1]. The right coronary artery and right ventricle are the most common origin and distal connection sites, respectively [2, 3]. Coronary sinus drainage has been found in 7% of surgical cases and multiple coronary artery fistulas in 5% of patients [2, 3]. The majority of the coronary artery fistulas were congenital. This may occur as an isolated finding or may appear in the context of other congenital cardiac anomalies or structural heart defects, most frequently in critical pulmonary stenosis or atresia with an intact interventricular septum and in pulmonary artery branch stenosis, tetralogy of Fallot, coarctation of the aorta, hypoplastic left-heart syndrome, and aortic atresia.

Acquired coronary artery fistula may rarely arise as a consequence of trauma such as a gunshot wound or a stab wound. It can also occur after cardiac surgery or invasive cardiac catheterization with percutaneous transluminal coronary angioplasty, pacemaker implantation, endomyocardial biopsy, atrial septal defect, or can be caused by an infection that weakens the wall of the coronary artery and the heart [1, 4, 5].

A CAF may arise from any branch of the coronary artery system and originate from the right coronary artery (RCA) in 60%, left anterior descending (LAD) artery in 35%, and from the right posterior descending artery, obtuse marginal and diagonal arteries in 0.5% to 1.9% of patients [6]. In congenital fistulae, drainage is most often to a low-pressure cardiac chamber; the right ventricle (RV), right atrium (RA), or the pulmonary arteries (PA), and less frequently to the superior vena cava, coronary sinus, and pulmonary veins [6–9]. Communication into the left ventricle (LV) is extremely rare. The angiographic classification of Sakakibara [10] divides CAF into two categories – type A, proximal coronary segment dilated to the origin of the fistula with distal end normal, and type B, coronary dilated over the entire length, terminating as a fistula in the right side of the heart (end-artery type). Our patient had a short left main coronary artery-derived three branches significant dilated over the entire length, terminating as fistula drainage into the left side of the heart. The right coronary artery was significantly dilated over the entire length, terminating as multiple fistula drainage into RV cavity. This type does not belong to Type A or Type B.

Although the course of this malformation is usually benign, significant complications can occur, such as congestive heart failure, bacterial endocarditis, myocardial ischemia, ventricular arrhythmia, or sudden death [6]. In the small fistulas, the myocardial blood supply is not compromised enough to cause symptoms, fistulas remain clinically silent and are recognized at routine echocardiography and autopsy. Spontaneous closure usually occurs; however, some can dilate over time.

Larger fistulae progressively enlarge over time, and complications, such as congestive heart failure, myocardial infarction, arrhythmias, infectious endocarditis, aneurysm formation, rupture, and death, are more likely to arise in older patients. Spontaneous closure has been rarely reported in the setting of large fistulas. The exertional dyspnea of our patient might be result from multiple coronary fistulas.

Coronary angiography remains the most common method for diagnosis of coronary fistula. Most of the fistula are small and found accidently during coronary angiography but sometimes the exact communication of the fistula with the adjacent cardiac chamber is difficult to determine by coronary angiography alone. Noninvasive methods, such as transthoracic echocardiography with Doppler and color flow imaging, magnetic resonance imaging (MRI) and contrast-enhancing multislice computed tomography can be used with coronary angiography [11].

Two-dimensional echocardiography may detect the proximal segment of a dilated coronary artery, as in our case. A color Doppler echocardiographic study also is helpful. Yoshikawa et al. studied 14 patients with CAF using two-dimensional echocardiography, verified by CA angiography [12]. Using two-dimensional echocardiography, the dilated arteries were visualized by the parasternal short-axis approach. These techniques can be helpful in the detection of CAF before cardiac catheterization. We detected the dilate proximal segment of LCA and RCA, and also found the fistula by two-dimensional and Doppler echocardiography, which was verified by coronary angiography and coronary CT angiogram.

Coronary CT angiography using Flash mode with a high pitch and an ECG-triggered spiral scanning revealed an extremely rare combination of coronary anomalies. In our case, CT demonstrated significantly dilated right coronary over its entire length, and three giant left anomalous coronary aneurysms were derived from the left main coronary forming multiple fistula connecting the left coronary artery and the left ventricle cavity, which was demonstrated by a coronary angiogram.

Clinical symptoms of ischemia or volume overload, such as exertional angina or dyspnea, are the primary indication for closure of a fistula. The treatment of asymptomatic lesions is controversial, with some authors recommending early surgical intervention while others recommend a more conservative approach [13, 14]. The choice of treatment method depends on the anatomy and morphologic features of the fistula. In 1947, Bjork and Crafoord [15] described the first successful surgical repair of a CAF. Twelve years later Swan et al. [16] reported the closure of a fistula using a cardiopulmonary bypass. The first report of percutaneous therapeutic embolization was in 1983, when Reidy and colleagues [17] reported successful transcatheter fistula occlusion. Various transcatheter occlusion techniques have been used with excellent outcomes for fistulas with shorter, less tortuous courses.

Surgical treatment results in a low mortality, from 0 to 4%, and morbidity from 10% to 15% [18–20]. Operative correction in patients younger than 10 years or older than 45 years of age is coupled with an increase risk of morbidity and mortality. In a review by McNamara et al. [21], 57% of patients were treated surgically with a 0.5% operative mortality rate.

Key Points

1. Coronary artery fistulas are rare anomalies and those presenting in late adult life are even more unusual.
2. They should always be considered in the differential diagnosis and diagnostic evaluations of patients with coronary artery disease and concomitant abnormalities.
3. Surgical coronary revascularization and operative fistula ligation can markedly improve ventricular function and symptom.

References

1. Vavuranakis, M., Bush, C.A. and Boudoulas, H. (1995). Coronary artery fistulas in adults: incidence, angiographic characteristics, natural history. *Cathet Cardiovasc Diagn.* 35 (2): 116–120.
2. Liberthson, R.R., Sagar, K., Berkoben, J.P. et al. (1979). Congenital coronary arteriovenous fistula: report of 13 patients, review of the literature and delineation of management. *Circulation* 59: 849–854.
3. Urrutia, S.C., Falaschi, G., Ott, D.A., et al. (1983). Surgical management of 56 patients with congenital coronary artery fistulas. *Ann Thorac Surg* 35: 300–307.
4. Chiu, S.N., Wu, M.H., Lin, M.T., et al. (2005). Acquired coronary artery fistula after open heart surgery for congenital heart disease. *Int J Cardiol* 103 (2): 187–192.
5. Sandhu, S.J., Uretsky, B.F., Zerbe, T.R. et al. (1989). Coronary artery fistula in the heart transplant. A Potential complication of endmyocardial biopsy. *Circulation* 79: 350–356.
6. Kirklin, J.W. and Barratt-Boyes, B.G. (1993). Congenital anomalies of the coronary arteries. *Cardiac Surgery*, 1167–1193. New York, NY: Churchill Livingstone.
7. Levin, D.C., Fellows, K.E. and Abrams, H.L. (1978). Hemodynamically significant primary anomalies of the coronary arteries: angiographic aspects. *Circulation* 58: 25–34.
8. Fernandes, E.D., Kadivar, H., Hallman, G.L. et al. (1992). Congenital malformations of coronary arteries: The Texas Heart Institute experience. *Ann Thorac Surg* 54: 732–740.
9. Yamanaka, O. and Hobbs, R.E. (1990). Coronary artery anomalies in 126,595 patients undergoing coronary arteriography. *Cathet Cardiovasc Diagn* 21: 28–40.
10. Sakakibara, S., Yokoyama, M., Takao, A. et al. (1966). Coronary arteriovenous fistula. *Am Heart J* 72: 307–314.
11. Armsby, L.R., Keane, J.F., Sherwood, M.C. et al. (2002). Management of coronary artery fistulae. Patient selection and results of transcatheter closure. *Am J Coll Cardiol* 39: 1026–1032.
12. Yoshikawa, J., Kata, H., Yanagihara, K. et al. (1982). Noninvasive visualization of the dilated main coronary arteries in coronary artery fistula by cross sectional echocardiography. *Circulation* 65: 600–603.
13. Liotta, D., Hallman, G.L., Hall, R.J. et al. (1971). Surgical treatment of congenital coronary artery fistula, *Surgery* 70: 856–864.
14. Kamiya, H., Yasuda, T., Nagamine, H. et al. (2002). Surgical treatment of congenital coronary artery fistulas: 27 years experience and a review of the literature. *J Card Surg* 17 (2): 173–177.
15. Biorck, G and Crafoord, C. (1947). Arteriovenous aneurysm on the pulmonary artery simulating patent ductus arteriosus botalli. *Thorax* 2: 65–74.
16. Swan, H., Wilson, I.N., Woodwark, G. et al. (1959). Surgical obliteration of a coronary artery fistula to right ventricle. *AMA Arch Surg* 879: 820–824.
17. Reidy, J.F., Jones, O.D.H., Tynan, M.J. et al. (1985). Embolisation procedures in congenital heart disease. *Br Heart J* 54: 184–192.
18. Sherwood, M., Rockenmacher, S., Colan, S. et al. (1999). Prognostic significance of clinically silent coronary artery fistulas. *Am J Cardiol* 83: 407–411.
19. Bogers, A.J.J.C., Quaegebeur, J.M. and Huysmans, H.A. (1987). Early and late results of surgical treatment of congenital coronary artery fistula. *Thorax* 42: 369–373. doi:10.1136/thx.42.5.369
20. Cooley, D.A. and Ellis, P.R. (1962). Surgical considerations of coronary arterial fistula. *Am J Cardiol* 10: 467–474.
21. McNamara, J.J. and Gross, R.E. (1969). Congenital coronary artery fistula. *Surgery* 65: 59.

7 Crista Terminalis Bridge Mimicking Right Atrial Mass

Jing Ping Sun, Alex Pui-Wai Lee, and Xing Sheng Yang

The Chinese University of Hong Kong, Hong Kong

History

An 85-year-old female with a history of hyperlipidemia. A mass was noted by echocardiographic examination.

Physical Examination

Blood pressure was 120/80 mmHg, pulse rate 82 bpm, respiration rate 18/min. All other physical findings were unremarkable.

Echocardiography

The left and right cardiac chambers were normal in size and systolic function. There were mild pulmonic, mitral and moderate tricuspid valvular regurgitation. A small mass/structure $(0.91 \times 0.9 \, cm^2)$ was noticed at the roof of right atrium (Figure 7-1, Video 7-1, and Video 7-2), which might represent a prominent crista terminalis or residual thrombi.

Magnetic Resonance Imaging (MRI)

Magnetic resonance imaging showed normal concordance of heart chambers, normal wall thickness and motion of the left ventricle. There was a linear bandlike structure in the roof of the right atrium with a signal identical to the myocardium (Figure 7-2, Video 7-3). No abnormal hyperenhancement was detected.

Discussion

The crista terminalis represents the junction between the sinus venosus and the heart in the developing embryo. In the development of the human heart, the right horn and transverse portion of the sinus venosus ultimately become incorporated with and form a part of the adult right atrium. The line of union between the right atrium and the right auricle is present on the interior of the atrium in the form of a vertical crest, known as the crista terminalis of His (Wilhelm His, Jr.). The crista terminalis originates from the atrial septal wall medially, passes anterior to the orifice of the superior vena cava, descends posteriorly and laterally, and then turns anteriorly to skirt the right side of the

Comparative Cardiac Imaging: A Case-based Guide, First Edition.
Edited by Jing Ping Sun, Xing Sheng Yang, and Bryan P. Yan.
© 2018 John Wiley & Sons Ltd. Published 2018 by John Wiley & Sons Ltd.
Companion website: www.wiley.com/sun/comparative_cardiac_imaging

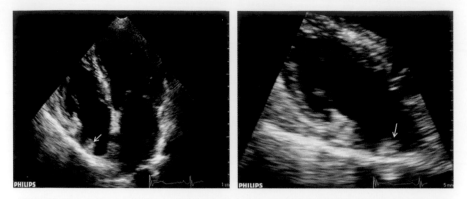

Figure 7-1   Two-dimensional echocardiography: A small mass/structure (1 × 0.9 cm, arrow) noted in the right atrial roof from an apical four-chamber view (left), and right ventricular inflow view (right).

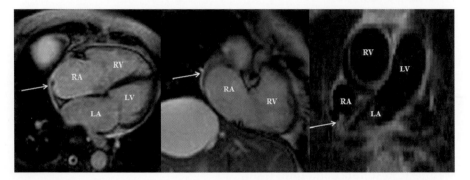

Figure 7-2   MRI images showed a linear band–like structure in the roof of the right atrium with signal identical to myocardium with no evidence of thrombus. Appearance is compatible with a prominent crista terminalis (arrow).

orifice of the inferior vena cava, generally a smooth-surfaced, thick portion of heart muscle in a crescent shape at the opening into the right auricle. On the external aspect of the right atrium, corresponding to the crista terminalis, is the sulcus terminalis. The crista terminalis provides the origin for the pectinate muscles [1, 2]. The crista terminalis is an important anatomical structure, shown to be the site of origin of right atrial tachyarrythmias referred to as "cristal tachycardias" [3]. It has been studied most extensively by electrophysiologists and its anatomic importance related to arrhythmogenesis is well documented. Atrial tachycardias commonly originate from the crista terminalis and can be eliminated by ablation of that area [4].

As the sensitivity of imaging equipment continues to improve and intracardiac structures can be more clearly visualized by echocardiography imaging, an appreciation of the appearance of a prominent crista terminalis on a transthoracic echocardiography will minimize the misdiagnosis of this right atrial structure. A better assessment of these structures using three-dimensional echocardiography was described [5].

Meier and Harnell's study reviewed 149 MRI examinations to determine the frequency of a prominent crista terminalis. Fifty-nine percent of the subjects were shown to have a prominent intra-atrial structure diagnosed as a prominent crista terminalis. In both studies, the conclusion was that an awareness of the location, anatomic, and MRI features of the crista terminalis would help prevent misdiagnosis of this structure as an intracardiac tumor [6].

Key Points

1. The crista terminalis represents the junction between the sinus venosus and the heart in the developing embryo.
2. Transesophageal echocardiography, CT/MRI, and 3D transthoracic imaging could be used to differentiate a prominent crista terminalis from a true right atrial mass.
3. Understanding of the right atrial anatomy is important to making an accurate diagnosis and to avoid unnecessary additional tests.

References

1. Sanchez-Quintana, D., Anderson, R.H., Cabrera, J.A. et al. (2002). The terminal crest: Morphological features relevant to electrophysiology. *Heart* 88: 406–411.
2. Ho, S.Y., Anderson, R.H., and Sanchez-Quintana, D. (2002). Gross structure of the atriums: More than an anatomic curiosity? *Pacing Clin Electrophysiol* 25: 342–350.
3. Kalman, J.M., Olgin, J.E., Karch, M.R. et al. (1998). "Cristal tachycardias": Origin of right atrial tachycardias from the crista terminalis identified by intracardiac echocardiography. *J Am Coll Cardiol* 31: 451–459.
4. Marchlinski, F.F., Ren, J.F., Schwartzman, D. et al. (2000). Accuracy of fluoroscopic localization of the crista terminalis documented by intracardiac echocardiography. *J Interv Card Electrophysiol* 4: 415–421.
5. Chan, K.L., Liu, X., Ascah, K.J. et al. (2004). Comparison of real-time three-dimensional echocardiography with conventional two-dimensional echocardiography in the assessment of structural heart disease. *J Am Soc Echocardiogr* 17: 976–980.
6. Meier, R.A. and Hartnell, G.G. (1994). MRI of right atrial pseudomass: Is it really a diagnostic problem? *J Comput Assist Tomogr* 18: 398–401.

8 A Criss-cross Heart with Double Outlet Right Ventricle

Lianghua Xia[1], Bo Zhang[1], Fanxia Meng[1], and Jing Ping Sun[2]

[1] Tongji University School of Medicine, Shanghai, China
[2] The Chinese University of Hong Kong, Hong Kong

History

A 30-year-old male presented with a history of cyanosis since childhood. There was no family history of congenital heart disease.

Examination

The patient appears lip cyanosis. His heart rate and respiratory rates were 84 bmp and 22/min, respectively. Blood pressure was 110/75 mmHg. All the peripheral pulses were clearly felt. Cardiac auscultation revealed normal first and second heart sound along with 3/6 ejection systolic murmur, which was most audible at the left upper parasternal area.

Transthoracic Echocardiography

Atypical apical view showed that the left atrium was connected with the right ventricle through tricuspid valve; aorta and pulmonary artery were arising from the right ventricle, but pulmonary valves were thickened with stenosis (arrow), the velocity of pulmonary artery was 4.7 m/s (maximal gradient was 88 mmHg). An apical view showed that the right atrium was connected with the left ventricle through the mitral valve. An apical four-chamber view showed double outlets right ventricle with a ventricular septal defect. A super sternum notch view showed collateral circulation between aorta and pulmonary artery (Figure 8-1, Video 8-1). Left and right ventricular function was normal.

Atypical apical view with color Doppler showed blood flow from the left atrium into right ventricle through tricuspid valve, and then flew into double outlets; but pulmonary valves were thickened with stenosis (Video 8-2). The color Doppler echocardiography showed blood flow from the right atrium into left ventricle through the mitral valve and into right ventricular cavity through a ventricular septal defect (Video 8-3).

Computed Tomography

Computed tomography multiplanar reconstruction images showed the right atrium connected with the left ventricle through the mitral valve, and a ventricular septal defect (Figure 8-2A); the left atrium connected with the right ventricle (Figure 8-2B); the left atrium was located at upper left of right atrium (Figure 8-2C); the right ventricle (RV) was superiorly and the left ventricle (LV) inferiorly located (Figure 8-2D). These images

Comparative Cardiac Imaging: A Case-based Guide, First Edition.
Edited by Jing Ping Sun, Xing Sheng Yang, and Bryan P. Yan.
© 2018 John Wiley & Sons Ltd. Published 2018 by John Wiley & Sons Ltd.
Companion website: www.wiley.com/sun/comparative_cardiac_imaging

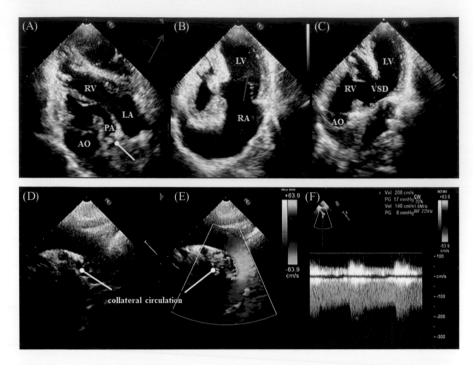

Figure 8-1 Transthoracic echocardiography. A. An atypical apical view showed that the left atrium was connected with right ventricle through the tricuspid valve; the aorta and pulmonary artery arose from the right ventricle, but the pulmonary valves were thickened with stenosis (arrow). B. An apical view showed the right atrium was connected with left ventricle through the mitral valve. C. An apical four-chamber view showed double outlets right ventricle with a ventricular septal defect. D and E. A super sternum notch view showed collateral circulation between aorta and pulmonary artery. F. The velocity of collateral circulation.

indicated that the atrioventricular (AV) connection is discordant in this case (Figure 8-3). Computed tomography 3D reconstructive image showed a plenty collateral circulation between aorta and pulmonary artery (Figure 8-4).

Discussion

The criss-cross heart is a rare congenital abnormality characterized by crossing of the inflow streams of two ventricles due to an apparent twisting of the heart along its long axis. The etiology and the development mechanism remains unknown. The right atrium is closely associated with the left ventricle in space, and the left atrium is closely associated with the right ventricle in criss-cross heart [1]. Most patients with criss-cross heart have other anomalies such as ventricular septal defect (VSD), transposition of great vessels, right ventricular hypoplasia, pulmonary stenosis, straddling AV and others [2].

The diagnosis should be suspected by echocardiography when the parallel arrangement of the AV valves and ventricular inlets cannot be obtained, and the two valves are not easily visualized simultaneously on apical four-chamber view. Color flow mapping

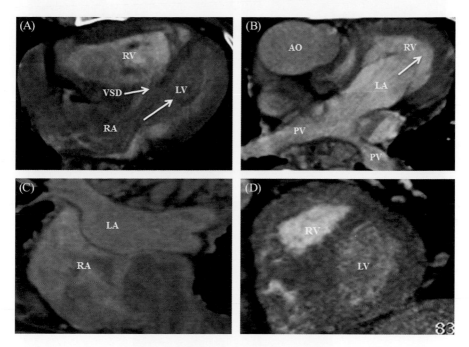

Figure 8-2 Computed tomography multiplanar reconstruction images showed: A. Right atrium connected with left ventricle through the mitral valve, and a ventricular septal defect. B. Left atrium connected with the right ventricle. C. Left atrium located at upper left of right atrium. D. Right ventricle (RV) superiorly located and the left ventricle (LV) inferiorly located. These images indicated that the AV connection is discordant in this case.

can help in assessing the AV connection, visualization of the direction of intracardiac blood flows and recognition of the crossover of the inflow streams [3, 4]. Echocardiography is the primary diagnostic tool, as for all forms of heart disease; CT and MRI could be used as supplement tools in some cases difficult to visualize with echocardiography.

The physiology is determined by the concordant or discordant AV and ventriculoarterial (VA) connection and the associated cardiac defects [2, 5]. We report a rare adult case of criss-cross with discordant AV connections, double outlet right ventricle and pulmonary stenosis, which was diagnosed by echocardiography and confirmed by cardiac CT. The physiology of our case is that the right ventricle received oxygenated blood from the left atrium and pumped into the body through aorta; even though the pulmonary raised from right ventricle, the amount of blood going to the pulmonary was limited due to stenosis. The ventricular defect and abundant collateral circulation between aorta and pulmonary artery are the compensation for pulmonary valve stenosis in this case. There might be a need for further intervention over time, because the right ventricle has been exposed to systemic intraventricular pressure for many years, though without any evidence of impaired systolic function. In addition, a long-term possibility of right-sided heart failure, there is the risk of paradoxical embolism. Tachyarrhythmias may also occur requiring intervention.

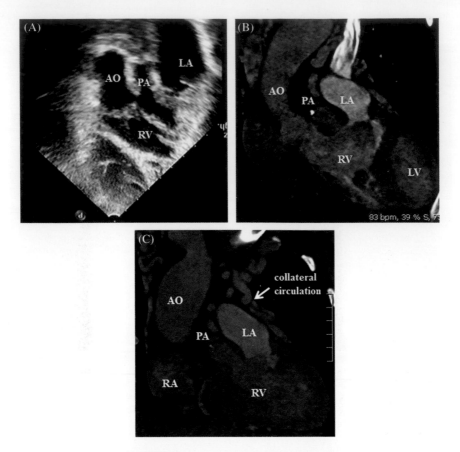

Figure 8-3 A. An echocardiography image showed that the left atrium was connected with the right ventricle through the tricuspid valve; the aorta and pulmonary artery arose from the right ventricle. B. The findings of CT images were consistent with echocardiography. C. Computed tomography image showed a plentiful collateral circulation between the aorta and the pulmonary artery.

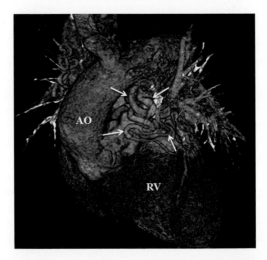

Figure 8-4 Computed tomography three-dimensional reconstruction image displaying the aorta, which originated from the right ventricle, and plentiful collateral circulation between the aorta and pulmonary artery (arrows).

Key Points

1. A criss-cross heart is a rare cardiac anomaly, which can be diagnosed by a transthoracic echocardiography, and by an alert echocardiographer to determine the relationships of the cardiac chambers and associated cardiac anomalies.
2. Computed tomography yielded more confidence in the preoperative understanding of this complex anomaly, helping the surgical team in planning the most appropriate surgical approach.

References

1. Fontes, V.F., de Souza, J.A. and Pontes Jùnior, S. C. (1990). Criss-cross heart with intact ventricular septum. *Int J Cardiol* 26 (3): 382–385.
2. Van Praagh, R., Weinberg, P.M. and Van Praagh, S. (1977). Malposition of the heart. In: *Heart Disease in Infants, Children and Adolescents* (ed. A.J. Moss, F.H. Adams, and G.C. Emmanouilides), 394–417. Baltimore, MD: Williams & Wilkins.
3. Robinson, J.P., Kumpeng, V. and MaCartney, J.F. (1985). Cross sectional echocardiographic and angiocardiographic correlation in crisscross hearts. *Br Heart J* 54: 61–67.
4. Araoz, A.P., Reddy, P.G., Thompson, D.P. et al. (2002). Magnetic resonance angiography of crisscross heart. *Circulation* 105: 537–538.
5. Cabrera, D.A., Alcíbar, V.J., Rienzu, I.M.-A. et al. (2000). Corazón en crisscross con discordancia auriculoventricular y ventrículo arterial. *Rev Esp Cardiol* 53: 1121–1122.

9 Double-Chambered Right Ventricle with Ventricular Septal Defect

Lei Zhang[1], Fanxia Meng[1], Ming Chen[1], and Jing Ping Sun[2]

[1] Tongji University School of Medicine, Shanghai, China
[2] The Chinese University of Hong Kong, Hong Kong

History

A 37-year-old female presented with heart murmur, which she has had since childhood. She was well developed with normal activity.Past medical history was unremarkable.

Physical Examination

Blood pressure 110 / 70 mmHg. Breathing: 28 times/min. Heart rate: 70 bpm. Lungs are clear to auscultation and percussion bilaterally. A grade 3/6 systolic decrescendo murmur is heard best at the third right intercostal space, which radiates to the apex.

Electrocardiogram

Sinus rhythm, right axis deviation of +120°, dominant R wave in V1 (>7 mm tall), dominant S wave in V5 or V6 (>7 mm deep), QRS duration < 120 ms, suggesting right ventricular hypertrophy.

Chest X-ray

Chest film showed an enlarged heart coupled with an increase in pulmonary vascular markings.

Two- dimensional Transthoracic Echocardiography with Color Doppler

The presence of hypertrophied muscle bundle in the right ventricular outflow region (arrows in Figure 9-1A, Video 9-1) along with color flow turbulence (Figure 9-1A, *). The peak velocity across stenosis pulmonary valve was 4.8 m/sec (peak and a mean gradient was 92 mmHg and 60 mmHg, respectively) (Figure 9-1B). Apical five-chamber view (Figure 9-2A) showed the presence of a 1.78 cm perimembranous ventricular septal defect (VSD) with bidirectional shunt (left to right predominant) and a subaortic mem- brane (Video 9-1).The parasternal long-axis view showed a ridgelike subaortic membrane (Figure 9-2B, Video 9-2). The subaortic membrane resulted in blood flow with higher peak velocity (1.96 m/s) in the left ventricular outflow tract. The pulmonary artery and aortic arch were normal. On the basis of this finding, a preliminary diagnosis of dou- ble-chamber right ventricle (DCRV) with VSD and subaortic membrane was made.

Comparative Cardiac Imaging: A Case-based Guide, First Edition.
Edited by Jing Ping Sun, Xing Sheng Yang, and Bryan P. Yan.
© 2018 John Wiley & Sons Ltd. Published 2018 by John Wiley & Sons Ltd.
Companion website: www.wiley.com/sun/comparative_cardiac_imaging

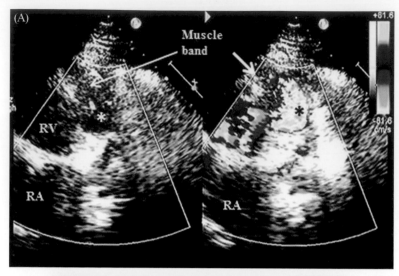

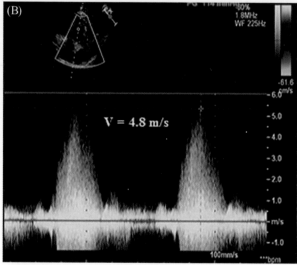

Figure 9-1   Echocardiographic findings (a modified view) in a patient with a double-chambered right ventricle. A. A modified view showed an anomalous RV muscle bundle (large and small arrows), turbulent Doppler color flow velocity pattern in the right ventricular outflow tract (RVOT, *), which suggested RV obstruction between RV and RVOT. B. The high velocity by continuous wave Doppler in RVOT indicated obstruction within the RV.
Notes: RV, right ventricle; RA, right atrium.

Cardiac Computed Tomography

Computed tomography ventriculography showed dilated RA and VSD with a left-to-right shunt; the thickness of the RV wall was significantly increased. A CT atypical short axis image showed that the RV wall exhibited significant hypertrophy; there was an obstruction between RV lower chamber and the right ventricular outflow tract (Figure 9-2).

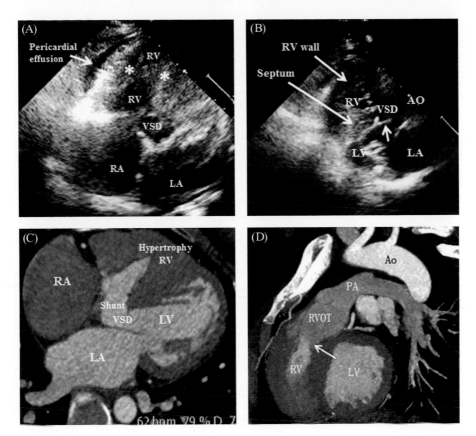

Figure 9-2   A. Atypical four-chamber view showed a dilated right atrium (RA), anomalous RV muscle bundle (*) from the RV free wall and septum hypertrophy resulting in RV obstruction. B. A parasternal long-axis view showed significantly hypertrophy of the ventricular septal and right ventricle wall, and a ventricular septal defect; the arrow pointed to the subaortic membrane. C. A computed tomography image showed dilated RA and VSD with a left-to-right shunt; the thickness of the RV wall was significant increased. D. A CT atypical short-axis image showed that RV wall was significantly hypertrophied; there is an obstruction (arrow) between the RV and the RVOT.
Notes: RV, right ventricle; LV, left ventricle; RVOT, right ventricle outflow tract; AO, aorta; and PA, pulmonary artery.

Surgical Operation

Surgical correction was performed for this patient with DCRV. Surgery consisted of a patch closure of the VSD, excision of subaortic membrane, and a resection of the anomalous muscle bundles through a right atriotomy and a right ventriculotomy.

Discussion

Double-chambered right ventricle is a rare congenital heart disease of the right ventricular outflow tract obstruction characterized by anomalous muscle bands (AMBs), that divide the right ventricle into two compartments, a high-pressure inflow chamber, and a low-pressure outflow chamber [1]. Here we describe a case of an adult male with DCRV associated with ventricular septal defect and subaortic membrane. Two-dimensional echocardiography with color flow clearly outlined all the three cardiac anomalies as well as their relationships with each other. The diagnosis was confirmed by cardiac CT. The patient underwent successful surgical resection of the anomalous muscle bundle along with repair of the associated anomalies.

Lesions frequently associated with double-chambered right ventricle include ventricular septal defect (VSD), pulmonic stenosis, and discrete subaortic stenosis [2]. Vogel et al [3] described 36 patients with membranous VSD and DCRV, of which 88% had echocardiographic evidence of subaortic stenosis.

Several subtypes of divided RV are observed. These subtypes include anomalous septoparietal band, anomalous apical shelf, hypertrophy of apical trabeculations, anomalous apical shelf with Ebstein malformation, and sequestration of the outlet portion of the ventricle from a circumferential muscular diaphragm in patients with tetralogy of Fallot [4]. The most common form of double-chambered right ventricle is the RV divided into two chambers by the presence of AMBs. However, no uniformity is observed in the position of these anomalous muscle bundles or in the manner in which the right ventricle is divided [5].

Diagnosis

Transthoracic echocardiography has its limitations for the diagnosis of DCRV owing to the proximity of the RVOT region to the transducer from the precordial planes, and other limitations encountered while studying adults, such as obesity and emphysema [6]. Three-dimensional echocardiography played a complementary role to two-dimensional echocardiography in making a diagnosis of DCRV with VSD and subaortic membrane. The anatomical relationship between the membranous VSD, subaortic membrane and the RVOT muscle bundle might be clearly delineated with 3DTTE [7]; but it faced a similar limitation of two-dimensional echocardiography in the evaluation of the RVOT muscle bundle due to transthoracic approach. Transesophageal echocardiography is an excellent supplementary tool to assist delineation of the RV abnormalities as well as to assess and quantify the severity of the RV cavitary obstruction. Recently, contrast computed tomography and CMR have been introduced in the identification of DCRV. Those diagnostic tools are now sufficiently mature to preclude the need for invasive testing [8–10].

Cases of DCRV should in general be treated surgically because the obstruction is progressive and ends in heart failure. In asymptomatic patients, where the peak gradient exceeds 40 mm Hg, surgical intervention is indicated [10, 11].

Key Points

1. Double-chambered right ventricle (DCRV) is a rare congenital heart disease of the right ventricular outflow tract obstruction characterized by AMBs that divide the right ventricle into a high-pressure inflow chamber and a low-pressure outflow chamber.
2. Double-chambered RV should be suspected in adults when there is a RV outflow tract obstruction with unusual symptoms.
3. Cases of DCRV should in general be treated surgically because the obstruction is progressive and ends in heart failure.

References

1. Alva, C., Ho, S.Y., Lincoln, C.R. et al. (1999). The nature of the obstructive muscular bundles in double-chambered right ventricle. *J Thorac Cardiovasc Surg* 117: 1180–1189.
2. Restivo, A., Cameron, A.H., Anderson, R.H. et al. (1984). Divided right ventricle: a review of its anatomical varieties. *Pediatr Cardiol* 5 (3):197–204.
3. Vogel, M., Smallhorn, J.F. and Freedom, R.M. (1988). An echocardio-graphic study of the association of ventricular septal defect and right ventricular muscle bundles with affixed subaortic abnormality. *Am J Cardiol* 61: 857–860.
4. Hubail, Z.J. and Ramaciotti, C. (2007). Spatial relationship between the ventricular septal defect and the anomalous muscle bundle in a double-chambered right ventricle. *Congenit Heart Dis* 2 (6): 421–423.
5. Byrum C.J., Dick, M. and Behrendt, D.M. (1982). Excitation of the double chamber right ventricle: electro- physiologic and anatomic correlation. *Am J Cardiol* 49 (5): 1254–1258.
6. Hoffman, P., Wojcik, A.W., Roaski, J. et al. (2004). The role of echocardiography in diagnosing double chambered right ventricle in adults. *Heart* 90: 789–793.
7. Kharwar, R.B., Dwivedi, S.K. and Sharma, A. (2016). Double-chambered right ventricle with ventricular septal defect and subaortic membrane – three-dimensional echocardiographic evaluation. *Echocardiography* 33 (2): 323–327.
8. Chang, R.Y., Kuo, C.H., Rim, R.S. et al. (1996). Transesophageal echocardiographic image of double-chambered right ventricle. *J Am Soc Echocardiogr* 9: 347 352.
9. Kilner, P.J., Sievers, B., Meyer, G.P. et al. (2002). Double-chambered right ventricle or sub-infundibular stenosis assessed by cardiovascular magnetic resonance. *J Cardiovasc Magn Reson* 4 (3): 373–379.
10. Darwazah, A.K., Eida. M., Bader, V. et al. (2011). Surgical management of double-chambered right ventricle in adults. *Tex Heart Inst J* 38: 301–304.
11. McElhinney, D.B., Chatterjee, K.M. and Reddy, V.M. (2000). Double chambered right ventricle presenting in adulthood. *Ann Thorac Surg* 70: 124–127.

10 Isolated Double-Orifice Mitral Valve

Jing Ping Sun

The Chinese University of Hong Kong, Hong Kong

History

A 52-year-old female was referred to our outpatients' clinic for follow up and to monitor progress of systemic lupus erythematosus (SLE).

Physical examination

The clinical examination and resting electrocardiogram were normal.

Echocardiography

The echocardiographic examination in the parasternal short-axis view showed a distinctive morphology of an isolated double-orifice mitral valve (DOMV) (Figure 10-1A and B). The two mitral orifices were located in the posteromedial and posterolateral positions and their estimated areas were 2.0 cm^2 and 1.9 cm^2, respectively (Figure 10-1; Video 10-1). There was a single mitral annulus with the two valvular orifices separated by a central fibrous bridge (Figure 10-1; Video 10-2). The echocardiographic two- and four-chamber views indicated separated subvalvular structures for each of the two orifices (Figure 10-1C; Video 10-3, and Video 10-4). Two-dimensional echocardiography with color Doppler examination demonstrated that the function of each orifice was normal without evidence of either systolic mitral regurgitation jets or diastolic turbulence (Figure 10-1D; Video 10-2). Moreover, the two peak and the mean transmitral gradients were normal. The resting echocardiographic examination excluded the presence of any sign of congenital morphological cardiac abnormalities. The right ventricle and atrium were mildly dilated with normal systolic function; pulmonary trunk was moderate dilated with moderate pulmonary regurgitation. The estimate pulmonary artery systolic pressure was 75 mmHg. The changes in the right heart resulted from the SLE.

Discussion

Isolated double-orifice mitral valve (DOMV) is an extremely rare congenital anomaly occurring in 0.05% of the general population [1]. DOMV was first described by Greenfield in 1876 [2]. This anomaly is characterized by the presence of a single mitral

Comparative Cardiac Imaging: A Case-based Guide, First Edition.
Edited by Jing Ping Sun, Xing Sheng Yang, and Bryan P. Yan.
© 2018 John Wiley & Sons Ltd. Published 2018 by John Wiley & Sons Ltd.
Companion website: www.wiley.com/sun/comparative_cardiac_imaging

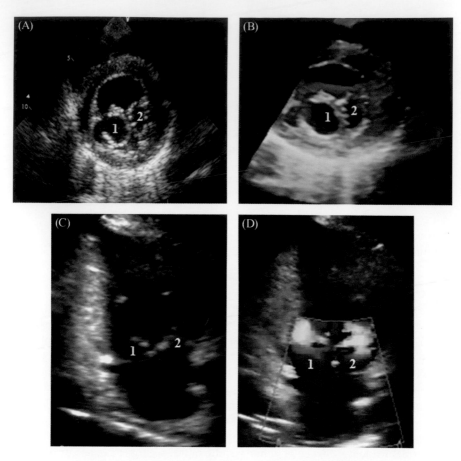

Figure 10-1 Transthoracic two-dimensional echocardiography. A parasternal short-axis view showed distinctive morphology of an isolated double orifice mitral valve; two orifices are equal in size (A and B). An apical two-chamber view showed that there was a single mitral annulus with the two valvular orifices separated by a central fibrous bridge (C). The same view with color Doppler showed that there are two normal laminar flows from double orifice into left ventricle separately (D).

annulus with two orifices, each having independent subvalvular apparatus and papillary muscles [3, 4]. The etiology of DOMV has been recognized in the abnormal fusion of the endocardial cushions and abnormal development of the mitral valve during the delamination process [3]. Transthoracic echocardiography is the modality of choice for the characterization of this anomaly; in this respect, the parasternal short-axis view allows a full morphologic characterization of the anomaly and should always be performed in the case of a meaningful clinical suspect [5].

Generally, the symptoms are related to mitral regurgitation or stenosis, but it can also present as an incidental finding in patients with normal-valve-function DOMV [5, 6] Three specific types of DOMV can be described at two-dimensional echocardiography: (i) Complete bridge type (about 15% of DOMVs), in which both openings are visible from the leaflet edge and both orifices appear circular (equal or unequal in size) with normal subvalvular apparatus and papillary muscles; (ii) incomplete bridge type, in which the connection is seen only at the leaflet edge; and (iii) hole type (the most frequent) characterized by a small accessory orifice situated at either the posteromedial or anterolateral commissure and identifiable only at the midleaflet level [3]. Accordingly, our patient presented the complete bridge-type DOMV, which is the rarest form of this anomaly.

Function of both components of the DOMV is mildly impaired in most cases but at times can be normal in some patients. Mild to severe regurgitation or significant stenosis of either or both orifices has been reported [7]. The DOMV can be an isolated anomaly, but in most cases, it is associated with other congenital malformations.

Two-dimensional echocardiography is the first choice to scan this abnormality. Theoretically, transesophageal echocardiography (TEE) defines the anatomy of the mitral valve better than transthoracic echocardiography and may help to differentiate DOMV from other conditions such as lesions of valvular leaflets provoked by endocarditis [8]. Three-dimensional echocardiography is generally useful to add anatomical details to those obtained by two-dimensional echocardiography. However, it should be performed only in case of uncertain findings from two-dimensional echocardiography, which is considered the screening test for DOMV.

Cardiac magnetic resonance imaging evaluation becomes a mandatory step to confirm the clinical suspicion, and to exclude any concurrent cardiac and vascular abnormalities.

The management of DOMV is related to the type and severity of mitral valve dysfunction. Asymptomatic DOMV usually requires no active intervention; surgical repair is needed in case of severe mitral regurgitation, stenosis, or associated cardiac anomalies [9]. In all cases of DOMV, a long-term follow up is required for the early detection of complications [9].

Double-orifice mitral valve as a cause of symptomatic mitral valve disease is also seen in middle aged/elderly people. Some of the patients may stay asymptomatic. Transthoracic echocardiography examination, especially in short-axis parasternal views, is a reliable method and in most cases, sufficient to confirm a diagnosis of DOMV and to determine its type. In any case, with DOMV, the presence of other coexistent cardiovascular abnormalities should be excluded.

Key Points

1. Isolated DOMV is an extremely rare congenital anomaly.
2. This anomaly is characterized by the presence of a single mitral annulus with two orifices, each having independent subvalvular apparatus and papillary muscles.
3. Double-orifice mitral valve might be a cause of symptomatic mitral valve disease, or have a normal valve function.
4. In any case, with DOMV, the presence of other coexistent cardiovascular abnormalities should be excluded.

References

1. Banerjee, A., Kohl, T. and Silverman, N.H. (1995). Echocardiographic evaluation of congenital mitral valve anomalies in children. *Am J Cardiol* 76 (17): 1284–1291.
2. Greenfield, W.S. (1876). Double mitral valve. *Trans Pathol Soc Lond* 27: 128–129.
3. Wójcik A., Klisiewicz A., Szymanski P. et al. (2011). Double-orifice mitral valve – echocardiographic findings. *Kardiol Pol* 69: 139–143.

4. Marcu, C.B., Beek, A.M., Ionescu, C.N. et al. (2012). Double orifice mitral valve visualized on echocardiography and MRI. *Neth Heart J* 20: 380–381.
5. Agarwal, A., Kumar, T., Bhairappa, S. et al. (2013). Isolated double-orifice mitral valve: An extremely rare and interesting anomaly. *BMJ Case Rep* 2013 Bcr2013008856. doi:10.1136/bcr-2013-008856
6. Zalzstein, E., Hamilton, R., Zucker, N. et al. (2004). Presentation, natural history, and outcome in children and adolescents with double orifice mitral valve. *Am J Cardiol* 93: 1067–1069.
7. Hoffman P, Stumper O, Groundstroem K. et al. (1993). The transesophageal echocardiographic features of double-orifice left atrioventricular valve. *J Am Soc Echocardiogr* 6 (1): 94–100.
8. Erkol, A, Karagöz, A., Ozkan, A. et al. (2009). Double-orifice mitral valve associated with bicuspid aortic valve: A rare case of incomplete form of Shone's complex. *Eur J Echocardiogr* 10: 801–803.
9. Mouine, N., Amri, R. and Cherti, M. (2014). Unusual findings in secondary hypertension: Double orifice mitral associated to aortic coarctation, bicuspid aortic valve, and ventricular septal defect. *Int Arch Med* 7: 14.

11 The Gerbode Defect: A Ventriculo-Atrial Defect

Xing Sheng Yang and Jing Ping Sun

The Chinese University of Hong Kong, Hong Kong

History

A 62-year-old female was admitted with a 2-week history of fever, and shortness of breath. There were no previous symptoms.

Physical Examination

On physical examination, she had a collapsing pulse and a grade 3/4 pansystolic murmur along the left sternal border, heard best in the second, third and fourth intercostal spaces. Body temperature: 38 °C. Blood pressure: 80/50 mmHg. The patient had mild peripheral edema.

Laboratory

Electrocardiogram showed sinus tachycardia (100 beats per minute). Blood culture was positive once (*Streptococcus bovis*), but three other blood cultures were negative. Chest X-ray showed normal heart size.

Transthoracic echocardiography (TTE) revealed that the size and systolic function of both ventricles were normal. The left-ventricle ejection fraction (LV EF) was 60%. The right atrium was moderately dilated. The structures of mitral and tricuspid were normal with mild tricuspid and mitral regurgitation. There was a perimembranous ventricular septal defect with a small aneurysm (Figure 11-1, Video 11-1) and a shunt from left ventricle to right atrium (Figure 11-1, Video 11-2, and Video 11-3). The continuance wave Doppler recording showed the high velocity of the left-ventricular to right-atrial shunt; the instantaneous gradient in this patient was 76 mm Hg (Figure 11-2).

Transesopheageal echocardiography showed that there was vegetation associated with the right and noncoronary cusps of aortic valves, about 0.5 cm in size (Figure 11-3, Video 11-4) with moderate to severe aortic regurgitation.

Computed Tomography

The right atrium was moderately dilated. There was no pericardial effusion. The pulmonary trunk appears prominent (3.2 cm). There was a Gerbode defect, with shunting of blood from the left ventricle into the right atrium via the membranous portion of the

Comparative Cardiac Imaging: A Case-based Guide, First Edition.
Edited by Jing Ping Sun, Xing Sheng Yang, and Bryan P. Yan.
© 2018 John Wiley & Sons Ltd. Published 2018 by John Wiley & Sons Ltd.
Companion website: www.wiley.com/sun/comparative_cardiac_imaging

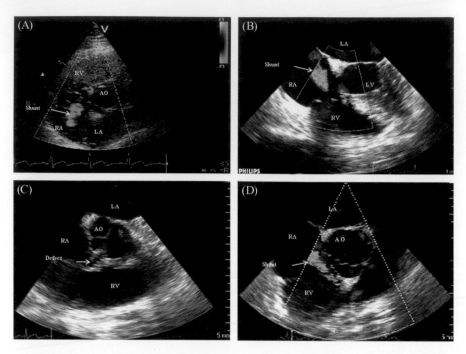

Figure 11-1   A. A transthoracic parasternal short-axis view showed the true or direct left-ventricular to right-atrial shunt. B. A transesopheageal four-chamber view showed the direct left-ventricular to right-atrial shunt. C. A transesopheageal short-axis view showed the ventricular septal defect. D. A transesopheageal short-axis view showed the direct left-ventricular to right-atrial shunt.

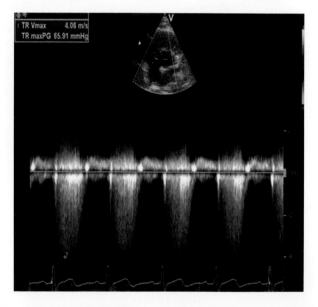

Figure 11-2   The continuance wave Doppler recording showed the high velocity of left ventricular-to-right atrial shunt; the instantaneous gradient in this patient was 76 mm Hg.

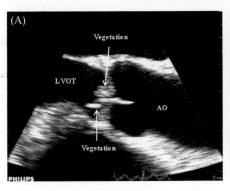
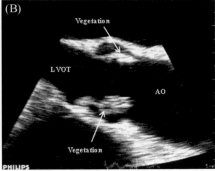

Figure 11-3 A transesopheageal long-axis view showed the vegetation attached to aortic valves during diastole (A), and systole (B).

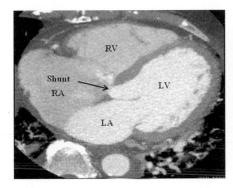
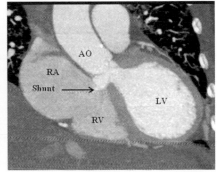

Figure 11-4 A computed tomography four-chamber view indicated there is a Gerbode defect with shunting of blood from the left ventricle into the right atrium, via the membranous portion of the interventricular septum and at a level above the tricuspid annulus plane (arrow). The defect size is estimated as 1.1 cm on CT.

interventricular septum and at level above the tricuspid annulus plane (Figure 11-4). The defect size is estimated 1.1 cm on CT.

Discussion

The Gerbode defect is a very rare congenital anomaly, which represents less than 1% of congenital cardiac defects [1]. The first description of a direct communication between the left ventricle and the right atrium was reported by Buhl in 1857 [2]. The first successful series of patients operated on with a left-ventricular to right-atrial shunt was reported by Frank Gerbode, a surgeon at Stanford University. There are two types known – direct and an indirect – as reported by Gerbode et al. [3]. Gerbode described three general varieties of communication that should be considered: (i) Fusion of the septal leaflet of the tricuspid valve to the edges of the ventricular septal defect associated with a perforation of the leaflet. The shunt occurs from the left ventricle directly into the right atrium; (ii) a defect or cleft of the tricuspid valve leaflet at its point of attachment directly overlying the ventricular defect – the shunt occurs from the left ventricle to the right ventricle and, by regurgitation, into the right atrium; (iii) a combination of these two lesions allowing a varying proportion of shunted blood to enter the right atrium and right ventricle. Acutely, there were two routes for blood to travel from the left ventricle to the right atrium. One is a perimembranous ventricular septal defect and in addition a defect in the tricuspid valve (fenestration) – the shunt is from left ventricle to right ventricle, through the tricuspid valve into the right atrium. This is also referred to as an indirect left-ventricular to right-atrial shunt. The second is the true or direct left-ventricular to right-atrial shunt. In the less common form, usually acquired in association with infective endocarditis, the shunt occurs between the left ventricle and the right atrium above the septal leaflet of the tricuspid valve, which remains intact [4–6]. Often there is an extension of the infection into the subannular region with involvement of the high membranous septum. This leads to a rupture of the portion of the septum that divides the LV from the RA and results in a LV to RA shunt with an intact tricuspid valve. In our case, the patient was admitted due to definite endocarditis. There was a perimembranous ventricular septal defect with a small aneurysm, an intact tricuspid valve by transthoracic echocardiography on admission. The patient was 62 years old, without previous characteristic symptoms or clinical signs; we hypothesized that the ventricular septal aneurysm might be intact before and ruptured due to the infection. The causative organism is usually a *Staphylococcus aureus*. Gerbode's defect has also been reported in association with trauma, following aortic valve replacement, mitral valve replacement, previous repair of an AV septal defect, and ischemic heart disease [7].

The membranous ventriculoatrial defect can be recognized echocardiographically on the basis of dilation of the right atrium in the setting of an unusually high Doppler echocardiogram gradient compared to the ventricular septal defect with shunting only at ventricular level. The high velocity of ventriculoatrial shunt may be misinterpreted as evidence of pulmonary hypertension. Transesophageal echocardiography has been demonstrated to be superior to transthoracic echocardiography in the detection of vegetation associated with endocarditis and complications such as abscess and fistula formation [7].

Most published articles have described typical cardiac catheterization features of this defect, with cardiac MR imaging reportedly offering better visualization of the defect and helping to quantify the amount of blood shunting across the defect [8].

Cardiac CTA allows for more detailed visualization of cardiac anatomy and can supplement or supplant TEE as the diagnostic test of choice for evaluation of patients with this rare defect [9].

Key Points

1. The Gerbode ventriculoatrial defect is a very rare congenital anomaly.
2. The membranous ventriculoatrial defect can be recognized echocardiographically on the basis of the dilation of the right atrium in the setting of an unusually high Doppler velocity.
3. The high velocity of ventriculoatrial shunt into the right atrium may be misinterpreted as tricuspid regurgitation and as evidence of pulmonary hypertension.

References

1. Wasserman, S., Fann, J., Atwood, J. et al. (2002). Acquired left ventricular–right atrial communication Gerbode-type defect. *Echocardiography* 19 (1): 67–72.
2. Meyer, H. (1857). Über angeborene Enge oder Verschluss der Lungenarterienbahn. *Virchow's Arch f Path Anat* 12: 532.
3. Gerbode, F., Hultgren, H., Melrose, D. et al. (1958). Syndrome of left ventricular–right atrial shunt. Successful repair of defect in five cases, with observation of bradycardia on closure. *Ann Surg* 148: 433–446.
4. Cantor, S., Sanderson, R. and Cohn, K. (1971). Left ventricular–right atrial shunt due to bacterial endocarditis. *Chest* 60 (6): 552–554.
5. Velebit, V., Schoneberger, A., Ciaroni, S. et al. (1995). Acquired left ventricular–right atrial shunt (Gerbode defect) after bacterial endocarditis. *Tex Heart Inst J* 22: 100–102.
6. Battin, M., Fong, L.V. and Monro, J.L. (1991). Gerbode ventricular septal defect following endocarditis. *Eur J Cardiothorac Surg* 5: 613–614.
7. Elian, D., Di Segni, E., Kaplinsky, E. et al. (1995). Tel-Hashomer, Israel. Acquired left ventricular–right atrial communication caused by infective endocarditis detected by transesophageal echocardiography: case report and review of the literature. *J Am Soc Echocardiogr* 8: 108–110.
8. Cheema, O.M., Patel, A.A., Chang, S.M. et al. (2009). Gerbode ventricular septal defect diagnosed at cardiac MR imaging: Case report. *Radiology* 252 (1): 50–52.
9. Dragicevic, N., Schmidlin, E., Hazelton, T.R. et al. (2011). Gerbode ventricular septal defect diagnosed using cardiac CTA imaging. *Radiol Case Rep* 6 (3): 530.

12 Intralobar Pulmonary Sequestration

Lei Zhang[1] and Jing Ping Sun[2]

[1] Tongji University School of Medicine, Shanghai, China
[2] The Chinese University of Hong Kong, Hong Kong

History

A 37-year-old male presented with minor hemoptysis, and complained of coughing and sputum persisting from childhood.

Physical Examination

Cardiovascular examination was unremarkable.

Chest X ray

An irregular solid mass was shown in the thoracic cavity behind the heart (Figure 12-1).

Computed Tomography (CT)

In his thorax enhancement CT, there was an area of consolidation in posterobasal segments of the left inferior lung lobe, and there was aberrant lung tissue, which received arterial blood supply from the descending aorta and venous drainage by pulmonary veins (Figures 12-2 and 12-3).

Hospital Course

Patient underwent segmentectomy of the left inferior lung lobe. The diagnosis of intralobar pulmonary sequestration was confirmed by histology.

Discussion

Pulmonary sequestration is a rare anomaly, which does not have a connection with the bronchial system and gets its blood supply, generally, from the aorta or its branches.

In the literature, a widely accepted hypothesis is the development of an accessory bud during development of the normal lung bud. The accessory bud, which develops independently from the normal tracheobronchial tree in embryogenesis, receives its arterial blood supply, generally from the aorta [1]. Current, more accepted theory suggests that obliterate bronchitis with lower lobe bronchial obstruction, caused by one, or more than one, necrotizing pneumonitis attack, results in pulmonary sequestration [2].

Pulmonary sequestration accounts for 0.15%–6.4% of all congenital pulmonary anomalies [3]. It's an area of dysplastic and nonfunctioning lung parenchyma [4].

Comparative Cardiac Imaging: A Case-based Guide, First Edition.
Edited by Jing Ping Sun, Xing Sheng Yang, and Bryan P. Yan.
© 2018 John Wiley & Sons Ltd. Published 2018 by John Wiley & Sons Ltd.
Companion website: www.wiley.com/sun/comparative_cardiac_imaging

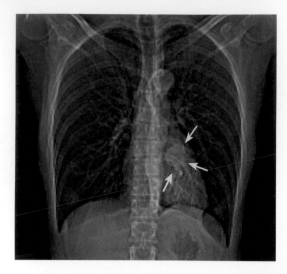

Figure 12-1 An irregular solid mass was shown in the thoracic cavity behind the heart.

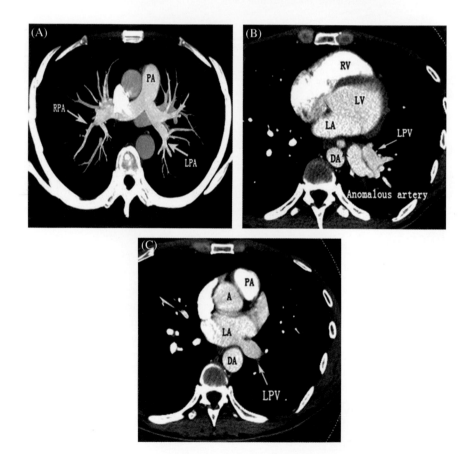

Figure 12-2 A. A maximal intensity projection (MIP) reconstructive image of thoracic CT scan shows normal main pulmonary artery (PA) and branches (yellow arrow). B. A transverse image of the venous phase showing dilated left inferior pulmonary vein and draining into the left atrium (yellow arrow). C. A transverse reconstructive image of thoracic CT scan shows the aberrant vascular structure originating from descending aorta (red arrow) and the dilated left inferior pulmonary veins (yellow arrow).

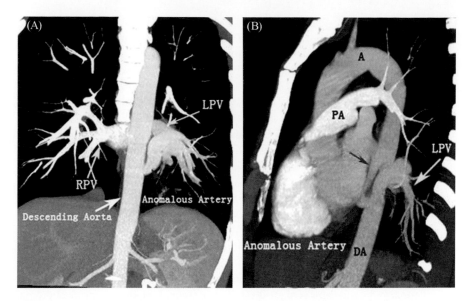

Figure 12-3   A. In coronal reconstruction, the aberrant vascular structure originating from the descending aorta (red arrow) extends to the left inferior pulmonary sequestration (red arrow). The draining vein of the pulmonary sequestration is the left inferior pulmonary veins (yellow arrow). B. A sagittal reconstructive image of thoracic CT scan shows the aberrant vascular structure originating from descending aorta (red arrow).

It is anatomically classified into two types: intralobar and extralobar. Intralobar pulmonary sequestration is located within the visceral pleura and is surrounded by normal lung, whereas extralobar pulmonary sequestration is separated from the lung by a pleural envelope.

It receives its vascular supply from a systemic artery. Seventy-four percent of intralobar pulmonary sequestrations receive their blood supply from the descending thoracic aorta. Venous drainage in pulmonary sequestration is provided by pulmonary veins, in 95% of the cases [5].

Imaging

An arteriogram has been considered vital in documenting the systemic blood supply, allowing definitive diagnosis as well as preoperative planning.

The advent of new noninvasive imaging techniques has provide more convenient tools to diagnosis pulmonary sequestration.

Chest Radiography

Sequestrations typically appear as a uniformly dense mass within the thoracic cavity or pulmonary parenchyma. Recurrent infection can lead to the development of cystic areas within the mass. Air-fluid levels due to bronchial communication can be seen. An irregular solid mass was seen in the thoracic cavity behind the heart in our case.

Ultrasound

The typical sonographic appearance of BPS is an echogenic homogeneous mass that may be well defined or irregular. Some lesions have a cystic or more complex appearance. Doppler studies are helpful to identify the characteristic aberrant systemic artery that arises from the aorta and to delineate venous drainage.

Computed Tomography

CT scans have 90% accuracy in the diagnosis of pulmonary sequestration. The most common appearance is a solid mass that may be homogeneous or heterogeneous, sometimes with cystic changes. Less frequent findings include a large cavitary lesion with an air-fluid level, a collection of many small cystic lesions containing air or fluid, or a well-defined cystic mass. Emphysematous changes at the margin of the lesion are characteristic and may not be visible on the chest radiograph. CT technique for the optimal depiction of lesions using state-of-the-art volumetric scanning requires a fast intravenous (IV) contrast injection rate and appropriate volume and delay based upon size.

Multiplanar and three-dimensional reconstructions are helpful. Visualization of the anomalous arteries and veins is of great significance in making the diagnosis of pulmonary sequestration and differentiating it from other lung parenchymal abnormalities. The ability of CT angiography to simultaneously image the arterial supply, venous drainage, and parenchymal changes in a single examination makes it the imaging modality of choice [6]. Our case showed a good example: CT imaging demonstrated the aberrant vascular structure originating from descending aorta extends to the left inferior pulmonary sequestration. The draining vein of the pulmonary sequestration is the left inferior pulmonary veins. The definite diagnosis lead to successful surgery.

Magnetic Resonance Imaging (MRI)

Contrast-enhanced magnetic resonance angiography (MRA) or even conventional T1-weighted spin-echo (SE) images may help in the diagnosis of pulmonary sequestration by demonstrating a systemic blood supply, particularly from the aorta, to a basal lung mass. In addition, MRA may demonstrate venous drainage of the mass and may obviate more invasive investigations.

However, CT allows sharper delineation of thin-walled cysts and emphysematous changes than MRI.

Treatment

Most extralobar sequestrations require lobectomy or segmentectomy of the involved lung, whereas the sequestered segment can be removed without resection of the normal lung tissue in extralobar sequestration.

Optimally defining an infradiaphragmatic anomalous vessel is important because it necessitates transabdominal surgery rather than transthoracic intervention [7]. Preoperative identification of anomalous venous drainage in a sequestered segment can prevent massive intraoperative hemorrhage due to accidental transection of an unanticipated vessel [8]. With advances in technology, video-assisted thoracoscopic surgery was used with success in the surgical management of sequestration with minimal invasiveness [9, 10].

In our case, the abnormal sequestered segment was successfully excised by the surgeon based on the vascular road map provided by the CT angiography images.

Key Points

1. Pulmonary sequestration is a rare anomaly, which does not have a connection with the bronchial system and gets its blood supply, generally, from the aorta or its branches.
2. CT angiography provides the opportunity to evaluate arterial blood supply, venous drainage and changes in lung parenchyma in a single test, and differential diagnosis and preoperative evaluation can also be done.
3. The treatment for this is a segmentectomy via a thoracotomy.

References

1. Corbett, H.J. and Humphrey, G.M. (2004). Pulmonary sequestration. *Paediatr Respir Rev* 5: 59 -68.
2. Prasad, R., Garg, R. and Verma, S.K. (2009). Intralobar sequestration of lung. *Lung India* 26: 159–161.
3. Halkic, N., Cuenoud, P.F., Corthesy, M.E. et al. (1998). Pulmonary sequestration: A review of 26 cases. *Eur J Cardiothorac Surg* 14: 127- 133.
4. Rosado-de-Christansen, M.L., Frazier, A.A., Stocker, J.T. et al. (1993). From the archive of the AFIP: Extralobar sequestration: Radiologic pathologic correlation. *Radiographics* 13: 425–441.
5. Franco, J., Aliaga, R., Domingo, M L, et al. (1998). Diagnosis of pulmonary sequestration by spiral CT *Angiography Thorax* 53: 1089–1092.
6. Kang, M., Khandelwal, N., Ogili, V. et al. (2006). Multidetector CT and pulmonary sequestration. *J Comput Assist Tomogr* 30: 926–932.
7. Lee, E. Y., Dillon, J F,, Callahan, M.J. et al. (2006). 3D Multidetector CT angiographic evaluation of extralobar pulmonary sequestration with anomalous venous drainage into the left internal mammary vein in a pediatric patient. *Br J Radiol* 79: e99 -102
8. Felkar, R.E. and Tonkin, I.L. (1990). Imaging of pulmonary sequestration. *AJR Am J Roentgenol* 154: 241–249.
9. Avgerinos, D., Reyes, A., Plantilla, E. et al. (2008). Video-assisted thoracoscopic surgery for intralobar pulmonary sequestration. *Cases J* 1: 269.
10. Gonzalez, D., Garcia, J., Fieira, E. et al. (2011). Video-assisted thoracoscopic lobectomy in the treatment of intralobar pulmonary sequestration. *Interact Cardiovasc Thorac Surg* 12: 77–79.

13 Partial Anomalous Pulmonary Venous Connection with Secundum Atrial Septal Defect

Liu Chen[1], Hong Tang[1], Yuan Feng[1], and Jing Ping Sun[2]

[1] West China Hospital of Sichuan University, Chengdu, China
[2] The Chinese University of Hong Kong, Hong Kong

History

A 39-year-old woman presented to hospital with exertional dyspnea and productive cough of 10 years.

Physical Examination

The thoracic cage is normal with symmetrical and clear breath sounds. Heart rate was 75 bpm. Blood pressure was 108/80 mmHg. There was a soft ejection systolic murmur over the base of the heart. No jugular venous distension was present.

Electrocardiography

Electrocardiography showed normal sinus rhythm.

Transthoracic Echocardiography

Transthoracic echocardiography showed that the right atrium and right ventricle are markedly dilated and an atrial septal defect (5 mm) of fossa ovalis type was noted. The coronary sinus was enlarged with a diameter of approximately 18 mm. The orifice of right lower pulmonary veins into the left atrium could be visualized; another three pulmonary veins could not be seen (Figure 13-1A and C). Saline contrast echocardiography showed that a few microbubbles entered the left atrium via the defect and there was a small contrast negative area in the RA, which was consistent with the left-to-right shunt through the atrial defect (Figure 13-1B). A suprasternal short-axis view and color Doppler flow images revealed that the superior vena cava is enlarged, there is a flow in red towards the left innominate vein and superior vena cava, suggesting that this flow is in a vertical vein (Figure 13-1D and E). Moderate tricuspid regurgitation showed a velocity$_{max}$ = 3.2 m/s, pressure gradient = 41 mmHg (Figure 13-1F). The biatrial view obtained from subcostal window showing super vena cava, inferior vena cava and atrial septal defect (Video 13.1).

Comparative Cardiac Imaging: A Case-based Guide, First Edition.
Edited by Jing Ping Sun, Xing Sheng Yang, and Bryan P. Yan.
© 2018 John Wiley & Sons Ltd. Published 2018 by John Wiley & Sons Ltd.
Companion website: www.wiley.com/sun/comparative_cardiac_imaging

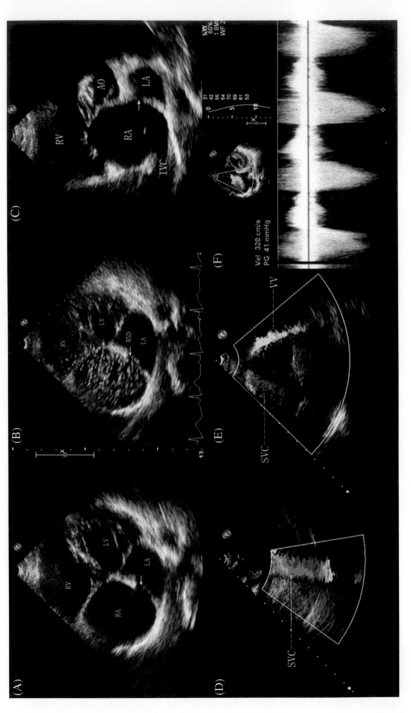

Figure 13-1 A. A two-dimensional image in the apical four-chamber view showing that the right ventricle and atrium are markedly dilated, a secundum atrial defect is seen (arrow), and the right lower pulmonary vein can be visualized. B. A saline contrast echocardiographic image demonstrates that a small contrast negative filling area in the RA, which is consistent with left to right shunt through the atrial septum defect. C. Parasternal short-axis view showing dilated RV and RA as well as the atrial septum defect (arrow). D. A suprasternal short-axis view and Doppler color flow images revealed the superior vena cava is enlarged. E. There is a flow in red towards the left innominate vein and superior vena cava, suggested this flow is in a vertical vein. F. Tricuspid regurgitation evaluated by continuous wave Doppler; the estimating pulmonary arterial systolic pressure is about 51 mmHg.

Computed Tomography

High-slice multidetector-row computed tomography provided more information, which confirmed the diagnosis. The right upper-lobe and middle-lobe veins drain into the SVC posteriorly, while the left upper pulmonary vein connects to the left brachiocephalic vein via a vertical vein. Both left and right pulmonary inferior veins are normal connected with the left atrium (Figure 13-2).

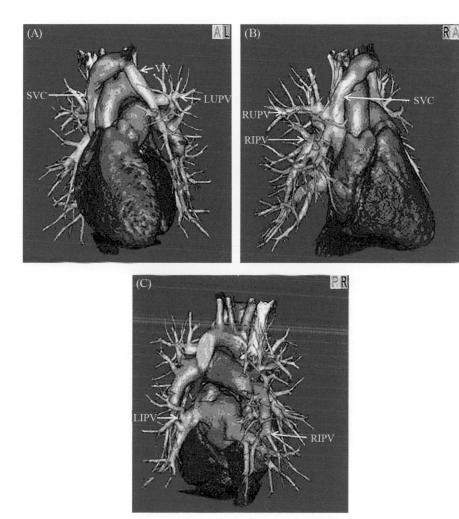

Figure 13-2 Three-dimensional reconstruction of MDCT. A. An anterior view reveals anomalous drainage of the left upper pulmonary vein via a vertical vein into the brachiocephalic vein. B. A right-anterior-oblique view shows anomalous drainage of the right upper and middle pulmonary veins to the SVC. C. The left and right inferior pulmonary veins are normal connected to the left atrium.
Notes: SVC, superior vena cava; VV, vertical vein; LUPV, upper pulmonary vein; RUPV, right upper pulmonary vein; RIPV, right inferior pulmonary vein; LIPV, left inferior pulmonary vein.

Hospital Course

The Warden procedure for partially anomalous pulmonary venous and anastomosis of anomalous left superior pulmonary vein to the left atrium were successfully performed on the patient without any early complication. Operative findings were consistent well with the CT and TTE diagnose.

Discussion

A partial anomalous pulmonary venous connection (PAPVC) is a congenital anomaly in which one or more of the pulmonary veins drain into the right atrium instead of the left atrium, creating a left-to-right shunt. Embryologically, PAPVC is similar to total anomalous pulmonary venous connection (TAPVC); however, TAPVC differs in that all or most pulmonary venous vessels connect to the right side of the heart in TAPVC. To date no evidence exists implicating common teratogens (e.g., drugs, infections) in the genesis of PAPVC. Partial anomalous pulmonary venous connection from the right lung is twice as common as PAPVC from the left lung. The most common form of PAPVC is one in which a right upper pulmonary vein connects to the right atrium or the superior vena cava. This form is almost always associated with a sinus venosus type of atrial septal defect (ASD).

The right pulmonary veins can also drain into the inferior vena cava. The left pulmonary veins can drain into the innominate vein, the coronary sinus, and, rarely, the cavae, right atrium, or left subclavian vein. Knowledge of the variation patterns of normal pulmonary venous drainage is necessary in order to diagnose PAPVC.

Most data regarding the prevalence of this condition have been garnered from autopsy series that estimates an incidence of 0.4–0.7% [1]. It has been argued, however, that autopsy series overestimate the clinical significance of this condition, as many of these cases were asymptomatic; thus the true incidence of patients presenting ante mortem with this condition is lower. Clinical diagnosis of isolated PAPVC is quite rare; it occurs in approximately 10% of patients with a proven atrial septal defect. In children with an atrial septal defect, additional partial anomalous pulmonary venous drainage is common.

Pathophysiology

Numerous factors determine the ratio of pulmonary blood flow (Qp) to systemic flow (Qs). The most important factor is the number of pulmonary veins that drain into the systemic circulation. The more veins that anomalously drain, the more blood returns to the right side of the heart. An associated cardiac defect, such as an ASD, may add to the left-to-right shunting. The shunt volume determines the symptoms and signs.

Over many years, excessive pulmonary venous return to the right side of the heart causes right atrial and ventricular dilation. This has numerous consequences, including risk of arrhythmia development, right-sided heart failure, and development of pulmonary hypertension. Some children are asymptomatic or show failure to develop, increased number of respiratory infections, and limitations of physical exercise. Our case is an adult; her right atrium and right ventricle are markedly dilated with moderate pulmonary hypertension, which cause exertional dyspnea and respiratory infection.

Diagnostic Evaluation

Clinical examination, the electrocardiogram, and a plain radiograph of the chest are unhelpful in this case, because the picture resembles a simple secundum atrial septal defect.

Echocardiography

Transthoracic ultrasound is a sensitive method of detecting anomalous venous connections in small children, who have good transthoracic ultrasound windows [2, 3]. However, in older children or in those with complex cardiac malformations, the transsthoracic approach is frequently limited in clinical practice. The definition of the site of connection of all four pulmonary veins by transthoracic ultrasound studies is difficult in children beyond infancy. Thus, the correct identification of partial nomalous pulmonary venous connections or the differentiation of total from mixed total anomalous pulmonary venous connection and the subsequent determination of the exact site of the venous connections is often impossible. In this case, echocardiography demonstrated a small atrial septal defect, which could not explain the significantly dilated RV and RA. There is a flow towards into the left innominate vein and enlarged superior vena cava, which suggest that this patient may associated with partial anomalous pulmonary venous connection. However, we cannot obtain a complete anatomic picture of anomalous pulmonary venous connection.

Transesophageal echocardiography is a newer method of assessing congenital heart disease: with the availability of dedicated pediatric transesophageal transducers it has now become a feasible and safe technique even in small children [4, 5]. Proximity of the transducer to the atrial chambers and to the sites of venous return potentially allows for an improved evaluation of these structures.

Cardiac Magnetic Resonance Imaging

Cardiac MRI may be useful and may give the same type of information that echocardiography can provide. It is seen as providing the "gold standard" for the assessment of right ventricular size and function, and it may help define whether the right heart chambers are in fact enlarged. Magnetic resonance imaging is also excellent at assessing pulmonary venous return [6]. In patients who cannot have an MRI, computed tomographic scanning and angiography can offer similar information.

Computed Tomographic Scanning

Three-dimensional MDCT image reconstructions were used to better clarify this rare type of disease and an adequate choice of surgical approach. A partial anomalous pulmonary venous connection was seen in 0.2% of adults on CT [7]. In our case, CT images provided clear anatomic pictures, which are very helpful for surgical correction.

Prognosis

Prognosis is excellent for patients with PAPVC. The perioperative mortality rate should be comparable to that for ASD repair (<0.1%). Prognosis becomes more guarded if the lesion is undetected for a long period of time and complications, particularly pulmonary hypertension. The patient should therefore be operated on as soon as the diagnosis is confirmed.

Key Points

1. A partial anomalous pulmonary venous connection (PAPVC) is a congenital anomaly; its prevalence has been garnered from autopsy series that estimate an incidence of 0.4–0.7%.
2. The markedly dilated right atrium and right ventricle are characteristics of this congenital anomaly.
3. Echocardiography is a useful tool for diagnosis but is difficult to detect all of the pulmonary veins.
4. Three-dimensional MDCT image reconstructions were used to clarify this rare type of disease better and to select an adequate choice of surgical approach.

References

1. Lucas, R.V. and Schmidt, R.E. (1999) Anomalous venous connections, pulmonary and systemic. In: *Heart Disease in Infants, Children and Adolescents*, 2nd edn (ed. A.J. Moss, F.H. Adams and G.C. Emmanoulides), 437–470. Baltimore, MD: Williams & Wilkins.
2. Sahn, D.J., Allen, H.D., Lange, L.W. et al. (1979). Crosssectional echocardiographic diagnosis of the sites of total anomalous pulmonary venous drainage. *Circulation* 60: 1317–1325.
3. Huhta, J.C., Gutgesell, H.P. and Nihill, M.R. (1985). Cross sectional echocardiographic diagnosis of total anomalous pulmonary venous connection. *Br Heart J* 53: 525–534.
4. Kyo, S., Koike, K., Takanawa, E. et al. (1989). Impact of transoesophageal Doppler echocardiography on paediatric cardiac surgery. *Int J Card Imaging* 4: 41–42.
5. Stumper, O., Elzenga, N.J., Hess, J. and Sutherland, G.R. (1990). Transoesophageal echocardiography in children with congenital heart disease – an initial experience. *J Am Coll Cardiol* 16: 433–441.
6. Prasad, S.K., Soukias, N., Hornung, T. et al. (2004). Role of magnetic resonance angiography in the diagnosis of major aortopulmonary collateral arteries and partial anomalous pulmonary venous drainage. *Circulation* 109: 207–214.
7. Haramati, L.B., Moche, I.E., Rivera, V.T. et al. (2003). Computed tomography of partial anomalous pulmonary venous connection in adults. *J Comput Assist Tomogr* 27 (5): 743–749.

14 Pulmonary Arteriovenous Malformation

Jing Ping Sun, Xing Sheng Yang, and Ka-Tak Wong
The Chinese University of Hong Kong, Hong Kong

History

A 38-year-old woman, presented with type 1 respiratory failure with no history of wheeze; oxygen flow rate was 6 L/min. Family history was unremarkable.

Physical Examination

Heart rate was regular at 65 bpm. Blood pressure was 94/77 mm Hg. Cardiac and chest examination was normal. Her lips and nails showed cyanosis. No ankle edema was noted.

Laboratory

- Hemoglobin level: 16.4. White blood cell count: 6.8. Oxygen saturation (SaO_2) was 95%. Oxygen flow rate: 6 L/min O_2, not in distress.
- Chest X ray: Chest clear.
- Electrocardiogram: Normal.
- Lung function test: Normal spirometry, no reversible components.
- Echocardiogram: The cardiac chambers were normal in size and function. There was trivial tricuspid regurgitation. The estimated pulmonary artery pressure was normal.
- Positive agitated saline bubble test. large amount of bubble appears from pulmonary vein into left heart after five cardiac cycles consistent with pulmonary arteriovenous malformations (Figure 14-1, Video 14-1).

Computed Tomography

No filling defect is detected in the main, right, and left pulmonary arteries down to the subsegmental level to suggest pulmonary embolism. Prominent serpiginous vessels are present in the mediobasal segment of the left lower lobe with arterial supply from a subsegmental branch of the pulmonary artery supplying the mediobasal segment, and venous drainage into a prominent vein that drains into the left inferior pulmonary vein. Features are compatible with pulmonary arteriovenous malformations (PAVM). The nidus measures 14×8 mm in size. Smaller clusters of prominent serpiginous vessels are also noted in the inferior aspect of the lateral segment of the right middle and the anterobasal segment of the right lower lobe. The right bronchial artery was tortuous with a

Comparative Cardiac Imaging: A Case-based Guide, First Edition.
Edited by Jing Ping Sun, Xing Sheng Yang, and Bryan P. Yan.
© 2018 John Wiley & Sons Ltd. Published 2018 by John Wiley & Sons Ltd.
Companion website: www.wiley.com/sun/comparative_cardiac_imaging

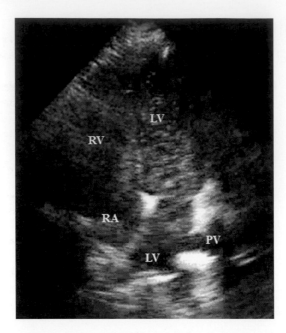

Figure 14-1 An apical four-chamber view showed a positive agitated saline bubble test. Large amounts of bubbles appear at the left heart after five cardiac cycles, consistent with pulmonary arteriovenous malformations.

focal fusiform ectasia (diameter 6 mm) at the proximal segment of the more anterior branch just after the common trunk bifurcates (Figure 14-2). The left bronchial artery appears unremarkable.

Discussion

A pulmonary arteriovenous malformations (PAVM) is a rare vascular abnormality of the lung. In an autopsy study in 1953 at Johns Hopkins Hospital [1], only three cases of PAVM were detected in 15 000 consecutive autopsies. However, it was noted by the same investigators that a small PAVM may easily be missed in routine autopsies. Most cases tend to be simple AVMs (single feeding arteries) although up to 20% of cases can have complex (two or more) feeding vessels [2]. They can be multiple in approximately one-third of cases.

Demographics and Clinical Presentation

There is a recognized female predilection. Cases of PAVM may be associated with hereditary hemorrhagic telangiectasia (HHT), the incidence of which varies. Although the AVMs in HHT are inherited and should be present at birth, they seldom manifest clinically until adult life, after the vessels have been subjected to pressure over several decades [3]. Most patients being asymptomatic, the connection between the venous and arterial system can lead to dyspnea (due to right-to-left shunting), as well as embolic events (due to paradoxical emboli). The most common complaint in symptomatic patients with PAVM is epistaxis, which is caused by bleeding from mucosal telangiectasia and reflects the high incidence of HHT in patients with PAVM. Epistaxis is characteristically spontaneous or precipitated by minor trauma.

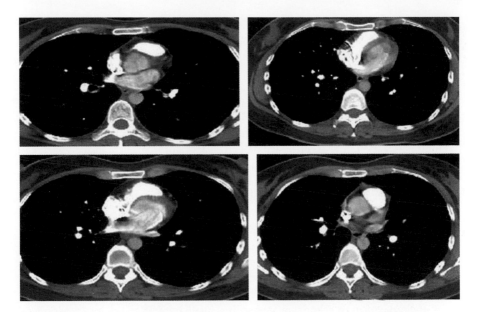

Figure 14-2 Computed tomography with contrast injection demonstrates enhancement of the feeding artery, the aneurysmal part (arrow), and the draining vein on early phase sequences.

Dyspnea is most common in patients with large or multiple PAVM, and is seen in almost all patients who have associated clubbing [4]. Interestingly, it has been noted clinically that symptoms such as dyspnea are sometimes strikingly minimal when compared with associated signs such as cyanosis and clubbing [5]. Some patients also have platypnea (improvement in breathing on reclining) [6]. This phenomenon is believed to be secondary to a decrease in blood flow through PAVM in the dependent portions of the lungs upon assuming the supine position. Hemoptysis is the third most common symptom but may be a more common presenting complaint. Massive hemoptysis may occur, but is rarely fatal [7].

Clinically a murmur or bruit may audible over the lesion (especially if it is peripheral). Digital clubbing and cyanosis were seen in 62–82% of patients reported in literature reviews [1, 8, 9]

Etiology and Pathology
The etiology of PAVM is unknown, but recent discoveries about the genetics of HHT may be relevant to the etiology of PAVM in patients with HHT—and perhaps in patients without HHT.

In congenital cases PAVM is considered to result from a defect in the terminal capillary loops, which causes dilatation and the formation of thin-walled vascular sacs. These are often unilateral. Although they can potentially affect any part of the lung, there is a recognized predilection towards the lower lobes (50–70%) [2].

Associations
PAVMs have been described in association with a number of conditions. Hereditary hemorrhagic telangiectasia (HHT) is frequently associated with PAVMs [1]. It is reported that at least 33% of those with a single PAVM and at least 50% of those with multiple PAVMs have HHT [6].

In addition, PAVMs have been found in hepatic cirrhosis (as part of the hepatopulmonary syndrome), schistosomiasis, mitral stenosis, trauma, and so forth.

Diagnosis

A number of modalities are available for the diagnosis of PAVMs, including contrast echocardiography, radionuclide perfusion lung scanning, computed tomography (CT), magnetic resonance imaging (MRI), and the gold standard is pulmonary angiography.

Pulmonary function tests: orthodeoxia is the laboratory correlate of platypnea and represents a decrease in PaO_2 or SaO_2 when going from the recumbent to the seated or upright position; it is probably present in most patients with PAVM [10, 11].

Chest radiography: the chest radiograph shows some abnormality in about 98% of patients from consecutive series of patients with PAVM. The classic roentgenographic appearance of a PAVM is that of a round or oval mass of uniform density, frequently lobulated but sharply defined, more commonly in the lower lobes.

Contrast echocardiography is an excellent tool for the evaluation of cardiac and intrapulmonary shunts, and is able to identify small right-to-left shunts even when they are not suggested by gas exchange data. This technique involves the injection of 5–10 ml of indocyanine green or saline (agitated with a small amount of air) into a peripheral vein while simultaneously imaging the right and left atria with two-dimensional echocardiography. Both liquids contain microbubbles, which are easily visualized during echocardiography as contrast compared with the normally echolucent blood. In patients without right-to-left shunting, the microbubbles are rapidly visualized in the right atrium and then gradually dissipate. In the case of intracardiac shunts, the contrast is visualized in the left heart chambers within one cardiac cycle following its appearance in the right atrium. In the case of PAVM, there is nearly always a delay of three to eight cardiac cycles before contrast is visualized in the left atrium, due to the time required for the contrast to traverse the pulmonary vasculature.

Our case is a typical example: the saline contrast could be visualized in the left atrium delay five cardiac cycles after contrast appearance in the right atrium, which indicated the present of right-to-left shunt and provided an important clue for diagnosis.

Computed tomography is often the diagnostic imaging modality of choice. The characteristic presentation of a PAVM on noncontrast CT is a homogeneous, well circumscribed, noncalcified nodule up to several centimeters in diameter or the presence of a serpiginous mass connected with blood vessels. Occasionally associated phleboliths may be seen as calcifications. Contrast injection demonstrates enhancement of the feeding artery, the aneurysmal part, and the draining vein on early phase sequences. The obvious advantages of three-dimensional helical CT scanning over angiography are its noninvasiveness and its avoidance of contrast injection; it is also more sensitive than angiography in picking up multiple lesions.

Magnetic Resonance Imaging

Magnetic resonance (MR) imaging of PAVM has been studied less than CT. If the MR techniques show conflicting images, however, additional methods of diagnosis should be sought. The main limitations of MR imaging in the routine evaluation of PAVM include expense, limited availability, and the highly specialized techniques required for accurate interpretation.

Pulmonary Angiography

Despite advances in the techniques mentioned thus far, contrast pulmonary angiography remains the gold standard in the diagnosis of PAVM, and is usually necessary if resectional or obliterative therapy is being considered.

Complications

Complications include cyanosis (due to the right to left shunt), high output congestive cardiac failure, polycythemia and paradoxical cerebral embolism.

Treatment and Prognosis

Embolization therapy, in which the AVM is occluded angiographically, is considered a first-line treatment for pulmonary AVM, with a procedural success rate (defined as involution of the AVM) of 97% [12]. Embolization therapy allows patients to avoid major surgery, with its potential complications, and it has a shorter recovery time.

Surgical procedures such as excision, vascular ligation, or lobectomy can be considered if the lesion cannot be treated by embolization or if the patient has an anaphylactic allergy to contrast dyes.

Once successfully treated (embolotherapy, surgical resection), prognosis is generally good for an individual lesion.

Differential Diagnoses

Including abnormal systemic vessels, highly vascular parenchymal mass, other congenital or acquired pulmonary arterial or venous lesions, and retroperitoneal varices.

Key Points

1. Patients considered at risk of PAVMs because of suspicious symptoms, signs, or radiological appearances should be investigated with at least measurement of arterial blood gas tensions and / or supine and erect oximetry, together with posterior-anterior and lateral chest radiographs.
2. Contrast echocardiography is a simple noninvasive tool to investigate the right-to-left shunting.
3. Computed tomography is a sensitive technique to detect the PAVM.

References

1. Sloan R.D. and Cooley, R.N. (1953). Congenital pulmonary arteriovenous aneurysm. *Am J Roentgenol Radium Ther Nucl Med* 70: 183–210.
2. Lee, E.Y., Boiselle, P.M. and Cleveland, R.H. (2008). Multidetector CT evaluation of congenital lung anomalies. *Radiology* 247, 632–648.
3. Hodgson, C.H., Burchell, H.B., Good, C.A. et al. (1959). Hereditary hemorrhagic telangiectasis and pulmonary arteriovenous fistula. *N Engl J Med* 261: 625–636.
4. Stringer, C.J., Stanley, A.L., Bates, R.C. et al. (1955). Pulmonary arteriovenous fistulas. *Am J Surg* 89: 1054–1080.

5. Chilvers, E.R., Whyte, M.K.B., Jackson, J.E. et al. (1990). Effect of percutaneous transcatheter embolization on pulmonary function, right-to-left shunt and arterial oxygenation in patients with pulmonary arteriovenous malformations. *Am Rev Respir Dis* 142: 420–425.

6. Robin, E.D., Laman, D., Horn, B.R. et al. (1976). Platypnea related to orthodeoxia caused by true vascular lung shunts. *N Engl J Med* 294: 941–943.

7. Hoffman, W.S., Weinberg, P.M., Ring, E. et al. (1980). Massive hemoptysis secondary to pulmonary arteriovenous fistula: treatment by a catheterization procedure. *Chest* 77: 697–700.

8. Stringer, C.J., Stanley, A.L., Bates, R.C. et al. (1955). Pulmonary arteriovenous fistulas. *Am J Surg* 89: 1054–1080.

9. Moyer, J.H., Glantz, G., and Brest, A.N. (1962). Pulmonary arteriovenous fistulas: physiologic and clinical considerations. *Am J Med* 32: 417–435.

10. Dutton, J.A.E., Jackson, J.E., Hughes, J.M.B. et al. (1995). Pulmonary arteriovenous malformations: Results of treatment with coil embolization in 53 patients. *Am J Roentgenol* 165: 1119–1125.

11. Terry, P.B., White, R.I., Barth, K.H. et al. (1983). Pulmonary arteriovenous malformations: physiologic observations and results of therapeutic balloon embolization. *N Engl J Med* 308: 1197–1200.

12. Pollak, J.S., Saluja, S., Thabet, A. et al. (2006). Clinical and anatomic outcomes after embolotherapy of pulmonary arteriovenous malformations. *J Vasc Interv Radio* 17: 35–44.

15 Right Pulmonary Agenesis associated with Congenital Heart Diseases

Junli Hu[1], Guiling Sui[1], and Jing Ping Sun[2]

[1] Affiliated Hospital of Jining Medical University, Jining, China
[2] The Chinese University of Hong Kong, Hong Kong

History

A 6-month-old boy was born preterm at $36 + 6$ gestational weeks and was admitted with cyanosis. There was systolic murmur 2/6 at the right second intercostal space. His artery blood oxygen saturation was 80–85%.

Laboratory

Chest X-ray. A postero-anterior view showed left pulmonary agenesis with mediastinal shift and right-lung hyperinflation, dextrocardia, and T3 vertebra anomaly (Figure 15-1A).
- Transthoracic echocardiography. The apical four-chamber view showed dextrocardia, a small secundum atrial septal defect, the left atrium was small without the entrances of pulmonary veins (Figure 15-1A). Left upper and lower pulmonary veins formed a left pulmonary vein draining into the right superior vena cava. The right pulmonary artery could not be identified. A 4 mm tunnel was visualized between left pulmonary artery and descending aorta, which was suspected to be patent ductus arteriosus (Figure 15-2B; Video 15-1).

Computed Tomography

Pulmonary artery and venous angiography by 64-slice spiral computed tomography minimum intensity projection (MinIP) reconstruction of air way showed a normal trachea and left bronchi, absence of right lung, bronchus and right pulmonary artery and veins (Figure 15-1B). Left pulmonary vein and the right pulmonary vein merged into one left common pulmonary vein and drain into the superior vena cava at the back area of left atrium. The end of the left common pulmonary vein was narrow and drains into the right superior vena cava (Figure 15-3A). There was a patent ductus arteriosus between beginning of descending aorta and main pulmonary artery; but right pulmonary artery was absent (Figure 15-3B and C).

Complete pulmonary venous drainage correction surgery was performed, patent ductus arteriosus was ligated, and the atrial septal defect was repaired for this patient. The patient was transferred to the intensive care unit after operation. The patient's SpO_2 and pressure of pulmonary artery were improved; he was discharged 15 days after operation.

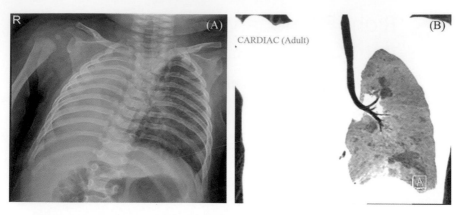

Figure 15-1   A. A chest X-ray showed right hemithorax opacity (lung agenesis), leftward deviation of the mediastinal structure, dextrocardia, and abnormal T3 vertebra. B. A MinMip reconstruction of the airway showed a normal trachea and left bronchus, and absence of right lung and bronchus.

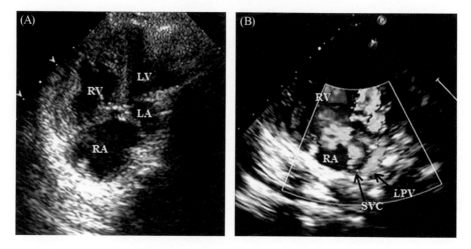

Figure 15-2   A. Echocardiography found dextrocardia; an apical four-chamber view showed the left atrial was small, and there was no pulmonary venous return. B. Left anomalous pulmonary venous drainage into the superior vena cava.
Notes: RV, right ventricle; RA, right atrium; LV, left ventricle; LA, left atrium; SVC, superior vena cava; LPV, left pulmonary vein.

Three months after operation, patient was readmitted due to severe pneumonia, and eventually developed multiple organ failure. His parents gave up the treatment.

On the basis of all findings, the patient was diagnosed with left-sided pulmonary agenesis with congenital heart abnormalities including dextrocardia, atrial septal defect, ̄̄s arteriosus, and anomalous left pulmonary venous drainage.

Discussion

Congenital malformations of the lung are rare and vary widely in their presentation and severity [1]. Pulmonary agenesis is defined as complete absence of the lung parenchyma, bronchus, and pulmonary vasculature [2]. We reported a case of unilateral pulmonary agenesis was associated with congenital cardiac abnormalities.

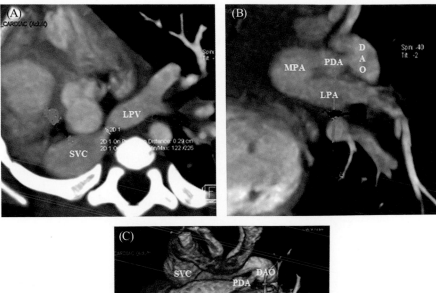

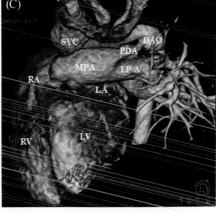

Figure 15-3 Pulmonary artery and venous angiography by 64-slice spiral computed tomography (CT) demonstrated: A. Both right pulmonary artery and right pulmonary vein were absent. The end of the left pulmonary vein was narrow and drained into the lower part of the right superior vena cava. B. There was a patent ductus arteriosus between the beginning of the descending aorta and the main pulmonary artery, but the right pulmonary artery was absent. C. Computed tomography reconstruction image showed dextrocardia; the left atrial was small, and the superior vena cava was dilated. There was a patent ductus arteriosus between the beginning of descending aorta and the main pulmonary artery, but the right pulmonary artery and vein were absent.
Notes: RV, right ventricle; RA, right atrium; LV, left ventricle; LA, left atrium; SVC, superior vena cava; LPV, left pulmonary vein; MPV, main pulmonary artery; PDA, patent ductus arteriosus, DAO, descending aorta. LPA, left pulmonary artery.

Pulmonary agenesis is a rare developmental defect of lung development, in which the clinical features may be variable: cyanosis, dyspnea, stridor, respiratory distress, pulmonary asymmetry; recurrent pulmonary infections or nonspecific pulmonary signs have also been reported [3]. The diagnosis was suggested by a routine chest X-ray showing hemithoracic opacity with mediastinal shift [3]. In recent years, progress achieved in obstetrical imaging has made early antenatal diagnosis possible. Zhang et al. reported 18 antenatal cases [4]. To confirm the diagnosis, additional investigations are necessary: Color Doppler of fetal vascular anatomy suggests the malformation when it shows absent pulmonary artery and veins on the same side as abnormal lung echogenicity.

In our case, diagnosed by X-ray and echocardiography, CT made a great contribution to the diagnosis. Three-dimensional reconstruction of the pulmonary artery and the collateral arteries are important for surgical planning. This tool allows the appreciation of lung structural anomalies but also permits the exclusion of other pathologies such as congenital heart diseases, which are detrimental to the outcome.

Prognosis of lung agenesis mainly depends on associated cardiac anomalies as well as respiratory complications.

There were cases where unilateral lung agenesis and total anomalous pulmonary venous return have been reported in the literature [5]. Surgical repair was performed in five, and only two patients survived after surgery. Surgery was performed successfully in our case but the patient suffered from severe pneumonia and multiple organ failure 3 months after the operation.

Patients with lung agenesis sometimes have tracheal stenosis [6] the left tracheal is normal in our case.

Key Points

1. Echocardiography is an important tool in the diagnosis of the pulmonary agenesis associated with congenital heart diseases.
2. Chest X-ray and intravenous contrast-enhanced CT of the chest confirmed the complete diagnosis of the pulmonary agenesis associated with congenital heart diseases.

References

1. Mohan, A., Guleria, R., Sharma, R. et al. (2005). Unilateral pulmonary agenesis: An uncommon cause of lower zone lung opacity. *Indian J Chest Dis Allied Sci* 47: 53–56.
2. Biyyam, D.R., Chapman, T., Ferguson, M.R. et al. (2010). Congenital lung abnormalities: embryologic features, prenatal diagnosis, and postnatal radiologic-pathologic correlation. *Radiographics* 30 (6): 1721–1738.
3. Maltz, D.L. and Nadas, A.S. (1968). Agenesis of the lung: Presentation of eight new cases and review of the literature. *Pediatrics* 42: 175–188.
4. Zhang, Y., Fan, M., Ren, W. et al. (2013). Prenatal diagnosis of fetal unilateral lung agenesis complicated with cardiac malposition. *BMC Pregnancy Childbirth* 13: 79.
5. Kaku, Y., Nagashima, M., Matsumura, G. et al. (2015). Neonatal repair of total anomalous pulmonary venous connection and lung agenesis. *Asian Cardiovasc Thorac Ann* 23 (6): 716–718.
6. Backer, C.L., Kelle, A.M., Mavroudis, C. et al. (2009). Tracheal reconstruction in children with unilateral lung agenesis or severe hypoplasia. *Ann Thorac Surg* 88 (2): 624–630.

16 Compressive Giant Right Atrial Diverticulum

Guozhen Yuan[1], Shaochun Wang[1], Bryan P. Yan[2], and Jing Ping Sun[2]

[1] Affiliated Hospital of Jining Medical University, Jining, China
[2] The Chinese University of Hong Kong, Hong Kong

History

An 18-year-old male with no past medical history presented with palpitations.

Physical Examination

On physical examination the patient did not appear ill. Blood pressure was 110/70 mmHg. Pulse was 85 bpm. The heart was enlarged to percussion but no precardial impulse could be felt. A systolic murmur could be heard at the right parasternal border.

Laboratory

Chest X-ray showed marked cardiomegaly (Figure 16-1) and 2D/3D transthoracic echocardiography revealed a giant diverticulum (13 cm × 8.9 cm × 13.8 cm) connected to the right atrial free wall by a large defect (5.8 cm × 3.2 cm) (Figure 16-2A). Spontaneous contrast but no thrombus could be seen within the diverticulum. There was free bidirectional flow between the right atrium and the diverticulum by color Doppler (Figure 16-2B, Video 16-1).

Computed tomography confirmed a giant diverticulum adjacent to the right side of the right atrium, compressing the right atrium and ventricle (Figure 16-3).

Hospital Course

The patient underwent surgical resection of the diverticulumsmoothly. He was doing well at 6 months after operation.

Pathology

Pathology showed a thin diverticulum wall consisting of fibrous tissue and intima without muscular tissue.

Comparative Cardiac Imaging: A Case-based Guide, First Edition.
Edited by Jing Ping Sun, Xing Sheng Yang, and Bryan P. Yan.
© 2018 John Wiley & Sons Ltd. Published 2018 by John Wiley & Sons Ltd.
Companion website: www.wiley.com/sun/comparative_cardiac_imaging

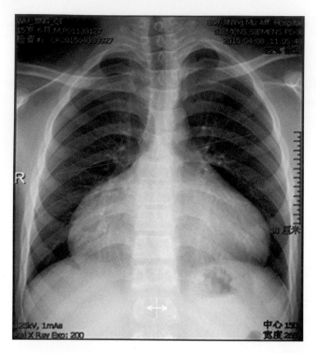

Figure 16-1   A chest X-ray showed marked cardiomegaly.

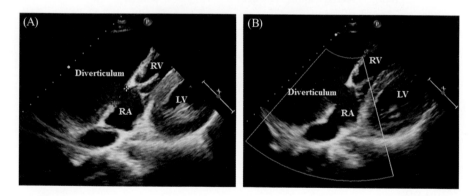

Figure 16-2   A. Echocardiography: two-dimensional transthoracic echocardiography revealed a giant diverticulum (13 cm × 8.9 cm × 13.8 cm) connected to the right atrial free wall by a large defect (5.8 cm × 3.2 cm). B. Spontaneous contrast but no thrombus could be seen within the diverticulum. There was free bidirectional flow between the right atrium and the diverticulum shown by color Doppler.

Discussion

Diverticulum is the third most frequent malformations of the RA, after congenital atrial enlargement and coronary sinus aneurysm [1], and a possible genetic cause has been proposed, based on a report of an affected family [2]. Bailey was the first to excise a diverticulum of the right atrium in 1953 [3]. The diverticulum does not contain all the layers of the atrial wall, it communicates with the RA via a defect in RA free wall as seen in our case.

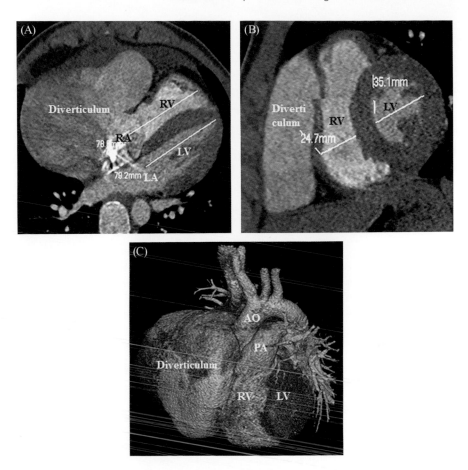

Figure 16-3 Computed tomography confirmed a giant diverticulum adjacent to the right side of the right atrium compressing the right atrium and ventricle (A and B). A three-dimensional reconstruction image shows the huge diverticulum adjacent to the right side of the heart (C).

The diagnosis of RA diverticulum can be confirmed by echocardiography. The use of contrast-enhanced ultrasound is very useful, it allows the relationship between the cavity and the RA to be established and provides information about the site and anatomical characteristics of the communication. Due to its accessibility, good tolerability and low cost, this technique can be considered the diagnostic procedure of choice.

In selected patients, high-resolution cardiac CT represents a unique tool to assess subtle anatomic cardiac variants. The CT imaging presented a clear morphology of the RA and diverticulum in our case. Magnetic resonance can help in differential diagnosis with pericardial cysts or mediastinal tumors [4].

The differential diagnosis includes right atrial aneurysms [5]; there are clear characteristics distinguishing these two entities. An aneurysm is defined as the dilatation of the atrium involving all layers of the atrial wall. In the patient reported here, the diverticulum wall consisting of fibrous tissue and intima without muscular tissue. This morphological pattern corresponds to the definition of a diverticulum, where communication through a defect has to be present. Atrial diverticula have been observed at any time from birth to adult life. Patients are frequently asymptomatic although progressive atrial dilatation and supraventricular arrhythmias may develop [6, 7]. Congestive heart failure rarely occurs and is usually related to impaired systolic left ventricular function caused by incessant tachycardia. Further complications include thrombus formation and rupture of the diverticulum. Surgical excision is the therapy of choice and has been shown to reduce the risk of atrial arrhythmia [8].

Key Points

1. Echocardiography is the first choice for diagnosis.
2. Giant atrial diverticulum is a rare congenital heart anomaly, which should be treated surgically because of the risk of thromboembolism, arrhythmia, and rupture of the diverticulum.

References

1. Binder, T.M., Rosenhek, R., Frank, H. et al. (2000). Congenital malformations of the right atrium and the coronary sinus: an analysis based on 103 cases reported in the literature and two additional cases. *Chest* 117: 1740–1748.
2. Agematsu, K., Okamura, T., Ishihara, K. et al. (2009). Remarkable giant right atrial diverticulum in asymptomatic patient. *Interact Cardiovasc Thorac Surg* 8: 705–707.
3. Bailley, C.P. (1955). *Surgery of the Heart*. Philadelphia, PA: Lea & Febiger, p. 413.
4. Juanpere, S., Cañete, N., Ortuño, P. et al. (2013). A diagnostic approach to the mediastinal masses. *Insights Imaging* 4 (1): 29–52.
5. Parker, J.O., Connell, W.F. and Lynn, R.B. (1967). Left atrial aneurysm. *Amer J Cardiol* 20: 579.
6. Shah, K. and Walsh, K. (1992). Giant right atrial diverticulum: an unusual cause of Wolff–Parkinson–White syndrome. *Br Heart J* 17: 874–882.
7. Scalia, G.M., Stafford, W.J., Burstow, D.J. et al. (1995). Successful treatment of incessant atrial flutter with excision of congenital giant right atrial aneurysm diagnosed by transesophageal echocardiography. *Am Heart J* 129: 834–835.
8. Binder, T.M., Rosenhek, R., Frank, H. et al. (2000). Congenital malformations of the right atrium and the coronary sinus. *Chest* 117: 1740–1748.

17 Shone's Syndrome

Weihua Wu[1], Bryan P. Yan[2], and Jing Ping Sun[2]

[1] Jiaotong University, Shanghai, China
[2] The Chinese University of Hong Kong, Hong Kong

History

Case 1 A 38-year-old male presented with high blood pressure for 6 years and recently has had shortness of breath. Family history was unremarkable for cardiovascular disease.

Case 2 A 24-year-old male presented with recurrent chest tightness. He had been given a diagnosis of congenital heart disease but no details were available. He has never received treatment for his heart condition

Physical Examination

Case 1 On physical examination, the patient was pale and febrile, with basilar crackles over both lung fields. Cardiac auscultation revealed tachycardia (100 beat per minute and irregular), a loud S2 and a diastolic murmur over the upper left parasternal border, a loud diastolic rumble at the apex, and a systolic murmur over the tricuspid area. The liver was enlarged and he did not have peripheral edema.

Case 2 Blood pressure was higher in the upper extremity (130/80 mmHg) than in the lower extremity (110/70 mmHg). There was a loud systolic murmur at the right second intercostal space.

Electrocardiogram

Case 1. EKG showed atrial fibrillation (100 beats per minute), biatrial enlargement, and signs of right ventricular (RV) hypertrophy.

Chest X-ray

Case 1. X-Ray showed a mildly increased cardiothoracic ratio.

Comparative Cardiac Imaging: A Case-based Guide, First Edition.
Edited by Jing Ping Sun, Xing Sheng Yang, and Bryan P. Yan.
© 2018 John Wiley & Sons Ltd. Published 2018 by John Wiley & Sons Ltd.
Companion website: www.wiley.com/sun/comparative_cardiac_imaging

Transthoracic Echocardiography (TTE)

Case 1. TTE revealed the following. The left atrium was significantly dilated. The left ventricle showed concentric left ventricle hypertrophy with normal wall motion and abnormal diastolic function (E' = 6 mm). The mitral valve was thickened with severe stenosis (mitral orifice area = 0.9 cm^2), mild mitral regurgitation and a small mitral annulus. All chordae tendinous were attached to a single posterior-lateral papillary muscle suggesting true parachute mitral valve (Figure 17-1A, B, Videos 17-1, 17-2, and 17-3). The right ventricle was normal in size and systolic function. There was mild tricuspid regurgitation with elevated peak velocity. The estimated pulmonary artery systolic pressure was 56 mm Hg. A small patent foramen ovale with left to right shunting was noted. The diameter of the ascending aorta was normal (2.9 cm). There was collateral circulation observed in the supersternal view.

Case 2. TTE showed: (i) a unicuspid aortic valve with mild aortic regurgitation (AR) (Video 17-4 and 17-5), severe aortic stenosis (peak gradient =104 mmHg) and a subaortic membrane (Figure 17-2A, Video 17-4, 17-5); (ii) supramitral valvular mitral ring with

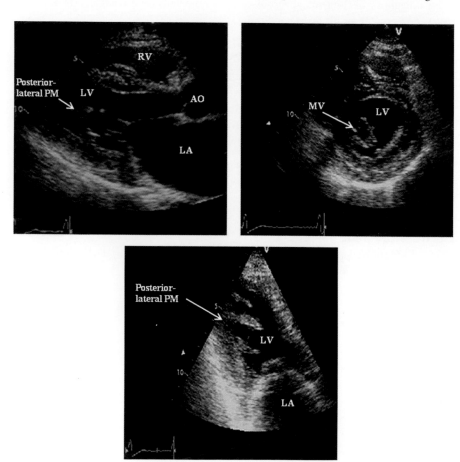

Figure 17-1   Case 1. Left: Parasternal long-axis view of a transthoracic echocardiogram showing the posterolateral papillary muscle. Middle: Parasternal short-axis view showing a small mitral annulus. Right: apical long axis view showing a prominent posterolateral papillary muscle.

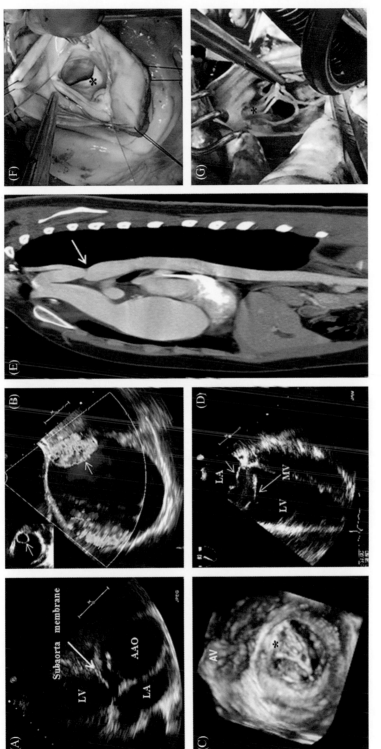

Figure 17-2 Case 2. A. Two-dimensional TTE apical three-chamber view showed subaortic membrane and unicuspid aortic valve. a unicuspid aortic valve (arrow). B. Two-dimensional TTE without (small one) and with color Doppler showed stenotic unicuspid aortic valve with high velocity (arrow). C. Three-dimensional TEE showed a supravalvular ring in left atrium. D. Two-dimensional TEE showed a supravalvular ring in left atrium (small arrow). E. Computed tomography aorta, long-axis view, and multiplanar reconstruction of aortic long-axis view showed that the ascending aorta was significantly dilated, and a mild to moderate coarctation of the descending aorta beyond the origin of the left subclavian artery (arrow) without poststenotic dilatation. F. The operative view showed subaorticvalvular membrane (*). G. The operative view showed the supravalvular ring (*).

mild stenosis, the anterolateral papillary muscle was smaller than the posteromedial one (Figure 17-2, Video 17-6); (iii) the ascending aorta was dilated (65 mm); (iv) left ventricular (LV) systolic function was normal (ejection function = 65 %).

Computed Tomography

Case 1. A CT scan showed the coarctation of the thoracic descending aorta (0.5 mm) just distal to the left subclavian artery. The multiple collateral vessels were present supplying the distal site of aortic coarctation (Figure 17-3).

Case 2. A CT multiplanar reconstruction of the aorta showed that the ascending aorta was significantly dilated with a mild to moderate coarctation of the descending aorta beyond the origin of the left subclavian artery without poststenotic dilatation (Figure 17-2E).

Case 2 was referred for surgical correction. Intraoperative transesophageal 2D and 3D echocardiography (TEE) confirmed all of the above malformations. The supravalvular mitral ring consisted of multiple fibers arranged like a hammock (Figure 17-2C). The supravalvular mitral ring and the subaortic membrane were excised, the mechanical aortic valve was implanted, and the aortic coarctation was corrected. The operation was successful, and the patient was discharged after 2 weeks.

Post-op TTE and TEE showed that the mechanical aortic valve was functioning well and the peak systolic gradient in the descending aorta was 27 mmHg.

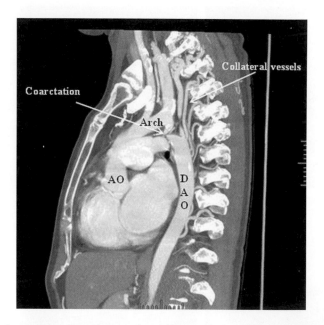

Figure 17-3 Computed tomography scan showed the coarctation of the thoracic descending aorta (0.5 mm) just distal to the left subclavian artery representing. The multiple collateral vessels were present, supplying the distal site of aortic coarctation.
Notes: AO, ascending aorta; DAO, descending aorta.

Discussion

Shone's complex is a very rare congenital heart disease. It also called Shone's anomaly, and consists of four cardiac defects: supravalvular mitral membrane, parachute mitral valve, subaortic stenosis (membranous or muscular), and coarctation of the aorta. Essentially, it is a syndrome characterized by both left ventricular inflow and outflow obstruction. It is diagnosed most frequently in its incomplete form.

We reported two cases. Case 1 had aortic coarctation, a small patent foramen ovale, a mitral supravalvular ring associated with a calcified mitral valve, and a single posterior-lateral papillary muscle that receives all chordae. The leaflets and chordae were thickened and shortened, causing severe mitral stenosis that resulted in severe pulmonary hypertension. Case 2 was a 24-year-old male who presented with recurrent chest tightness. Transthoracic echocardiogram (TTE) revealed (i) a unicuspid aortic valve with mild aortic regurgitation (AR) and severe left ventricular-aortic stenosis; (ii) supravalvular mitral ring with mild stenosis, and the antero-lateral papillary muscle was smaller than the posteromedial one; (iii) the ascending aorta was dilated (65 mm). Computed tomography multiplanar reconstruction of the aorta showed that the ascending aorta was significantly dilated with a mild to moderate coarctation of the thoracic aorta beyond the origin of the left subclavian artery (arrow) without poststenotic dilatation. The abnormalities found by TTE and CT were consistent with Shone's complex. Depending on the diagnostic criteria, this case could be classified as complete Shone's complex with unicuspid aortic valve. The patient received a successfully operation and recovered well. To the best of the authors' knowledge, this is the first case of an adult patient diagnosed as Shone's complex with unicuspid aortic valve.

Parachute mitral valve is a condition in which all mitral chordae arise from a single papillary muscle. Often only a single papillary muscle is present, usually in the posterior position [2]. The hemodynamic significance of PMV is variable and depends on mitral annular size and chordal structure [2]. Currently, the presence of a PMV is no longer a required component for the diagnosis of Shone's complex, as long as some other congenital abnormality of the MV is present [2, 4]. Bicuspid AV is frequently reported in cases of Shone's complex. The incidence of bicuspid AV was 87% among 46 children [2, 4].

The TTE is a cost effective diagnostic tool for the diagnosis of complex congenital heart disease. The diagnosis of Shone's complex was made by routine TTE in our cases. Computed tomography is an important supplemental study to illustrate aortic coarctation.

Shone et al. [1] noted that mitral valve obstruction appeared to be the most critical lesion. Other studies confirmed that the severity of mitral valve obstruction correlates with poor long-term outcome. Patients with the most severe form of mitral obstruction present with severely elevated pulmonary artery pressure and the poorest prognosis [2].

Mitral valve obstruction during early embryogenesis is considered the first pathological event in Shone's syndrome, causing underdevelopment of the left ventricular cavity, leading to various degrees of left-ventricular outflow tract obstruction and aortic coarctation. In their first description of the syndrome, the partial disappearance of elastic tissue at the level of aortic media in patients with aortic coarctation was to be an important feature. Aortic coarctation occurs in 20–59% of cases with mitral valve anomalies, whereas mitral supravalvular ring is associated with other defects in almost

90% of cases [3]. Therefore, the finding of either of these defects should prompt a search for other cardiac and vascular anomalies.

In one study, a bicuspid aortic valve was present in 50% of patients with parachute mitral valve [4]. In contrast to true parachute mitral valve, a parachute-like asymmetric mitral valve has two separate papillary muscles, with one being more dominant, as in our case 2. The dominant papillary muscle is usually located higher in the left ventricle and is attached to the ventricular wall from both the base and the lateral side [5]. The papillary muscle anatomy is normal in rheumatic valvular heart disease, in which the leaflets and subvalvular apparatus are thickened and fused. Transthoracic echocardiography is the primary modality used in the differential diagnosis. The parasternal short axis view is the main window for the evaluation of the number and orientation of the papillary muscles. However, in cases of poor echocardiographic acoustic quality, transthoracic echocardiography may not yield a definite diagnosis. The transesophageal echocardiography may provide valuable information. In some situations, MRI is a reasonable alternative with which to evaluate the mitral valve. Although multidetector-row computed tomography (MDCT) of the heart is used largely to evaluate the coronary arteries, there is accumulating evidence for its utility in the evaluation of heart valves and chambers [6, 7]. In our case, MDCT gave complementary information about the coarctation of aorta and helped in the final diagnosis.

Conclusions

Shone's syndrome consists of a set of congenital cardiac anomalies. Transthoracic echocardiography is the primary modality used to make a diagnosis. Multidetector-row computed tomography can be a complementary imaging technique for the evaluation of subvalvular mitral apparatus and papillary muscles, especially in patients with poor echocardiographic acoustic quality.

Key Points

1. These cases study raises awareness about this rare syndrome.
2. Parachute mitral valve is usually associated with a set of other congenital cardiac defects. A carefully performed echocardiogram is very important to avoid missing coexisting congenital heart lesions.
3. Multidetector-row computed tomography is an important complementary laboratory study to evaluate this syndrome.

References

1. Shone, J.D., Sellers, R.D., Anderson, R.C. et al. (1963). The developmental complex of "parachute mitral valve," supravalvular ring of the left atrium, subaortic stenosis and coarctation of the aorta. *Am J Cardiol* 11: 714–725.
2. Ikemba, C.M., Eidem, B.W., Fraley, J. et al. (2005). Mitral valve morphology and morbidity / mortality in Shone's complex. *Am J Cardiol* 95: 541–543.
3. Serra, W., Testa, P. and Ardissino, D. (2005). Mitral supravalvular ring: a case report. *Cardiovasc Ultrasound* 3: 19–22.

4. Konstantinov, I., Yun, T.J., Calderone, C.J. et al. (2004). Supramitral obstruction of left ventricular inflow tract by supramitral ring. *Oper Tech Thoracic Cardiovasc Surg* 9: 247–251.
5. Bolling, S.F., Iannettoni, M.D., Dick, M. II et al. (1990) Shone's anomaly: operative results and late outcome. *Ann Thorac Surg* 49: 887–893.
6. Pannu, H.K., Jacobs, J.E., Lai, S. et al. (2006). Gated cardiac imaging of the aortic valve on 64-slice multidetector row computed tomography:preliminary observations. *J Comput Assist Tomogr* 30: 443–446.
7. Vogel-Claussen, J., Pannu, H., Spevak, P.J. et al. (2006). Cardiac valve assessment with MR imaging and 64-section multi-detector row CT. *Radiographics* 26: 1769–1784.

18 Subaortic Membrane in the Adult

Jing Ping Sun and Alex Pui-Wai Lee

The Chinese University of Hong Kong, Hong Kong

History

A 48-year-old female presented with a 2-year history of increased exertional chest pain radiating to the shoulder. She had a history of heart murmur during childhood but otherwise she was well. She denied having a previous diagnosis of rheumatic fever.

Physical Examination

A systolic murmur was heard in the aortic valve area.

Echocardiogram

Transthoracic echocardiography showed normal LV systolic function and a pressure gradient (maximal gradient was 27 mmHg) within the left ventricular outflow tract (LVOT). A subtle tissue attached to ventricular septum in LVOT was seen in parasternal and apical three-chamber views (Figure 18-1, Video 18-1), which was suspected subaortic membrane. Transesophageal echocardiography (TEE) was performed to identify the tissue in LVOT. A subaorta incomplete membrane was clearly seen in TEE 2D and 3D imaging from long and short axis views (Figure 18-2, Videos 18-2, 18-3, and 18-4).

A treadmill stress echocardiography was performed. The patient complained of chest tightness during exercise. The echocardiography showed the pressure gradient increasing to 64 mmHg within the left ventricular outflow tract (Figure 18-3).

According to the findings of echocardiography, a mild subaortic membrane stenosis was made. The operation was suggested according to the symptoms of patient and the findings of stress echocardiography.

The subaortic membrane was resected down to the muscular septum during the operation. Postoperation TEE showed peak gradient within the left ventricular outflow tract reduced from 26 to 16 mmHg.

Pathology

The diagnosis of subaortic membrane was confirmed by histology.

Comparative Cardiac Imaging: A Case-based Guide, First Edition.
Edited by Jing Ping Sun, Xing Sheng Yang, and Bryan P. Yan.
© 2018 John Wiley & Sons Ltd. Published 2018 by John Wiley & Sons Ltd.
Companion website: www.wiley.com/sun/comparative_cardiac_imaging

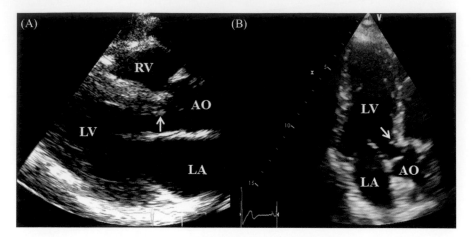

Figure 18-1   A subtle tissue (arrow) attached to the ventricular septum in LVOT was seen in parasternal (A) and apical three-chamber views (B).
Notes: LV, left ventricle; LA, left atrium; RV, right ventricle; AO, ascending aorta.

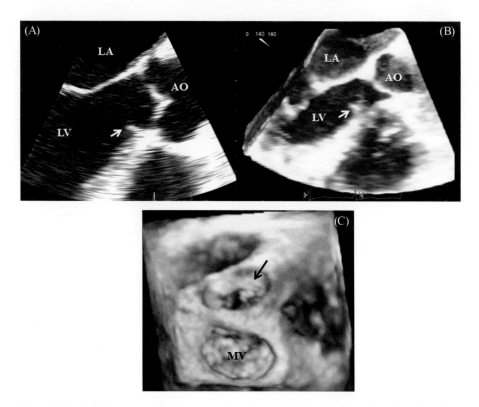

Figure 18-2   A. The long-axis view of transesophageal two-dimensional echocardiography showed a subaortic membrane attached to ventricular septum. B. The long-axis view of transesophageal three-dimensional echocardiography showed a subaortic membrane attached to ventricular septum. C. Three-dimensional transoesophageal echocardiography examination showing a pyramidal volume on the LV outflow tract and the subaortic membrane (arrow) in the short-axis view.
Notes: LV, left ventricle; LA, left atrium; RV, AO, ascending aorta; MV, mitral valve.

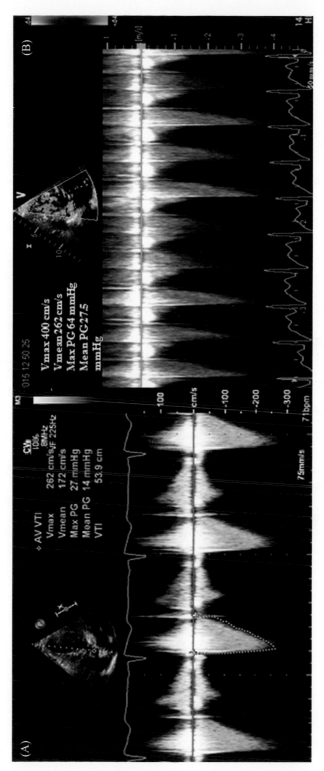

Figure 18-3 The continue wave Doppler spectrum showed. A. The maximal gradient was 27 mmHG during rest. B. The maximal gradient was 64 mmHG after treadmill exercise.

Follow up

The transesophageal echocardiography was performed after 40 days postoperation. The peak gradient was 18 mmHg. No residual membrane was noted on 3DTEE. The treadmill stress was repeated for this patient 4 months after surgery. The maximal heart rate was 162 bpm and the peak gradient was 35 mmHg.

Discussion

Discrete subaortic stenosis (DSS) is a manifestation of a geometric anatomic alteration in the LVOT. This endocardial abnormality involves not only the subaortic ridge but also the leaflets of the adjacent valves [1]. Although substantial pressure gradient and aortic regurgitation are the main indications for surgery, controversy persists about the timing of surgical repair and the surgical technique [2, 3].

Discrete subaortic stenosis is sometimes associated with various other cardiac malformations [1, 4–6], which must be monitored and treated surgically when necessary.

Although the most common symptom in patients with DSS is diminished exercise tolerance, they may also have syncope or angina pectoris [1, 2, 4]. It should be remembered that most patients are asymptomatic, even in the presence of important gradients that indicate surgery [1, 2, 6]. Rayburn and colleagues [2] confirmed that 70% of their patients had no symptoms, but the proportion varies from series to series. Kuralay and co-workers [7] reported that 64.4% of their patients had exertional dyspnea.

Subvalvular aortic obstruction is usually formed by a thin fibrous or occasionally muscular membrane of the LV outflow tract. Careful high-pulse repetition-frequency Doppler allows localization of the level of obstruction by detection of the site of maximum velocities. Transoesophageal imaging is usually needed to demonstrate the presence of the often subtle membrane. Live real-time 3D TEE may provide super 3D visualization quality of the subaortic membrane, as in our case. The size of the probe used is similar to that of standard probes making widely acceptable live 3D TEE in clinical practice. The early diagnosis is important to making decision of surgery. Echocardiography is the key tool for diagnosis; the stress echocardiography may be needed in patients with relative lower pressure gradient within the left ventricular outflow tract for making surgery decisions.

Acquired aortic insufficiency is the most common lesion found in association with subaortic stenosis, and it can be progressive. The thick fibrous tissue on the left ventricular surface of the valve leaflets appears to be the cause of aortic regurgitation. The fibrosis is caused by repetitive trauma from a jet of blood through the stenosis or by the proliferation of the fibroelastic membrane itself. This fibrous tissue can play an important role in the retraction of the valve leaflets [8]. Although an important study found no benefit in early surgery and a higher prevalence of aortic regurgitation in surgically treated patients [9], we think that early surgery may preserve the integrity of the aortic valve, to prevent aortic regurgitation and ventricular dysfunction. The aortic regurgitation progress in discrete subaortic stenosis can be slowed or stopped with adequate resection of DSS. This has been affirmed by various other studies [1, 2, 4, 10, 11].

Although DSS has been treated surgically for many years [1, 5], the optimal operative management and the timing of surgery remain controversial [12, 13]. Many authors have suggested surgery for patients who have left ventricle–aorta gradients that exceed

30 mmHg or a coexisting cardiac defect that requires surgical correction [1, 3, 6], while others advocate surgical resection for DSS of any degree because subaortic stenosis may play the developmental role in aortic insufficiency [9, 13].

Radical excision of all diseased tissue, which attains a minimal early postoperative gradient, may reduce the occurrence of late aortic regurgitation [14]. However, this more aggressive approach increases the risk of iatrogenic damage to the conduction tissue, ventricular septum (VSD), and mitral valve. Kuralay and co-workers [7] have reported fewer complications, such as conduction tissue injury, when myectomy is guided by transesophageal echocardiography.

Limited septal muscle resection can relieve obstruction of the LVOT in some patients, but a more aggressive approach must be taken when the pathologic condition requires it. Persistent dynamic obstruction was found in 44% of patients after removal of discrete subaortic obstruction [15].

Early results after surgery for DSS are usually good. The left ventricle–aorta gradient was decreased significantly in many studies [2–6].

In our case, the subaortic membrane was resected during surgery. The histopathology confirmed the diagnosis. The patient had an uneventful postoperative course and no residual membrane 4 months after membrane resection.

Key Points

1. Discrete subaortic stenosis (DSS) is a manifestation of a geometric anatomic alteration in the LVOT.
2. Echocardiography is the key tool for diagnosis; stress echocardiography may be needed in patients with relative lower pressure gradient within the left ventricular outflow tract for making the decision about surgery.
3. Surgery is indicated in order to relieve the obstruction and to prevent secondary complications due to longstanding ventricular hypertrophy, aortic valve damage, or infective endocarditis.

References

1. Kirklin, J.W. and Barratt-Boyes, B.G. (1993). *Cardiac Surgery: Morphology, Diagnostic Criteria, Natural History, Techniques, Results, and Indications*, 2nd edn. New York, NY: Churchill Livingstone, p. 1212–1224.
2. Rayburn, S.T., Netherland, D.E. and Heath, B.J. (1997). Discrete membranous subaortic stenosis: improved results after resection and myectomy. *Ann Thorac Surg* 64: 105–109.
3. Lupinetti, F.M., Pridjian, A.K., Callow, L.B. et al. (1992). Optimum treatment of discrete subaortic stenosis. *Ann Thorac Surg* 54: 467–471.
4. Kleinert, S., Ott, D.A. and Geva, T. (1993). Critical discrete subaortic stenosis in the newborn period. *Am Heart J* 125: 1187–1189.
5. de Leval, M. (1994). Surgery of the left ventricular outflow tract. In: *Surgery for Congenital Heart Defects*, 2nd ed (ed. J. Stark J, and M. de Levaltors.), 511–537. Philadelphia, PA: W.B. Saunders.
6. Rohlicek, C.V., del Pino, S.F., Hosking, M. et al. (1999). Natural history and surgical outcomes for isolated discrete subaortic stenosis in children. *Heart* 82 (6): 708–713.
7. Kuralay, E., Ozal, E., Bingol, H. et al. (1999). Discrete subaortic stenosis: assessing adequacy of myectomy by transesophageal echocardiography. *J Card Surg* 14 (5): 348–353.
8. Feigl, A., Feigl, D., Lucas, R.V. Jr, et al. (1984). Involvement of the aortic valve cusps in discrete subaortic stenosis. *Pediatr Cardiol* 5: 185–189.

9. Oliver, J.M., Gonzalez, A., Gallego, P. et al. (2001). Discrete subaortic stenosis in adults: in creased prevalence and slow rate of progression of the obstruction and aortic regurgitation. *J Am Coll Cardiol* 38: 835–842.

10. Jahangiri, M., Nicholson, I.A., del Nido, P.J. et al. (2000). Surgical management of complex and tunnel-like subaortic stenosis. *Eur J Cardiothorac Surg* 17: 637–642.

11. Kuralay, E., Ozal, E., Bingol, H. et al. (1999). Discrete subaortic stenosis: assessing adequacy of myectomy by transesophageal echocardiography. *J Card Surg* 14 (5): 348–353.

12. Lupinetti, F.M., Pridjian, A.K., Callow, L.B. et al. (1992). Optimum treatment of discrete subaortic stenosis. *Ann Thorac Surg* 54: 467–471.

13. Douville, E.C., Sade, R.M., Crawford, F.A. Jr et al. (1990). Subvalvar aortic stenosis: Timing of operation. *Ann Thorac Surg* 50: 29–34.

14. Parry, A.J., Kovalchin, J.P., Suda, K. et al. (1999). Resection of subaortic stenosis; can a more aggressive approach be justified? *Eur J Cardiothorac Surg* 15: 631–638.

15. Somerville, J., Stone, S. and Ross, D. (1980). Fate of patients with fixed subaortic stenosis after surgical removal. *Br Heart J* 43: 629–647.

19 Supracardiac Total Anomalous Pulmonary Venous Connection

Fanxia Meng[1], Ming Chen[1], and Jing Ping Sun[2]

[1] Tongji University School of Medicine, Shanghai, China
[2] The Chinese University of Hong Kong, Hong Kong

History

A 6-year-old boy was admitted due to a heart murmur found 4 years earlier.

Physical Examination

Patient's lips were mild cyanosis, clubbing fingers, and toes. There was a whole systolic murmur at the third intercostal space of the left parasternal border.

Echocardiogram

Transthoracic echocardiography showed that the right atrium and ventricle were significantly enlarged; the left atrium was small without a pulmonary vein entrance (Figure 19-1A). There was a atrial septal defect with right-to-left shunt (Figure 19-1B); the superior vena cava was significantly dilated (Figure 19-1C). A supersternal notch view showed four pulmonary veins converging into a common pulmonary vein connected with the vertical vein and entering into an innominate vein draining into the superior vena cava (Figure 19-2A, B, C). The velocity of tricuspid regurgitation was elevated (346 cm/s).

Computed Tomography

Computed tomography showed that four pulmonary veins entered into a common pulmonary vein (Figure 19-3A) connected with vertical vein, and an innominate vein entered into a significantly enlarged superior vena cava (Figure 19-3B). The relations among vertical vein, innominate vein, superior vena cava and right atrium are shown clearly in Figure 19-3C and D.

Surgical Findings

The four pulmonary veins merged into a common pulmonary vein connected with a vertical vein and entered into the innominate vein draining into the superior vena cava. The pulmonary artery was dilated, and the superior vena cava was significantly enlarged. The left atrium was small with a $3 \times 4\,cm^2$ atrial septal defect.

Comparative Cardiac Imaging: A Case-based Guide, First Edition.
Edited by Jing Ping Sun, Xing Sheng Yang, and Bryan P. Yan.
© 2018 John Wiley & Sons Ltd. Published 2018 by John Wiley & Sons Ltd.
Companion website: www.wiley.com/sun/comparative_cardiac_imaging

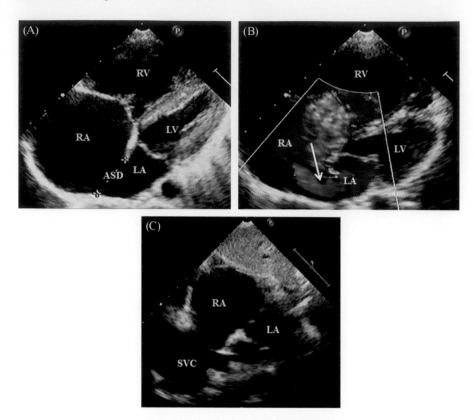

Figure 19-1   Echocardiography: A. An apical four-chamber view showed that the right atrium and ventricle were significantly enlarged, the left atrium was small without pulmonary vein entrance. The entrances of pulmonary veins were not seen in the roof of left atrium. B. An apical four-chamber view showed an atrial septal defect with right-to-left shunt. C. The subcostal view showed that the superior vena cava was significantly enlarged.
Notes: RV, right ventricle; RA, right atrium; LA, left atrial; LV, left ventricle; ASD, atrial septal defect; SVC, superior vena cava.

Postoperative Diagnosis

Congenital heart disease, total anomalous pulmonary venous drainage (supracardiac), atrial septal defect.

Discussion

Abnormal development of the pulmonary veins may result in either partial or complete anomalous drainage back into the systemic venous circulation. Total anomalous pulmonary venous connection (TAPVC) consists of an abnormality of blood flow in all four pulmonary veins draining into systemic veins or the right atrium with or without pulmonary venous obstruction. Systemic and pulmonary venous blood mix in the right atrium. This complete mixing of venous blood produces cyanosis. An atrial defect or foramen ovale (part of the complex) is important in the left ventricular output, both in fetal and in newborn circulation. In contrast, partial anomalous pulmonary venous

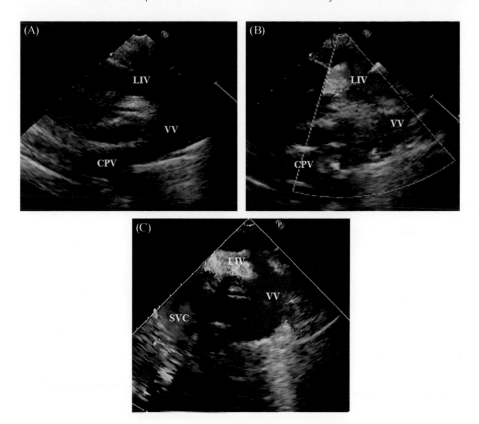

Figure 19-2 Ehocardiography: A. A supersternal notch view showed four pulmonary veins converging into a common pulmonary vein connected with the vertical vein and enter into innominate vein draining into the superior vena cava. B and C. Supersternal notch views with color Doppler showed the blood-flow directions.
Notes: CPV, common pulmonary vein; VV, vertical vein; LIV, left innominate vein.

return (PAPVR) is usually an acyanotic condition [1–3]. The incidence of this rare entity is approximately 1 in 17 000 live births [4] or 1–5% of all cardiovascular congenital anomalies [5].

Classification

Based on the location of pulmonary venous drainage, TAPVC is classified into four major types. In all four types, complete drainage of pulmonary venous blood is directed to the right heart [6].

Type I: Supracardiac (approximately 50%) [4]. As in our case, four pulmonary veins converge into a common pulmonary vein connected with the vertical vein and enter into the innominate vein draining into the superior vena cava (Figure 19-2A, B, C) and finally flow into the right atrium (RA). Rarely, the confluence may drain directly to the right SVC, the left SVC, or the azygous system [7].

Type II: Cardiac (approximately 25%): the pulmonary venous confluence drains either to the coronary sinus or directly into the RA [6, 8].

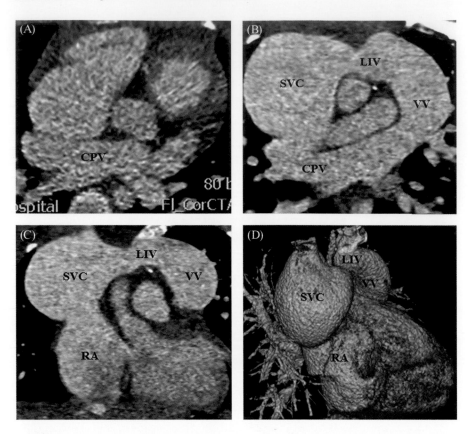

Figure 19-3   Computed tomography imaging: A. Four pulmonary veins entered into a common pulmonary vein. B. The common pulmonary vein connected with vertical vein; an innominate vein entered into a significantly enlarged superior vena cava. C. The relation among vertical vein, innominate vein, superior vena cava and right atrium was clearly presented. D. Three-dimensional cardiac CT image showed the vertical vein, innominate vein, huge superior vena cava, and right atrium.
Notes: CPV, common pulmonary vein; VV, vertical vein; LIV, left innominate vein; RA, right atrium.

Type III: Infracardiac (approximately 25%): the pulmonary venous confluence may drain into IVC, hepatic vein, azygous system, or portal venous system [6, 8].

Type IV: Mixed type (approximately 9%): usually no midline pulmonary confluence is present; thus, the right and left PVs may have different drainages. Almost any combination of drainage may occur into the SVC, innominate veins, coronary sinus, RA, azygous vein [6], or infradiaphragmatic veins [8].

Pulmonary venous obstruction may occur in any type but it is most commonly seen in infracardiac type which may be present in up to 78% of cases [7, 8].

Imaging Diagnosis

Echocardiography is the first and safest imaging modality for cardiovascular abnormalities but may fail in complete depiction of some complex feature of TAPVC [8]. Computed tomography angiography is then a noninvasive and sensitive choice for mapping the PVs without need for invasive cardiac catheterization [5]. Contrast-enhanced magnetic resonance (MR) angiography [8] is the radiation-free alternative for CT angiography but needs general anesthesia in younger children.

Echocardiography   In cases of anomalous pulmonary venous return, the characteristics of echocardiogram are: (i) a large right ventricle and atrium; (ii) a pattern of abnormal pulmonary venous connections is usually seen; (iii) shunting presents almost exclusively from right to left at the atrial level. As seen in our case, significantly enlarged right atrium; the left atrium was small with a defect, but without pulmonary vein entrance. A supersternal notch view showed four pulmonary veins converging into a common pulmonary vein connected with the vertical vein and entering into innominate vein, draining into the superior vena cava and final into the RA. The degree of confidence is high for anomalous pulmonary venous return. False-positive and false-negative results are rare in anomalous pulmonary venous return.

Computed Tomography   Fast CT is useful for indicating pulmonary drainage. The degree of confidence is good for anomalous pulmonary venous return. False-positive and false-negative results are rare in anomalous pulmonary venous return. As in our case, the relation among vertical vein, innominate vein, superior vena cava, and right atrium was clearly demonstrated by CT imaging, which is a good compensation for echocardiography.

Treatment

Surgery is the mainstay of treatment. Accurate diagnosis is the key point for successful operation. Improvements in diagnostic imaging result in accurate descriptions of complex abnormalities, which can assist the clinicians in planning the operative strategy and postoperative care. Advanced surgical techniques will decrease the postoperative mortality rates.

Prognosis

Generally speaking, patients with type I and II TAPVC can live for older age than those with type III and IV lesions [9]. The most important factors affecting the survival period are large ASDs and normal to near normal pulmonary artery pressure [1]. Several cases of adult untreated TAPVC have been reported, even few cases were diagnosed after 60 years of age [4, 10].

Key Points

1. Anomalous pulmonary venous connection is a rare congenital heart disease. Based on the location of pulmonary venous drainage, TAPVC is classified into four major types. In all four types, complete drainage of pulmonary venous blood is directed to the right heart.
2. Echocardiography is the first and safest imaging modality for diagnosis. Computed tomography imaging is good compensation for echocardiography.
3. Surgery is the mainstay of treatment.

References

1. Huddleston, C.B., Exil, V., Canter, C.E. et al. (1999). Scimitar syndrome presenting in infancy. *Ann Thorac Surg* 67 (1): 154–159; discussion 160.
2. Mullen, J.C., Waskiewich, K., Bhargava, R. et al. (1997). Bilateral partial anomalous pulmonary venous return. *Can J Cardiol* 13 (6): 567–569.
3. Rostagno, C., Diricatti, G., Galanti, G. et al. (1999). Partial anomalous venous return associated with intact atrial septum and persistent left superior vena cava: A case report and literature review. *Cardiologia* 44 (2): 203–206.
4. Ogawa, M., Nakagawa, M., Hara, M. et al. (2013). Total anomalous pulmonary venous connection in a 64-year-old man: a case report. *Ann Thorac Cardiovasc Surg* 19 (1): 46–48.
5. Lakshminrusimha, S., Wynn, R.J., Youssfi, M. et al. (2009). Use of CT angiography in the diagnosis of total anomalous venous return. *J Perinatol* 29 (6): 458–461.
6. Hines, M.II. and Hammon, J.W. (2001). Anatomy of total anomalous pulmonary venous connection. *Oper Tech Thorac Cardiovasc Surg* 6 (1): 2–7.
7. White, C.S., Baffa, J.M., Haney P.J. et al. (1997). MR imaging of congenital anomalies of the thoracic veins. *Radiographics* 17 (3): 595–608.
8. Dillman, J.R., Yarram, S.G. and Hernandez, R.J. (2009). Imaging of pulmonary venous developmental anomalies. *Am J Roentgenol* 192 (5): 1272–1285.
9. Feng, Q., Wu, S. and Yu, G. (2010). Surgical treatment of a 56-year-old woman with an intracardiac type of total anomalous pulmonary venous connection. *Thorac Cardiovasc Surg* 58 (3): 175–176.
10. McMullan, M.H. and Fyke, F.E. (1992). Total anomalous pulmonary venous connection: surgical correction in a 66-year-old man. *Ann Thorac Surg* 53 (3): 520–521.

20 Tricuspid Atresia

Jing Ping Sun

The Chinese University of Hong Kong, Hong Kong

History

A 18-year-old male with a history of tricuspid atresia, left cerebral embolism, and atrial fibrillation presented with shortness of breath on exertion, and palpitations.

Physical Examination

On physical examination his heart rate was 106 bpm. He had prominent neck veins, and swollen, cyanotic hands.

Echocardiography

An echocardiography apical four-chamber view showed (i) significantly dilated left and right atrium with spontaneous contrast and a large thrombus in the right atrium; (ii) a thick echogenic and immobile tricuspid valve without flow through the tricuspid valve on color flow mapping; (iii) a hypoplastic right ventricle and severe mitral valve regurgitation; (iv) an occluded pulmonary artery; (v) a ventricular septal defect; (vi) double outlet of the left ventricle (Figure 20-1, Videos 20-1 and 20-2).

Cardiac Computed Tomography

A CT scan of the four cardiac chambers demonstrated the muscular structure of the tricuspid valve (TV) and occluded pulmonary artery. The right ventricle appears hypoplastic. Left and right atriums were grossly dilated and a ventricular septal defect was noted (Figure 20-2). A large filling defect was seen in the right atrium, which might be RA thrombus.

Discussion

Tricuspid atresia may be defined as congenital absence or agenesis of the tricuspid valve [1]. It is the third most common cyanotic congenital heart defect; the other two frequently observed cyanotic congenital cardiac anomalies are transposition of the great arteries and tetralogy of Fallot. Although the true incidence of tricuspid atresia is not well defined, the prevalence of tricuspid atresia among congenital heart defects was estimated to be 2.9% in an autopsy series and 1.4% in a clinical series after extensive review. According to US data, tricuspid atresia may be estimated to occur in approximately 1 per 10 000 live births [2].

Comparative Cardiac Imaging: A Case-based Guide, First Edition.
Edited by Jing Ping Sun, Xing Sheng Yang, and Bryan P. Yan.
© 2018 John Wiley & Sons Ltd. Published 2018 by John Wiley & Sons Ltd.
Companion website: www.wiley.com/sun/comparative_cardiac_imaging

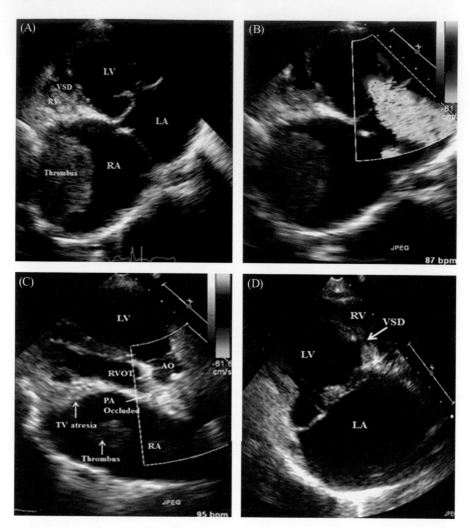

Figure 20-1 Transthoracic echocardiography four-chamber views without (A) and with color Doppler (B) showed: significantly dilated left (LA) and right atrium (RA) with spontaneous contrast, a large thrombus in right atrium and severe mitral valve regurgitation; tricuspid atresia and a hypoplastic right ventricle (RV). A modified view (C) showed tricuspid atresia (arrow), an occluded pulmonary artery (PA). A four-chamber view (D) showed ventricular septal defect (VSD) and dilated left atrium.

Tricuspid atresia has been classified according to the morphology of the valve [3], the radiographic appearance of pulmonary vascular markings [4, 5] and the associated cardiac defects [6–9].

Although these classifications are generally good, their exclusion of some variations in great-artery relationships and the lack of consistency in subgroups are problematic. Therefore, the following comprehensive-yet-unified classification was proposed [9].

The principal grouping continues to be based on the following interrelationships of the great arteries:

- Type I – normally related great arteries.
- Type II – D-transposition of the great arteries.

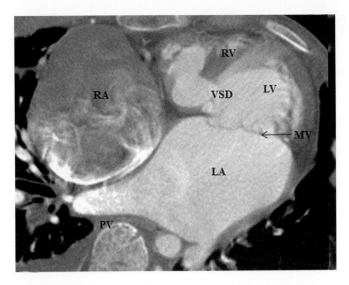

Figure 20-2 Computed tomography scan indicated a significantly dilated left atrium (LA) and right atrium (RA), and ventricular septal defect (VSD).

- Type III – great artery positional abnormalities other than D-transposition of the great arteries: [1] subtype 1 involves L-transposition of the great arteries, (ii) subtype 2 involves double outlet right ventricle, (iii) subtype 3 involves double outlet left ventricle, (iv) subtype 4 involves D-malposition of the great arteries (anatomically corrected malposition), and (v) subtype 5 involves L-malposition of the great arteries (anatomically corrected malposition).
- Type IV – Persistent truncus arteriosus.

All types and subtypes are subdivided into the following subgroups:

- Subgroup a – pulmonary atresia.
- Subgroup b – pulmonary stenosis or hypoplasia.
- Subgroup c – no pulmonary stenosis (normal pulmonary arteries).

After the above categorization, the status of the ventricular septum (intact or VSD) and the presence of other associated malformations are described.

This unified classification includes all the previously described abnormalities in the positions of the great arteries and can be further expanded if new variations are revealed [9].

Transthoracic echocardiography (TTE) is the first-line cardiovascular imaging modality in all types of tricuspid atresia patients. A computed tomography scan can provide the 3D spatial resolution imaging.

Poor prognosis of untreated tricuspid atresia patients is well known; only 10–20% of infants may live through the first year of life [10]. Considerable early mortality occurs and may be related to hypoxemia, cardiac failure, surgical intervention, or their combination. Surgical palliation to normalize pulmonary blood flow by means of systemic-to-pulmonary artery shunts in neonates with pulmonary oligemia and banding of the pulmonary artery in infants with markedly increased pulmonary flow improves survival rates.

Key Points

1. Tricuspid atresia is a complex congenital heart disease, its prognosis is poor without surgery.
2. According the interrelationships of the great arteries, tricuspid atresia has been classified into four types.
3. Echocardiographic features include an absent or atretic tricuspid valve, VSD, and a small RV.

References

1. Rao, P.S. (1997). Tricuspid atresia: Anatomy, imaging, and natural history. In: *Atlas of Heart Disease: Congenital Heart Disease* (ed. F. Braunwald and R. Freedom), vol. 12, 14.1. Philadelphia, PA: Current Medicine.
2. Mitchell, S.C., Korones, S.B. and Berendes, H.W. (1971). Congenital heart disease in 56 109 births. Incidence and natural history. *Circulation* 43 (3): 323–332.
3. Van Praagh, R. (1992). Discussion after paper by Vlad P: Pulmonary atresia with intact ventricular septum. In: *Heart Disease in Infancy: Diagnosis and Surgical Treatment*, 2nd edn. (ed. B.G. Barrett-Boyes, J.M. Neutze and E.A. Harris), 236. London: Churchill Livingstone.
4. Astley, R., Oldham, J.S. and Parsons, C. (1953). Congenital tricuspid atresia. *Br Heart J* 15 (3): 287–297.
5. Dick, M., Fyler, D.C. and Nadas, A.S. (1975). Tricuspid atresia: clinical course in 101 patients. *Am J Cardiol* 36 (3): 327–337.
6. Edwards, J.E. and Burchell, H.B. (1949). Congenital tricuspid atresia: a classification. *Med Clin North Am* 33: 1117.
7. Keith, J., Rowe, R.D. and Vlad, P. (1967). *Heart Disease in Infancy and Childhood. Tricuspid Atresia*, 2nd edn. New York, NY: Macmillian.
8. Vlad, P. (1977). Tricuspid atresia. In: Heart Disease in Infancy and Childhood, 3rd edn (ed. J.D. Keith, R.D. Rowe and P. Vlad), 518–541. New York, NY: Macmillian.
9. Rao, P.S. (1980). A unified classification for tricuspid atresia. *Am Heart J* 99(6): 799–804.
10. Dick, M. and Rosenthal, A. (1982). The clinical profile of tricuspid atresia. In: *Tricuspid Atresia*, 2nd edn. (ed. P.S. Rao), 83–111. Mount Kisco, NY: Futura.

21 Isolated Congenital Tricuspid Valve Dysplasia in a 38-year-old Adult

Ligang Fang[1] and Jing Ping Sun[2]

[1] Affiliated Hospital of Peking Union Medical College, Beijing, China
[2] The Chinese University of Hong Kong, Hong Kong

History

A 38-year-old female was admitted due to intermittent palpitations, shortness of breath, which she had been experiencing for 4 years.

Physical Examination

Her blood pressure was 110/68 mmHg, heart rate 74 bpm. The jugular vein was distended. Her heart was extended to the right side and a 3/6 systolic murmur was heard in tricuspid valve area. There was mild edema in the lower limbs

Laboratory

B-type brain natriuretic peptide: 142 pg/ml.

Electrocardiogram: atrial fibrillation, ventricular rate 108 bpm, complete right bundle branch block.

Abdomen ultrasound showed liver congestion, hepatic vein dilated.

Right ventricular catheterization: right atrial pressure 25/6 mmHg, right ventricular pressure 25/7 mmHg, the main pulmonary artery pressure 23/14 mmHg, pulmonary capillary pressure 9 mmHg, cardiac output 4.4 L/min.

Coronary Computed Tomography Angiography (CCTA)

The coronary arteries were normal. The right ventricle was significantly dilated with tricuspid regurgitation. Anterior tricuspid valve was pulled by papillary muscle traction. The inferior vena cava and hepatic vein were dilated. The pericardial effusion and bilateral pleural effusion were noted.

Echocardiography

Right heart was significantly enlarged with significantly decreased systolic function, the left heart is relatively small with normal systolic function The tricuspid valve annulus was significantly dilated with severe regurgitation. The septal leaflet of the tricuspid valve was short, but in the normal position (Figure 21-1 and Video 21-1, and Video 21-2). The inferior vena cava was dilated and diminished inspiratory collapse.

Comparative Cardiac Imaging: A Case-based Guide, First Edition.
Edited by Jing Ping Sun, Xing Sheng Yang, and Bryan P. Yan.
© 2018 John Wiley & Sons Ltd. Published 2018 by John Wiley & Sons Ltd.
Companion website: www.wiley.com/sun/comparative_cardiac_imaging

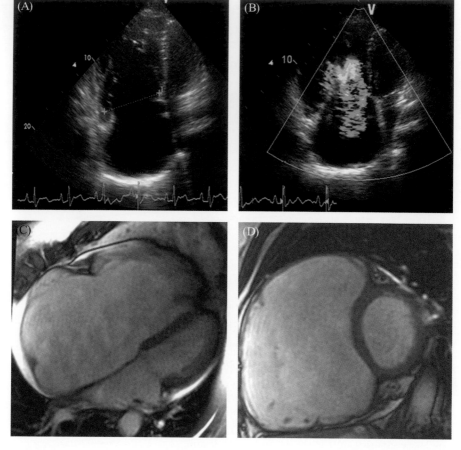

Figure 21-1 Transthoracic echocardiography: A and B. Apical four-chamber view showed significantly dilated right atrium and ventricle and enlarged tricuspid valve annulus with severe tricuspid regurgitation (color Doppler). C and D. Magnetic resonance imaging indicated: The right ventricle and atrial were significantly dilated.

Magnetic Resonance Imaging The right ventricle and atrial was significantly dilated (Figure 21-1), right ventricular wall was thin with decreased ventricular wall motion (right ventricular EF was 31%), with severe tricuspid regurgitation. The tricuspid valve and annulus were in right position, the activity of tricuspid valves was decreased; the anterior papillary muscle was thick. The pericardial and bilateral pleural effusion was seen. Delayed scan showed no significant abnormal myocardial enhancement,

Hospital Course
After hospitalization, the operation was performed. Surgical inspection showed the tricuspid valve annulus was significantly enlarged (the diameter was about 40 mm). The valve development was very poor: three leaflets were small and flimsy, and the anterior valve was slightly larger but its tendon was pulled to the anterior wall. The septal leaflet was small, its tendon was short, attached to the interventricular septum. A tricuspid

valvuloplasty (autologous pericardial patch widening, artificial chordae, artificial valve ring St Jude 31 # Tailor) was performed. The patient recovered well after the operation.

Discussion

Isolate congenital tricuspid valve dysplasia is a rare form of congenital heart disease, which is characterized by early onset of congestive heart failure, massive cardiomegaly, and profound hypoxemia [1–4]. This condition may be difficult to differentiate from persistent pulmonary hypertension of the newborn (PPHN), as both share many common hemodynamic and clinical feature [1, 3]. The tricuspid valve dysplasia was precisely defined on pathological examination: (i) thickened valve, (ii) hypoplastic chordae and papillary muscles, (iii) incomplete separation between the leaflets and ventricular wall, (iv) focal agenesis of valvular tissues. An associated pulmonary artery stenosis in the newborn may explain the severity of symptoms in this age group. This hypothesis, based only on pathological studies, cannot be confirmed [5].

Two congenital anatomical defects are commonly recognized, namely Ebstein's anomaly, and dysplastic tricuspid valve with or without abnormal chordal attachment in the absence of annulus displacement [1, 6, 7]. However, patients with valvular dysplasia will, in addition, have hepatomegaly; a massively enlarged cardiac silhouette on the chest radiograph should be differentiated. The two-dimensional and Doppler echocardiogram is the most useful investigation in confirming the structural abnormalities of the tricuspid valve [6]. We report an isolated tricuspid valve atresia without any associated congenital abnormality. A cross-sectional apical four chamber view showed a dilated right ventricle and atrium with that leaflet of the tricuspid valve could not close properly. But the tricuspid valve is in the correct position and is not thickened. In our case, the features of echocardiography are easy to make a distinction from diagnosis of Ebstein's anomaly, and the carcinoid tricuspid disease, in which the tricuspid valve should be thickened with tricuspid stenosis and regurgitation. CT and MRI discovered similar information. The final diagnosis is made by surgery.

Key Points

1. Isolated tricuspid valve atresia is a rare congenital heart disease.
2. Echocardiography is important for the diagnosis and differential diagnosis for this disease.
3. Tricuspid valve atresia is often associated with another congenial abnormalities. One should investigate this possibility carefully.

References

1. Boucek, R.J. Jr, Graham, T.P., Morgan, J.P. et al. (1976). Spontaneous resolution of massive congenital tricuspid insufficiency. *Circulation* 54: 795–800.
2. Freedom, R.M. (1992). Congenital valvular regurgitation. In *Neonatal Heart Disease* (ed. R.M. Freedom, L.N. Benson, and J.F. Smallhorn), 679–692. Berlin: Springer-Verlag.
3. Marsh, T.D. and Shelton, L.W. Jr. (1993). Neonatal tricuspid insufficiency with abnormal tricuspid valve treated with extracorporeal membrane oxygenation (ECMO): Possible extension of ECMO use. *Am J Perinatol* 10: 36–38.

4. Reisman, M., Hiaona, F.A., Bloor, C.M. et al. (1965). Congenital tricuspid insufficiency. J Pediatr 66: 869–876.

5. Lagarde, O., Garabedian, V., Coignard, A. et al. (1980). Congenital tricuspid insufficiency due to valvular dysplasia. Review of the literature in light of a case in a 40-year-old adult. *Arch Mal Coeur Vaiss* 73 (4): 387–396.

6. Gewillig, M., Dumoulin, M., and Vander Hauwaert, L.G. (1988). Transient neonatal tricuspid regurgitation: A Doppler echocardiographic study of three cases. *Br Heart J* 60: 446–451.

7. Becker, M.J., Edwards, J.E. (1971). Pathologic spectrum of dysplasia of the tricuspid valve. *Arch Pathol* 91: 167–178.

22 Unroofed Coronary Sinus Defect

Ran Guo¹, Jing Ping Sun², and Alex Pui-Wai Lee²

¹ Affiliated Hospital of Dalian Medical University, Dalian, China
² The Chinese University of Hong Kong, Hong Kong

History

A 44-year-old male presented with a history of two strokes. He did not have chest discomfort.

Physical Examination

Blood pressure was 110/70 mmHg. Heart rate was 88 bpm with a regular rhythm. Cardiac examination was unremarkable.

Electrocardiogram

Electrocardiogram showed a broadened P (>0.12 s) in lead II.

Echocardiography

On transthoracic echocardiography (TTE), the parasternal long-axis view showed a significantly enlarged left atrium (LA) and the drainage of unroofed coronary sinus into the left atrium, constituting a bidirection shunt–coronary sinus ASD (atrial septal defect) (Figure 22-1A), with a LA-to-CS shunt (Figure 22-1B) during LA contraction, and CS-to-LA (Figure 22-1C) during LA relaxation (Video 22-1). A three-dimensional (3D) transesophageal echocardiographic (TEE) en face view of the mitral valve from the LA perspective showed a large entrance from a dilated mid-cardiac vein in the CS (Figure 22-2A). The apical four-chamber view of TTE revealed a severely enlarged LA, the defect (arrow) between the LA posterio-lateral wall and dilated CS (*) (Figure 22-2B). An atypical parasternal short-axis view showed a defect between the CS and LA floor, and the stenosis entrance of the CS (Figure 22-2C, arrow).

A three-dimensional TEE basal short-axis view showed the long axis of the CS and the defect between the LA posterior wall and CS (Figure 22-3 left; Video 22-2), and a defect between LA posterior lateral wall and CS, and the significantly dilated orifice of mid coronary vein in CS and a narrow entrance flow from CS to right atrium (Figure 22-3 right, Video 22-3).

Comparative Cardiac Imaging: A Case-based Guide, First Edition.
Edited by Jing Ping Sun, Xing Sheng Yang, and Bryan P. Yan.
© 2018 John Wiley & Sons Ltd. Published 2018 by John Wiley & Sons Ltd.
Companion website: www.wiley.com/sun/comparative_cardiac_imaging

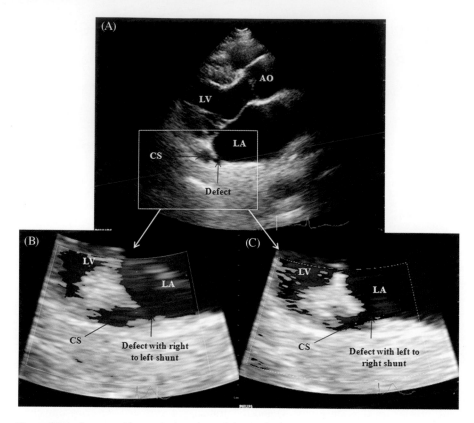

Figure 22-1 Parasternal long-axis view showed the significantly enlarged left atrium and the drainage of unroofed coronary sinus into the left atrium, constituting a bidirection shunt – coronary sinus ASD (atrial septal defect) (A), with a LA-to-CS shunt (B) during LA contraction, and CS-to-LA (C) during LA relaxation.

Computed Tomography (CT)

A coronal view of CT image showed that the junction of mid vein and unroofed CS was significantly dilated, and communicated with the LA before entering the right atrium (Figure 22-4A). The 3D rendered image showed that the mid cardiac vein was aneurysmal and the entrance of coronary sinus draining into the RA (arrow) was narrow. The coronary sinus was not significantly dilate (Figure 22-4B, arrow).

Discussion

An unroofed coronary sinus defect (UCSD) is a very rare type of atrial septal defect. An unroofed coronary sinus defect is seen in over 70% of patients with a left superior vena cava (LSVC) that drains into the LA [1]. The morphological type can be classified as: Type I, completely unroofed with LSVC; type II, completely unroofed without LSVC; type III, partial unroofed mid portion; and type IV, partial unroofed terminal portion [1]. In patients with persistent LSVC and a history of paradoxical embolism or brain abscess, UCSD should be suspected. It has been reported that UCSD can occurred with

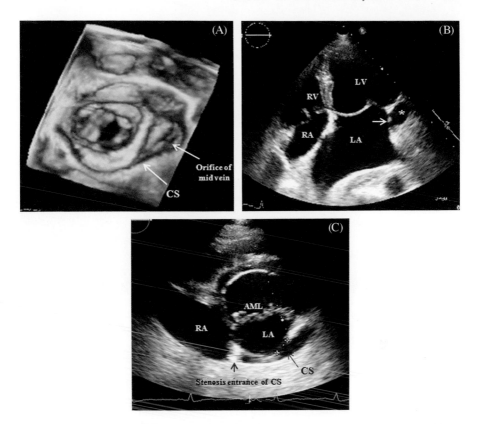

Figure 22-2 A. From three-dimensional full-volume imaging, a short-axis surgical view obtained by cropping showed the long axis of the coronary sinus and the ostium of the significantly dilated middle coronary vein. B. A four-chamber view of TTE presents a significantly enlarged LA, the defect (arrow) between the LA posterior-lateral wall and the coronary sinus (*). C. An atypical parasternal short-axis view indicated the long axis of CS and the defect between CS and LA and stenosis entrance of CS.

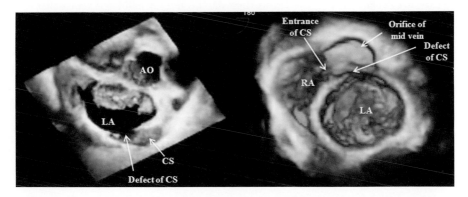

Figure 22-3 Left: From three-dimensional full-volume imaging, short-axis surgical views obtained by cropping showed a defect between the LA posterior lateral wall and the CS, as well as part of the CS long-axis view. Right: A narrow entrance flow from CS to right atrium, the significantly dilated ostium of mid coronary vein, and the defect between the LA posterior wall and the CS.

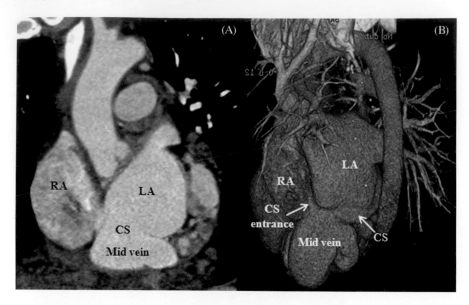

Figure 22-4 A. CT coronal view showed LA, RA and coronary sinus connected with LA. B. A three-dimensional reconstructive image presents a significantly enlarged LA and a huge midcoronary vein, a narrow entrance of CS (arrow), and the coronary sinus (arrow).

other congenital heart diseases, such as tetralogy of Fallot, cor triatriatum, pulmonary atresia, and anomalous pulmonary venous drainage [2].

A communication between the LA and a prominent CS could be identified easily on transverse cropping of the three-dimensional echocardiography with three-dimensional color Doppler flow signals moving from the LA into the CS and then into the RA. A definitive diagnosis of UCSD could be made using three-dimensional echocardiography because off-axis image planes can be reconstructed from the three-dimensional data set to allow us to follow the continuation of different structures and flow [3].

Cardiac MRI provides a high contrast view of the internal cardiac structures and can be used to calculate the effective left-to-right shunt (QP/QS), and right ventricular volumes. A multislice CT scan can offer 3D reconstructions of cardiac structures and require less time, making this imaging modality a favorable choice for uncooperative patients or pediatric patients [4]. Cardiac catheterization can also confirm the presence of an LSVC associated with an unroofed coronary sinus atrial septal defect via selective angiography of the coronary sinus and the left atrium [5].

In our case, the significantly enlarged LA with normal-size right ventricle and atrium could not be explained by an unroofed coronary sinus defect, which lead us to check the associated congenital abnormality. The CT study found an aneursymal mid-cardiac vein and a stenotic CS entrance, which impeded blood flow from the CS into the RA; due to the proximity of the defect very close to the ostium of mid cardiac vein, blood drains preferentially from the LA into this vein. The longstanding volume and pressure overload from the shunt resulted in an aneursymal mid-cardiacoronary venous aneurysm.

All of these results suggested that this is an unroofed coronary sinus defect associated with a stenotic entrance; a huge mid coronary vein with high pressure leading to bidirectional shunt from the defect; the long-term preload lead to LA enlarged. The sinus unroofed position is close the entrance of the coronary sinus, and direct to the ostium of ostium of mid cardiac vein.

Key Points

1. An unroofed coronary sinus defect (UCSD) is a very rare type of atrial septal defect. The morphological type can be classified as: Type I, completely unroofed with LSVC; type II, completely unroofed without LSVC; type III, partial unroofed mid portion; and type IV, partial unroofed terminal portion.
2. A UCSD can occur with other congenital heart diseases, such as tetralogy of Fallot, cor triatriatum, pulmonary atresia, and anomalous pulmonary venous drainage.
3. A definitive diagnosis of UCSD could be made using 3DTEE.
4. If the diagnosis of unroofed coronary sinus defect could not detected by echocardiography, further examination should be performed use newer modalities. Cardiac MRI provides high contrast of the internal cardiac structures, which will be help in complete diagnosis. The computed tomographic scanners can offer three-dimensional reconstructions of cardiac structures and require less time.

References

1. Ootaki, Y., Yamaguchi, M., Yoshimura, N. et al. (2003). Unroofed coronary sinus syndrome: diagnosis, classification, and surgical treatment. *J Thorac Cardiovasc Surg* 126: 1655–1656.
2. Gonzalez-Juanatey, C., Testa, A., Vidan, J. et al. (2004). Persistent left superior vena cava draining into the coronary sinus: report of 10 cases and literature review. *Clin Cardiol* 27: 515–518.
3. Singh, A., Nanda, N.C., Romp, R.L. et al. (2007). Assessment of surgically unroofed coronary sinus by Live/Real time three-dimensional transthoracic echocardiography. *Echocardiography* 24: 74–76.
4. Brancaccio, G., Miraldi, F., Ventriqlia, F. et al. (2003). Multidetector-row helical computed tomography imaging of unroofed coronary sinus. *Int J Cardiol* 91: 251–253.
5. Huang, X.S. (2007). Imaging in cardiovascular medicine. Partially unroofed coronary sinus. *Circulation* 116: 373–376.

Part II
Artery Disease

23 Acute Aortic Regurgitation caused by Spontaneous Aortic Valve Rupture

Li-Tan Yang, Ping-Yen Liu, Cheng-Han Lee, and Wei-Chuan Tsai

National Cheng Kung University, Taiwan

History

A 51-year-old woman complained of acute respiratory distress and received immediate intubation for acute respiratory distress in the emergence room. She was a smoker, without other medical conditions.

Physical Examination

On admission her blood pressure was 140/60 mm Hg, pulse rate was 90 bpm. Temperature was 37.5 °C, and respiration rate was 20 breaths per minute with support of a ventilator. A grade III/VI early diastolic murmur with a loud pulmonic component of the second heart sound was heard along the left sternal border.

X-ray

The chest roentgenogram showed a bilateral ground-glass pattern, which was consistent with pulmonary edema (Figure 23-1).

Transthoracic Echocardiography (TTE)

The left ventricle (LV) was hyperdynamic. The end-diastolic dimension was 5.5 cm, and left atrium was enlarged. Transesophageal echocardiography (TEE) short-axis view showed (i) prolapsed left coronary cups (LCC, arrow), (ii) the regurgitant flow through the dissected LCC (arrow), (iii) TEE long-axis view showing severe prolapse of the LCC, which mimicked a wreath drifting chaotically into the left ventricular outflow tract with severe aortic regurgitation (AR) (Figure 23-2, Videos 23-1, 23-2, and 23-3). There was no obvious vegetation, no sinus Valsalva aneurysm, no shunted flow communicating with other cardiac chambers, and no evidence of type-A aortic dissection was noted based on the transesophageal echocardiographic findings.

Angiogram

The coronary arteries were normal. Based on test results, the diagnosis of spontaneous aortic valve rupture was hypothesized.

Comparative Cardiac Imaging: A Case-based Guide, First Edition.
Edited by Jing Ping Sun, Xing Sheng Yang, and Bryan P. Yan.
© 2018 John Wiley & Sons Ltd. Published 2018 by John Wiley & Sons Ltd.
Companion website: www.wiley.com/sun/comparative_cardiac_imaging

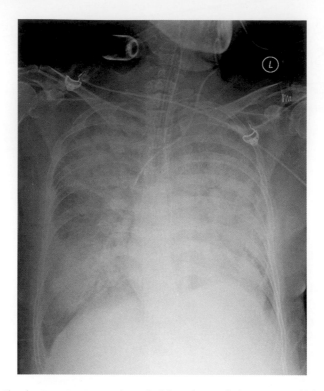

Figure 23-1   The chest roentgenogram showed a bilateral ground-glass pattern, which was consistent with pulmonary edema.

The patient received an operation. Surgical inspection revealed the left coronary cups was prolapsed with a rupture hole near its junction to the aortic wall (Figure 23-3A). The dissected LCC was redundant, clean, and transparent without vegetation.

Pathology

The dissected LCC was transparent with another two pieces of rupture structures (Figure 23-3B). Microscopically, the structures of aortic valve (AV) showed myxomatous degeneration without evidence of infection.

The culture results of both the operative tissue and the blood sample were negative. The patient recovered well and was discharged 9 days after an uneventful postoperative course.

Discussion

Rupture of an aortic leaflet was diagnosed either at surgery or at necropsy in patients with and without infective endocarditis.

In our patient, aortic regurgitation was acute, as supported by the sudden onset of symptoms and by the clinical, radiologic, and echocardiographic findings. There were no signs of previous or actual infectious or rheumatic endocarditis. In such a case presenting as frank pulmonary edema and severe AR, the first diagnostic challenge for clinicians is to determine the course of the AR because there are different causes and treatment strategies. Our patient was totally symptom free before this event.

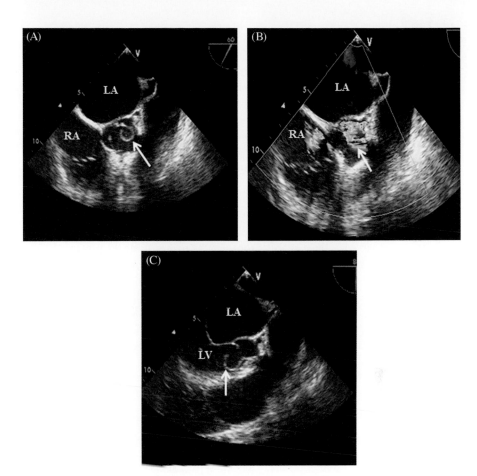

Figure 23-2 Transesophageal echocardiography short axis view showed. A. prolapsed left coronary cusp (LCC, arrow); B. the regurgitant flow through the dissected LCC (arrow); C TEE long axis view showing the prolapsed LCC, which mimicked a wreath drifting chaotically into the left ventricular outflow tract with severe aortic regurgitation (AR) (arrow).

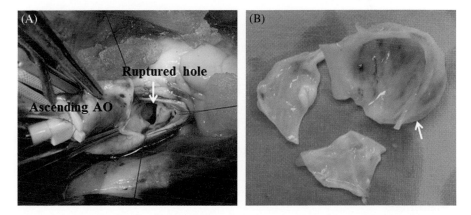

Figure 23-3 A. The intraoperative picture demonstrates the laceration at the bottom of left coronary (arrow shows point of laceration). B. The dissected LCC was transparent with another two pieces of rupture structures.

In clinical situations of acute severe AR, aortic dissection, infective endocarditis, and sinus of Valsalva aneurysm rupture are on the list of differential diagnoses. Lacking evidence supporting these diagnoses, AV rupture should be considered. Although one might be impressed by the prolapsed pattern of the AV in our case when first viewing the echocardiographic images, searching for the underlying mechanisms causing the valvular prolapse is more critical. The transesophageal images in our case demonstrated the striking finding of a ruptured defect on the LCC, which indicated this rare diagnosis to us. Without a history of trauma and infectious processes, spontaneous AV rupture was favored as the cause of the acute severe AR.

The pathologic link between spontaneous AV rupture and myxomatous transformation has scarcely been mentioned in the literature. We were able to find only five cases in a review of the literature [1–4]. Before two-dimensional echocardiography was available, M-mode images served as the diagnostic tool [1, 2] to demonstrate the prolapsed AV as thick bands of echoes occupying the aortic root throughout the diastole or as the abnormal echogenicity in the left ventricular outflow tract; this simulated the M-mode findings in our case. In the present case, we hypothesized that the myxomatous degeneration of the AV led to the prolapse. The combination of the progress of the disease per se and the effect of the shear force of the blood flow created a weak point where the rupture occurred. Subsequently, the AR jet dragged the AV down and resulted in a more severe prolapse, thus causing a more severe AR.

In conclusion, in the absence of clinically identifiable secondary causes for acute AR, such as infective endocarditis, aortic dissections, sinus Valsalva aneurysm rupture, or trauma, an uncommon diagnosis of spontaneous AV rupture should be considered and recognized.

Surgical intervention should not be delayed, and intraoperative tissue pathologic examination is important to provide an insight into the mechanisms of this rare disease.

Two-dimensional real-time echocardiography has the advantage of differentiating between a prolapse leaflet and vegetation by revealing the hinge point of the left ventricular outflow tract diastolic echo density, which in our case was seen. Prompt imaging evaluation, especially TEE, is also crucial in such a critical situation for the accurate diagnosis and appropriate management.

Key Points

1. Rupture of a fenestrated aortic valve represents a noninfectious cause of acute aortic regurgitation. It may affect congenitally bicuspid valves or tricuspid aortic valves with age-related fenestrations.
2. As the number of elderly citizens in the world continues to increase, the number of cases of acute aortic regurgitation due to rupture of fenestrated cusps may also increase, particularly in subjects with chronic hypertension.
3. Timely diagnosis can save patients from acute heart failure or death.

References

1. Estevez, C.M., Dillon, J.C., Walker, P.D. et al. (1976). Echocardiographic manifestations of aortic cusp rupture in a myxomatous aortic valve. *Chest* 69: 685–687.

2. Das, G., Lee, C.C. and Weissler, A.M. (1977). Echocardiographic manifestations of ruptured aortic valvular leaflets in the absence of valvular vegetations. *Chest* 72: 464–468.

3. Ide, H., Ino, T., Yamada, S. et al. (1991). Spontaneous aortic cusp rupture. *Nihon Kyobu Geka Gakkai Zasshi* 39: 1816–1820.

4. O'Brien, K.P., Hitchcock, G.C., Barrat-Boyes, B.G. et al. (1968). Spontaneous aortic cusp rupture associated with valvular myxomatous transformation. *Circulation* 37: 273–278.

24 Bicuspid Aortic Valve Complicated by Pseudo-aneurysm of Aortic Root Abscesses

Shuran Huang[1], Zhanguo Sun[1], and Jing Ping Sun[2]

[1] Affiliated Hospital of Jining Medical University, Jining, China
[2] The Chinese University of Hong Kong, Hong Kong

History

A 58-year-old male presented with the paroxysmal heart palpitations for 2 years, persistent chest pain for 3 days. He had fever one year ago and received unformal antibacterial therapy.

Physical Examination

Temperature 36.5 °C, heart rate was 114 bpm, respiration was 21/min, and BP was 122/79 mmHg. There was a 4/6 systolic murmur and an early diastolic murmur best heard at the second intercostal space of the left sternal border. The patient had moderate edema of the lower limbs. The other aspects of physical examination were unremarkable.

Transthoracic Echocardiography

The study was difficult. The interventricular septum and left ventricular walls were thickened with normal wall motion. The left atrium was mildly dilated. The parasternal short axis view at great vessel level showed that: (i) the configuration of aortic leaflets was not clear but they were thickened with calcification; (ii) there was an aortic right coronary sinus aneurysm (about 19 mm × 42 mm), which pressed the right ventricular outflow tract (the narrower width was 6 mm); (iii) there was moderate pericardial effusion (Figure 24-1). The velocity of the right ventricular outflow tract and pulmonary valve was 3 m/s, and the velocity of aortic valve was 4 m/s with diastolic Doppler flow spectral. The E/A ratio from mitral valve was < 1. The diagnosis of echocardiography was: (i) left ventricular hypertrophy with normal size and systolic function; (ii) right coronary sinus aneurysm and oppressed right ventricular outflow tract; (iii) aortic valvular stenosis and regurgitation; and (iv) moderate pericardial effusion (Figure 24-1).

Comparative Cardiac Imaging: A Case-based Guide, First Edition.
Edited by Jing Ping Sun, Xing Sheng Yang, and Bryan P. Yan.
© 2018 John Wiley & Sons Ltd. Published 2018 by John Wiley & Sons Ltd.
Companion website: www.wiley.com/sun/comparative_cardiac_imaging

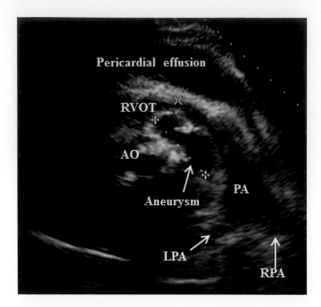

Figure 24-1   Transthoracic echocardiogram. Parasternal short axis view at great vessel level showed that the configuration of aortic leaflets was not clear but they were thickened with calcification; there was an aortic right coronary sinus aneurysm (about 19 mm × 42 mm), which pressed the right ventricular outflow tract (the narrower width was 6 mm). There was moderate pericardial effusion.

Computed Tomography

Multiplanar reconstruction of the aortic root short-axis view showed that there were two aneurisms from the valve junction points of the bicuspid annulus, which were filled with the contrast agent; the cross-section of larger one (Figure 24-2A; Δ, about 17 × 47 mm) was located at front left of the aortic root and pressed the right ventricular outflow tract (RVOT); the smaller one was located at the right rear of the aortic root (*, about 11 × 19 mm) and communicated with the right coronary sinus (Figure 24-2A). The oblique-coronal of the maximum intensity projection showed that the ascending aorta (AA) was dilated, two aneurysms (Figure 24-2B, Δand *) from the bicuspid annulus could be seen in this view. Computed tomography volume rendering imaging also showed the dilated ascending aorta (AA), two aneurysms (Δand *) from the bicuspid annulus between right and left coronary sinus, and the right coronary artery (RCA) originated from the superior margin of the right coronary sinus (Figure 24-2C).

Computed tomography virtual endoscopy (CTVE) imaging showed aortic bicuspid deformity with valve thickening, calcification; there was a small defect at right anterior sinus (arrow) (Figure 24-3A). The right coronary artery originated from the superior margin of the right coronary sinus, and the left coronary artery originated from the left coronary sinus (arrow). The opening of bicuspid aortic valves was restricted, which was consistent with stenosis (☆) (Figure 24-3B). A CT study also found coronary atherosclerosis presented as mixed plaque in (i) the proximal right coronary artery with mild luminal stenosis, (ii) the left anterior descending coronary artery with mild to moderate luminal stenosis, and (iii) the proximal left circumflex branch with mild luminal stenosis. There was left pleural effusion and moderate pericardial effusion.

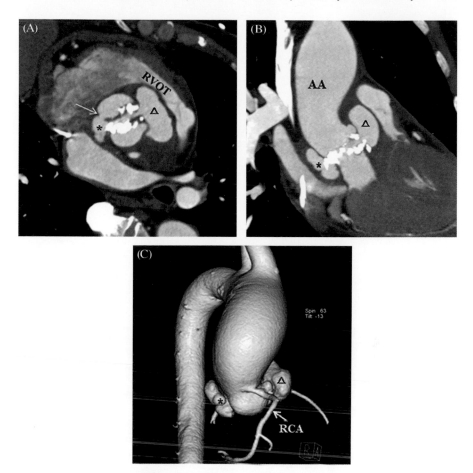

Figure 24-2 A. Multiplanar reconstruction of aortic root short-axis view showed that there were two aneurisms from the valve junction points of the bicuspid annulus respectively, which were filled with contrast agent. The cross-section of larger one (Δ, about 17 × 47 mm) was located at the front left of the aortic root, which oppresses right ventricular outflow tract (RVOT); the smaller one was located at the right rear of the aortic root (*, about 11 × 19 mm) and communicated with the right sinus. B. The oblique-coronal of maximum intensity projection showed ascending aorta (AA) was dilated. Two aneurysms (Δ and *) from the bicuspid annulus could be seen in this view. C. Computed tomography volume rendering imaging showed that the ascending aorta (AA) was dilated. Two aneurysms (Δ and *) from the bicuspid annulus could be seen and the right coronary artery (RCA) originated from the superior margin of the right coronary sinus.

Operation

The patient underwent Bentall's operation. The surgeon repaired aortic root, and performed aortic valve replacement. The operation was performed successfully without any complication. The diagnosis was aortic root abscess, aortic stenosis, and ascending aorta dilation.

The pathology result was that the aortic valve contained fibrosis with hyalinization, myxoid degeneration and calcification, a large amount of neutrophils and lymphocytes infiltrating connective tissue; the results were consistent with chronic inflammation (Figure 24-4).

The patient was discharged 20 days after operation.

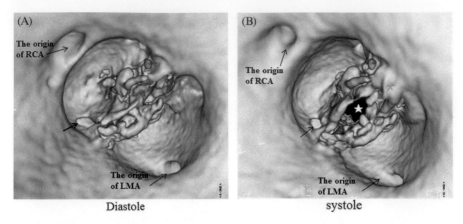

Figure 24-3 Computed tomography virtual endoscopy (CTVE). A. The imaging showed an aortic bicuspid deformity with valve thickening and calcification. There was a small defect at the right anterior sinus (arrow). The right coronary artery originated from the superior margin of right anterior sinus, and the left coronary artery originated from the left coronary sinus (arrow). B. The opening of valves was restricted, which was consistent with stenosis (☆).

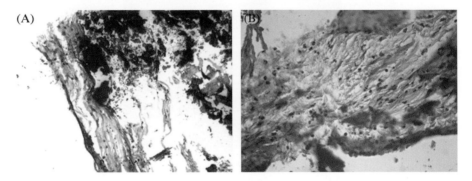

Figure 24-4 The pathology result. The aortic valve contain fibrosis with hyalinization, myxoid degeneration and calcification, a large amount of neutrophils and lymphocytes infiltrating connective tissue; the results were consistent with chronic inflammation.

Discussion

A bicuspid aortic valve (BAV) is the most common congenital heart disease, affecting 1–2% of the population [1]. Aortic stenosis, regurgitation and infective endocarditis are the most common complications of bicuspid aortic valve [2]. Infective endocarditis (IE) is a potentially life-threatening condition. Congenital structural anomalies such as BAV [3], prosthetic valves and intravenous drug use are the major risk factors for IE. Infection commonly spreads into the periannular soft tissues and can cause abscesses, pseudoaneurysms and fistulas with the incidence of these complications reported to be 30–50% for aortic valve IE [3]. Early detection of abscesses is particular important because it has been shown that the surgery may improve the prognosis by preventing widespread tissue disruption. The transthoracic echocardiography and color Doppler mapping have become the most popular noninvasive, cost-effective choice for detection of the IE complications [3]. However, perivalular pseudoaneurysms can be very difficult to define with TTE and TEE due to limited soft-tissue resolution.

The preoperative recognition of an infected pseudoaneurysm thus has important therapeutic implications requiring much more extensive surgical intervention, with the need for debridement and often annulus reconstruction, and multidetector computed tomography (MDCT) has an emerging role in this setting. An infected pseudoaneurysm appears as a contrast medium filling lesion in direct communication with the aortic root or left ventricular output [4, 5]. Computed tomography angiography has the advantage of simultaneous evaluation of valvular structures, coronary arteries, thrombi, and the precise relationship of the pseudo aneurysm with other cardiac chambers, the aortic root, and the pulmonary artery. The exact localization of the opening and neck of aneurysm is also essential; MDCT provides excellent multiplanar and 3D images of the aneurysm, its relationship with coronaries, aortic root, and cardiac chambers. This information is invaluable to the operating surgeon.

Magnetic resonance imaging also has advantages of CT; however, patient cooperation in holding their breath can limit the study in severely symptomatic or uncooperative patients.

In our case, the transthoracic echo only detected one larger aneurysm; even bicuspid aortic abnormality was not defined due to the imaging's limitations. A CT detector provided beautiful, clearer images to show all of the above information.

Our case had aortic stenosis, regurgitation, ascending aorta dilation and multiple aneurysms of an aortic root abscess. Surgical intervention was the best choice to prevent the dissection and rupture.

Key Points

1. Pseudo-aneurysm of aortic root abscesses is a complication of infective endocarditis. It should be kept in mind in patients who are suspected of an abscess in the region of the sinus of Valsalva.
2. Computed tomography angiography has the advantage of the simultaneous evaluation of aortic root aneurisms and their precise relationship of their surrounding structures.

References

1. Fedak, P.W., Verma, S., David, T.E. et al. (2002). Clinical and pathophysiological implications of a bicuspid aortic valve. *Circulation* 106 (8): 900–904.
2. Ward, C. (2000). Review. Clinical significance of the bicuspid aortic valve. *Heart* 83: 81–85.
3. Kahveci, G., Bayrak, F., Pala, S. et al. (2009). Impact of bicuspid aortic valve on complications and death in infective endocarditis of native aortic valves. *Tex Heart Inst J.* 36 (2): 111–116.
4. Feuchtner, G.M., Stolzmann, P., Dichtl, W. et al. (2009). Multislice computed tomography in infective endocarditis: comparison with transesophageal echocardiography and intraoperative findings. *J Am Coll Cardiol* 53: 436–444.
5. Gahide, G., Bommart, S., Demaria, R. et al. (2010). Preoperative evaluation in aortic endocarditis: Findings on cardiac CT. *Am J Roentgenol* 194: 574–578.

25 Coronary Artery Vasculitis in Patient with Systemic Lupus Erythematosus

Ligang Fang[1], Yining Wang[1], and Jing Ping Sun[2]

[1] Affiliated Hospital of Peking Union Medical College, Beijing, China
[2] The Chinese University of Hong Kong, Hong Kong

History

A 16-year-old female was admitted with systemic lupus erythematosus because of recurrent fever, chest tightness, and shortness of breath for 7 months.

Physical Examination

Blood pressure 145/88 mmHg, regular heart rate 62 bpm. Body temperature: 38 °C. There was a grade 3/4 diastolic murmur along the sternal left border. The patient had mild peripheral edema.

Biochemical Tests

Triglycerides (TG) 0.53 mmol/L, cholesterol (TC) 3.11 mmol/L, low-density lipoprotein cholesterol (LDL-C) 1.62 mmol/L, high density lipoprotein cholesterol (HDL-C) 1.28 mmol / L, high-sensitivity C-reactive protein 0.69 mg / L, fasting blood glucose 3.8 mmol / L, blood gas analysis: pH 7.428, PaO_2 92.3 mmHg, $PaCO_2$ 35.9 mmHg. N-terminal B type natriuretic peptide (NT-proBNP) 919 pg/ml. B-type natriuretic peptide (BNP) 84.5 pg/ml.

Endomyocardial Biopsy

There was a small amount of neutrophils as group infiltration in endocardial surface. The derangement of myocardial cells were noted with cardiomyocyte hypertrophy and interstitial hyperplasia. Special staining: Masson (+), PTAH (+), Congo red (−).

Electrocardiogram

Sinus rhythm, Q-wave presented with T-wave inversion in leads II, III, aVF, V6-V9 (Figure 25-1).

Coronary Intravascular Ultrasound

Coronary intima of left main, left anterior descending artery, left circumflex artery and right coronary artery was concentrically thickened, which was consistent with the change of vasculitis (Figure 25-2).

Comparative Cardiac Imaging: A Case-based Guide, First Edition.
Edited by Jing Ping Sun, Xing Sheng Yang, and Bryan P. Yan.
© 2018 John Wiley & Sons Ltd. Published 2018 by John Wiley & Sons Ltd.
Companion website: www.wiley.com/sun/comparative_cardiac_imaging

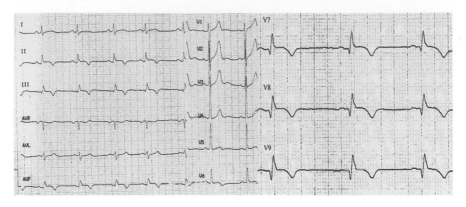

Figure 25-1   Electrocardiogram: sinus rhythm, Q-wave presented with T-wave inversion in leads II, III, aVF, V6-V9.

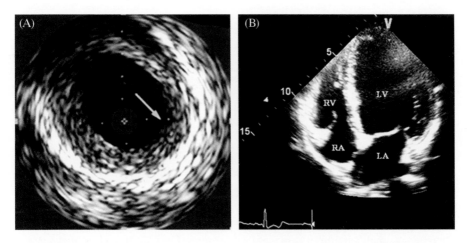

Figure 25-2   Coronary intravascular ultrasound imaging: A. Coronary artery intima were concentrically thickened, which was in line consistent with the change of vasculitis. B. Transthoracic echocardiography four chamber view showed that the left ventricle and atrium were enlarged.

Echocardiography

The left ventricle and atrium were enlarged (Figure 25-2). The end-diastolic LV internal diameter was 66 mm. The left ventricular systolic function was reduced, with ejection fraction 38%; the posterior wall, basal segment of inferior wall, and the middle and basal segments of post wall were thin and akinetic (Videos 25-1 to 25-4). The left ventricular diastolic dysfunction was in stage I. Moderate mitral, mild tricuspid, and aortic valvular regurgitation was detected.

Cardiac Magnetic Resonance Imaging (MRI)

The left ventricle and atrium were enlarged. The left ventricular systolic function was reduced, ejection fraction was 38%; the posterior wall, basal segment of inferior wall, the middle and basal segments of post wall were thin and akinetic. Moderate mitral, mild tricuspid and aortic valvular regurgitations were detected. The myocardial perfusion

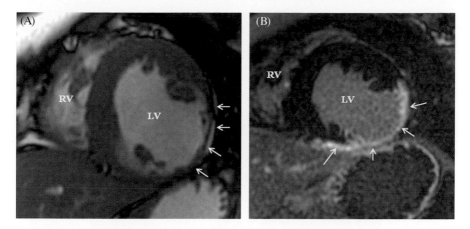

Figure 25-3   Cardiac magnetic resonance imaging (MRI). The ventricular short-axis view showed the myocardial perfusion was significantly reduced (arrows) in the lateral and inferior walls of left ventricle (A). Gadolinium-DTPA delayed-enhancement magnetic resonance imaging identified the left ventricular multiple abnormal enhancement, consistent with myocardial fibrosis (arrows) (B).

was significantly reduced in the lateral and inferior walls of the left ventricle (Figure 25-3A). Gadolinium-DTPA delayed-enhancement magnetic resonance imaging identified the left ventricular multiple abnormal enhancement consistent with myocardial fibrosis (Figure 25-3B).

Cardiac Tomography

The wall of all coronary arteries appeared diffusely thickened in various ways with mild calcification, which caused 30–40% stenosis in multiple segments (Figure 25-4). The distal segment of the left circumferential branch was totally occluded.

Discussion

Women with lupus in the 35 to 44 years age group were over 50 times more likely to have a myocardial infarction than those of similar age in the Framingham Offspring Study (rate ratio = 52.43, 95% confidence interval 21.6–98.5) [1]. The pathogenesis of cardiovascular disease in lupus is likely multifactorial because of an interaction between inflammation-induced and antiphospholipid antibody-related vascular injury/thrombosis from the underlying disease and traditional cardiovascular risk factors. Corticosteroid treatment and renal disease with secondary hypertension may accelerate atherosclerotic process in women with lupus.

The asymptomatic coronary-artery atherosclerosis, as detected by electron-beam CT, is more common in patients with lupus than in the general population. However, it is not associated with traditional coronary risk factors, lupus disease activity, or corticosteroid therapy.

Lupus should be added to the list of conditions that raise cardiovascular risk independent of conventional risk factors [2].

Patients with systemic lupus erythematosus (SLE) and those with arteritis are usually at the same age when the disease starts to develop, and there is clearly predominance of

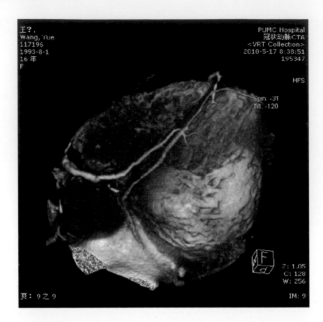

Figure 25-4   Computed tomography three-dimensional reconstruction imaging showing that all coronary arteries are thinner than normal.

females. Coronary vasculitis is rare [3]. However, Nagaoka et al. reported a case with SLE who had normal coronary artery when AMI occurred [4]. Fukai et al. reported that endothelial dysfunction and coronary vasospasm may play an important role in the pathogenesis of MI in patients without significant coronary stenosis [5]. Circulating immune mediators may give rise to perturbation in the endothelium-dependent vasodilation [6]. Such impairment is related to the reduction in vasodilator bioavailability, mainly nitric oxide [6].

The current case is a young girl with a history of myocardial infarction, which was well established by ECG, echocardiography and MRI. The coronary vasculitis was the definite cause of myocardial infarction, which was confirmed by endomyocardial biopsy and coronary intravascular ultrasound. The CT imaging indicated the patient had diffuse coronary vasculitis.

Key Points

1. Patients with SLE are at a high risk of cardiovascular events due to early subclinical atherosclerosis, endothelial dysfunction leading to coronary spasm or embolism, and coronary vasculitis.
2. Computed tomography is a good noninvasive technique to diagnose coronary diseases.

Reference

1. Manzi, S., Meilahn, E.N., Rairie, J.E. et al. (1997). Age-specific incidence rates of myocardial infarction and angina in women with systemic lupus erythematosus: comparison with the Framingham Study. *Am J Epidemiol* 145: 408–415.
2. Asanuma, Y., Oeser, A., Shintani, A.K. et al. (2003). Premature coronary-artery atherosclerosis in systemic lupus erythematosus. *N Engl J Med* 18 (25): 2407–2415.

3. Follansbee, W.P. (1992). The heart in vascuutis. In: *Systemic Vasculitis: The Biological Basis* (ed. E.C. LeRoy), 303–379. New York: Marcel Dekker, Inc.

4. Nagaoka, H., Funakoshi, N., Innami, R. et al. (1993). Left ventricular aneurysm, normal coronary arteries and embolization in a patient with systemic lupus erythematosus. *Chest* 103: 287–288.

5. Fukai, T., Koyanagi, S., Takeshita, A. et al. (1993). Role of coronary spasm in the pathogenesis of myocardial infarction: study in patients with no significant coronary stenosis. *Am Heart J* 126: 1305–1311.

6. Suwaidi, J.A., Hamasaki, S., Higano, S.T. et al. (2000). Long-term follow-up of patients with mild coronary artery disease and endothelial dysfunction. *Circulation* 101: 948–954.

26 Aortic Dissection

Jing Ping Sun and Xing Sheng Yang

The Chinese University of Hong Kong, Hong Kong

History

A 37-year-old male presented in the emergency room because of the sudden onset of severe chest pain radiating to the back. It was associated with diaphoresis. He has had hypertension for many years.

Physical examination

Blood pressure was 180/100 mmHg, pulse rate 102 bpm, respiration rate 30 breaths/min. He was conscious, and cooperative. Apex impulse was in normal location with presystolic and sustained. The peripheral pulses were normal bilaterally. All other physical findings were unremarkable.

The electrocardiogram showed QRS axis +2°, LVH. Chest X-ray revealed a widening in the aortic knob and the lateral margin of the ascending aorta.

Echocardiography

The LV displayed mildly concentric hypertrophy with normal size and systolic function (EF 55%). There was tricuspid valvular regurgitation with an estimated RV systolic pressure of 45 mmHg. The size and function of the RV were normal. The ascending aorta dilated to 4.2 cm; an aortic intramural hematoma is seen just above aortic valve (Figure 26-1). Supersternal notch long- and short-axis views with color Doppler showed linear echo densities within the lumen of the aortic arch parallel to the wall of the aorta compatible with an intimal flap (Figure 26-2B and C; Video 26-1 and Video 26-2), aortic dissection at beginning of descending aorta formed true and false lumens (Figure 26-2A, D, and F). The image of the abdomen aorta with the color Doppler showed true and false lumens with communications in between (Figure 26-3A).

Computed Tomography (CT)

Type A aortic intramural hematoma complicated with Type B aortic dissection. The intramural hematoma proximally to aortic root, maximum thickness was 13 mm. The aortic dissection was from beginning of descending aorta dawn to abdominal aorta and formed true and false lumens (Figure 26-2E, Figure 26-3, and Figure 26-4).

Comparative Cardiac Imaging: A Case-based Guide, First Edition.
Edited by Jing Ping Sun, Xing Sheng Yang, and Bryan P. Yan.
© 2018 John Wiley & Sons Ltd. Published 2018 by John Wiley & Sons Ltd.
Companion website: www.wiley.com/sun/comparative_cardiac_imaging

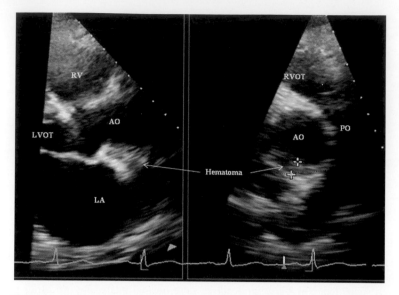

Figure 26-1   Parasternal long-axis view (left) and short-axis view (right) showed aortic intramural hematoma.

Discussion

An aortic dissection (dissecting aneurysm, dissecting hematoma) is a commonly fatal disorder in which the inner layer (lining) of the aortic wall tears because the artery's wall deteriorates. Most cases are associated with hypertension, which is present in more than two-thirds of patients who have an aortic dissection. Aortic dissection may be caused by hereditary connective-tissue disorders, especially Marfan syndrome and Ehlers–Danlos syndrome (a defect in collagen synthesis). Age-related structural changes of the aortic media, and "cystic medial necrosis," are also felt to contribute. Aortic dissections are also associated with defects of the heart and blood vessels, such as coarctation of the aorta, patent ductus arteriosus, and bicuspid aortic valves. Other causes include arteriosclerosis and injury [1]. Dissections may rarely be seen in younger women in the third trimester of pregnancy, and following cardiac surgery.

Conventional transthoracic echocardiography has limited diagnostic value in the evaluation of the thoracic aorta, particularly in its descending segment, because of a limited field of view but is most useful in ascending aortic dissections, especially within a few centimeters of the aortic valve; sensitivity is highest in this location [2]. The subcostal and suprasternal views may be particularly helpful. The apical five-chamber view may also provide usefulness in a very proximal dissection.

The sensitivity of transesophageal echocardiography for the diagnosis of acute aortic dissection is excellent; particularly for dissections that do not involve the very proximal aorta. False-positive results secondary to artificial images or extensive atherosclerotic plaque formation may occur.

Magnetic resonance imaging (MRI) has been demonstrated to be accurate for the diagnosis of aortic dissection. Advantages of this imaging modality include localization of the entry site, visualization of intra- and extraluminal thrombi and extension of dissection to the branch vessels, and the provision of additional data about the surrounding

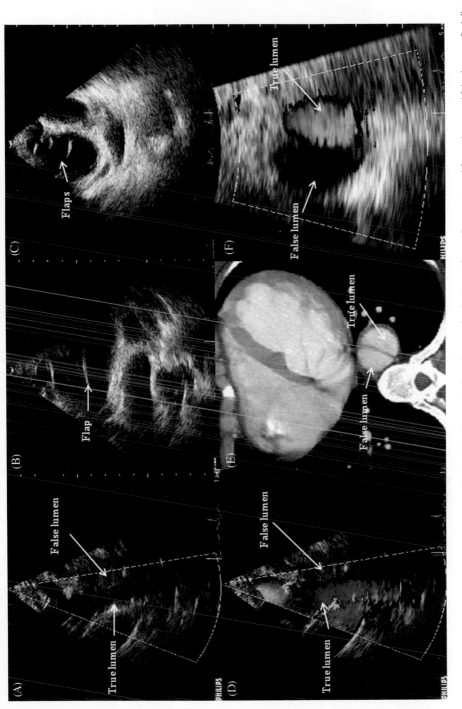

Figure 26-2 A. Supersternal notch aortic long-axis view showed that the aortic dissection was beginning at descending aorta, and formed true and false lumens. B. A flap was noted in the aortic arch. C. Supersternal notch short-axis view showed flaps in aortic arch. D. Long-axis views with color Doppler showed true and false lumens. Computed tomography imaging of descending aorta (E) and descending aorta short axis view by echocardiography (F) showed true and false lumens.

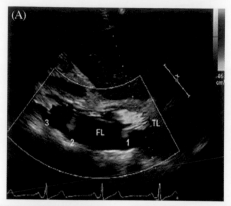

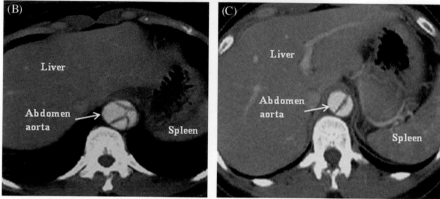

Figure 26-3 A. Echocardiographic abdominal aortic long-axis view with color Doppler showed three color flows from true lumen into false lumen. B and C. Computed tomograpy imaging showed the dissection of abdominal aorta with true and false lumina.

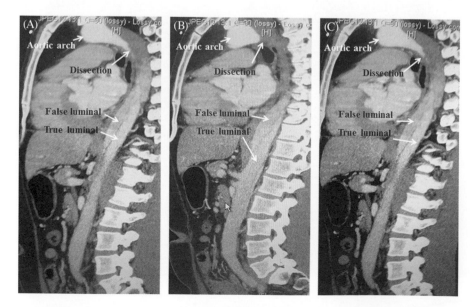

Figure 26-4 Computed tomography images (different phase) showed the aortic dissection from beginning of descending aorta dawn to abdominal aorta (A, B, and C).

mediastinal structures [3]. However, MRI is less sensitive than TEE for diagnosing the presence of aortic regurgitation, and is time-consuming to perform in unstable patients. Magnetic resonance imaging should be used in hemodynamically stable patients and TEE in unstable patients. Chest CT is less reliable than both TEE and MRI for the diagnosis.

Spiral CT can be used to create three dimensional reconstructions of excellent quality, and these reconstructions proved useful for visualization of the course of the dissection membrane in the aortic arch relative to the origin of the left subclavian artery in type B dissection. This information is especially important for the exclusion of retrograde dissection into the aortic arch, which was recently shown to occur in 27% of type B dissections, and is associated with substantially higher mortality rates of up to 43% [4]. In patients with retrograde dissection of the aortic arch, early surgery is recommended by some authors [4]. Spiral CT is fast and easy to perform and is probably the least operator-dependent imaging modality of the three studies. However, spiral CT requires intravenous administration of contrast medium, which may be a limiting factor in patients with severe cardiac failure and impaired renal function, or intolerance for contrast medium. Another important limitation of spiral CT is its inability to provide information about aortic regurgitation. Spiral CT and MR imaging do allow better comparison of follow-up studies because they provide measurements in well-defined planes.

The main disadvantages of MR imaging are its long examination time (compared with that of spiral CT and TEE), limited access to the patient, and impaired monitoring of vital signs. Furthermore, patients with cardiac pacemakers, ferromagnetic aneurysmatic or haemostatic clips, and ocular or topologic implants cannot undergo MR imaging. The main limitations of multiplane TEE are the strong dependence on the investigator's experience and the difficulty in objectively documenting pathologic findings for follow-up studies. The field of view is limited to the thoracic and proximal abdominal aorta; distal extension of aortic dissection below the celiac trunk cannot be visualized. Furthermore, TEE cannot be performed in patients with esophageal varicosis or stenosis. The main advantages of TEE are that it is widely available and can be performed quickly and easily at the bedside, which makes it ideal for use in patients with unstable conditions.

In one study [5], 49 symptomatic patients with clinically suspected aortic dissection were examined with contrast material-enhanced spiral CT, multiplanar TEE, and 0.5-T MR imaging. Imaging results were confirmed at autopsy. Sensitivity in the detection of thoracic aortic dissection was 100% for all techniques. Specificity was 100%, 94%, and 94% for spiral CT, multiplanar TEE, and MR imaging, respectively. In the assessment of aortic arch vessel involvement, sensitivity was 93%, 60%, and 67%, respectively, and specificity was 97%, 85%, and 88%, respectively.

The authors concluded that spiral CT and multiplanar TEE are as valuable as MR imaging in the detection of thoracic aortic dissection. In the assessment of the supraaortic branches, spiral CT is superior.

The key points of echocardiographic phenomenon in the diagnosis of aortic dissection are: (i) The presence of two vascular lumens separated by an undulating intimal flap; (ii) thrombus in the false lumen is consistent with the inability to detect blood flow in the false lumen of the aortic arch with color-Doppler imaging; (iii) the entry site of the dissection is commonly defined as a tear of the dissected membrane with blood flow demonstrated by color-Doppler imaging between the two aortic lumina; (iv) the direction of blood flow across the entry tear of the aortic dissection follows the pressure gradient between the false and true lumina.

The Stanford classification is the simplest of the various aortic dissection classification systems. It divides aortic dissections into two types, type A and B. Type A dissections involve the ascending aorta; the tear occurs in the proximal ascending aorta and can extend into descending thoracic aorta, or is confined to the ascending aorta. Type B originates in the descending aorta distal to the left subclavian artery and extends mostly above the diaphragm; occasionally, they may track into abdominal aorta or back into the ascending aorta [6].

A dissecting aneurysm is an acute hemorrhage into the media of the aorta, usually associated with an intimal tear. The clinical features emerge as the hematoma dissects along the plane of the media proximally and distally in the aorta. Cystic medial necrosis of the aorta sets the stage for this acute event. The pain of aortic dissection is very characteristic. It is tearing, most severe at its inception, is unremitting, and can migrate as the dissection propagates. The mechanisms producing pain in aortic dissection include dilation and stretch of the aorta or extravasation of blood into surrounding tissue.

A penetrating aortic ulcer is defined as a deep ulcerated lesion in the thickest part of the intramural hematoma (IMH) within the involved aorta. Erosion of the internal elastic membrane that lies beneath an inflammatory atherosclerotic plaque may allow luminal blood to burrow into the aortic media and thus lead to the formation of a penetrating aortic ulcer. These lesions occur most commonly in the descending thoracic aorta, usually in elderly patients with hypertension and atherosclerosis. They may stabilize with conservative therapy or progress to form a saccular aneurysm, pseudo aneurysm, dissection, or frank rupture.

In patients with an aortic dissection a vasodilator such as nitroprusside plus a beta-blocker, are given intravenously as soon as possible to reduce the heart rate and blood pressure to the lowest level that can maintain a sufficient blood supply to the brain, heart, and kidneys. The lower heart rate and blood pressure help limit the spread of the dissection. In acute type A dissections, immediate surgery is generally recommended. unless comorbidities preclude operative intervention. Type B dissections are most often treated with medical therapy but stent grafting or surgery may be recommended depending on the clinical circumstance [7].

Key Points

1. Dissection should be suspected if a patient has simultaneous pain in more than one location – for example, chest and back, or chest and abdomen – and it reaches maximal intensity immediately.
2. Aortic regurgitation and pericardial effusion +/– tamponade are sequelae.
3. If the patient is under age 40, consider Marfan syndrome or pregnancy likely contributors.
4. TEE is the diagnostic test of choice, especially if the patient is unstable; spiral CT is superior in the assessment of the supra-aortic branches.
5. Prognostic classification: proximal (type A) – ascending aorta involved best treated surgically; distal to the left subclavian (type B) – initially treated medically.

References

1. Goldman, L. and Ausiello, D.C. (2004). *Textbook of Medicine*, 22nd edn. Philadelphia, PA: WB Saunders Co.
2. Erbel, R., Engberding, R., Daniel, W. et al. (1989). Echocardiography in diagnosis of aortic dissection. *Lancet* 1: 457–461.
3. Tatli, S., Yucel, E.K. and Lipton, M.J. (2004). CT and MR imaging of the thoracic aorta: Current techniques and clinical applications. *Radiol Clin North Am* 42: 565–585.
4. Erbel, R., Oelert, H., Meyer, J. et al. (1993). Effect of medical and surgical therapy on aortic dissection evaluated by transesophageal echocardiography. *Circulation* 87: 1604–1615.
5. Sommer, T., Fehske, W., Holzknecht, N. et al. (1996). Aortic dissection: A comparative study of diagnosis with spiral CT, multiplanar transesophageal echocardiography, and MR imaging. *Radiology* 199 (2): 347–352.
6. Chen, K., Varon, J., Wenker, O.C. et al. (1997). Acute thoracic aortic dissection: The basics. *J Emerg Med* 15: 859–867.
7. Verhoye, J.P., Miller, D.C., Sze, D. et al. (2008). Complicated acute type B aortic dissection: Midterm results of emergency endovascular stent-grafting. *J Thorac Cardiovasc Surg* 136: 424–430.

27 Large Thrombus in Giant Unruptured Noncoronary Sinus of Valsalva Aneurysm

Weihua Wu[1] and Jing Ping Sun[2]

[1] Jiaotong University, Shanghai, China
[2] The Chinese University of Hong Kong, Hong Kong

History

A 52-year-old male presented with dyspnea on exertion (NYHA class II) for 3 years.

Physical Examination

An examination revealed normal systolic and diastolic blood pressures and a grade 3/6 diastolic murmur on the left side of the sternum.

Echocardiography

From the transthoracic echocardiogram, the parasternal long-axis with and without color Doppler showed mild aortic regurgitation and a giant cystic mass significantly pressed the left atria. The left ventricular inflow tract was almost obstructed by cystic mass, resulting in high velocity inflow through the mitral valve. A two-dimensional atypical apical four-chamber view showed a cystic mass (with spontaneous contrast and a big thrombus) compressing the right and left atria. The mass blocked both ventricle inflow tracts. A three-dimensional apical five-chamber view showed the cystic mass compressing right and left atria blocking mitral inflow tract (Figure 27-1, Videos 27-1 to 27-4). A two-dimensional apical four-chamber with color Doppler view showed the giant cystic mass was in position between the right and left atria, the velocity of tricuspid inflow was high with color Doppler (Figure 27-2A). With the transesophageal echocardiography (TEE), the long-axis view showed that the left atrium was significantly compressed by the aneurysm and the mitral inflow tract was blocked by the aneurysm (Figure 27-2B, Video 27-5).

An angiogram showed that the patient had normal coronary arteries. The patient was referred for surgical repair of the lesion. The surgeon found an unruptured giant Valsalva aneurysm of the noncoronary sinus with a large thrombus within the aneurysm, and repaired the Valsalva wall of the noncoronary sinus with the

Comparative Cardiac Imaging: A Case-based Guide, First Edition.
Edited by Jing Ping Sun, Xing Sheng Yang, and Bryan P. Yan.
© 2018 John Wiley & Sons Ltd. Published 2018 by John Wiley & Sons Ltd.
Companion website: www.wiley.com/sun/comparative_cardiac_imaging

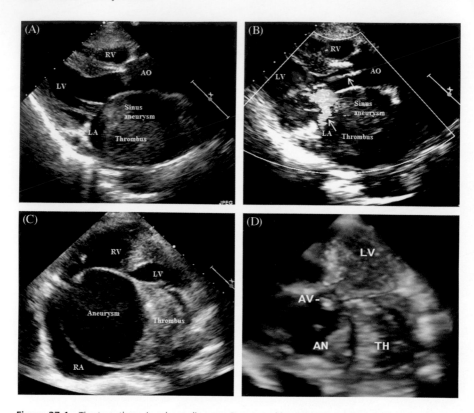

Figure 27-1 The transthoracic echocardiogram. Parasternal long axis view without (A) and with color Doppler (B) showed mild aortic regurgitation (arrow) and a giant cystic mass significantly pressed the left atria: the left ventricular inflow tract was almost obstructed by cystic mass resulting in high velocity inflow of the mitral valve. A two-dimensional atypical apical four-chamber view (C) showed a cystic mass (with spontaneous contrast and a big thrombus) compressing the right and left atria. The mass blocked both ventricle inflow tracts. A three-dimensional apical five-chamber view (D) showed the cystic mass compressing the right and left atria blocking mitral inflow tract.

pericardium. After operation, the TEE longitudinal view showed the mitral inflow tract and mitral valve were normal with a normal laminar flow (Figure 27-2C and D, Video 27-6).

The patient recovered well without any complications.

Discussion

Sinus of Valsalva aneurysm (SVA) is a rare cardiac abnormality occurring in 0.09–0.15% of cases with cardiac anomalies [1]. It can be either congenital or acquired. Congenital SVAs are usually encountered in young patients and may be associated with other congenital heart diseases such as a ventricular septal defect, coarctation of aorta, or bicuspid aortic valve [2]. Congenital aneurysm may result from localized weakness of the elastic lamina or an underlying deficiency of normal elastic tissue, with lack of continuity between the aortic media and the aortic annulus, leading to weakening and subsequent aneurysm formation. Sinus of Valsalva aneurysm can sometimes be associated with

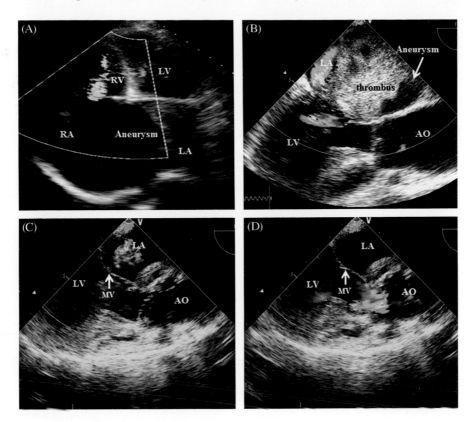

Figure 27-2 A, A two-dimensional apical four-chamber view with color Doppler showed the giant cystic mass was in position between the right and left atria, the velocity of tricuspid inflow was high by color Doppler. B. With the transesophageal echocardiography (TEF), the long-axis view showed that the left atrium was significantly compressed by the aneurysm and the mitral inflow tract was blocked by the aneurysm. C and D. After operation, the TEE longitudinal view showed the mitral inflow tract and mitral valve were normal with a normal laminar flow.

congenital diseases like Marfan's syndrome, Ehlers–Danlos syndrome, or Loeys–Dietz syndrome [3]. Acquired SVAs are more common in middle-aged and old patients, and are caused by infectious diseases like bacterial endocarditis and syphilis, or degenerative conditions like atherosclerosis and cystic medial necrosis or aortic root injury from deceleration chest trauma [3, 4].

The right coronary sinus is the most commonly involved, followed by the noncoronary sinus [4]. The characteristic diagnostic features of SVA include aneurysmal sac originating above the aortic annulus, the saccular shape of the aneurysm, and the normal diameter of the aortic root and ascending aorta [3].

A sinus of Valsalva aneurysm is most commonly diagnosed after rupture, frequently resulting in an aorto-cardiac shunt to the right ventricle. A ruptured aneurysm most commonly originates from the right coronary sinus (70%), followed by the noncoronary sinus (28%) [5, 6]. An unruptured sinus of Valsalva aneurysm usually remains clinically silent. They are rarely discovered unless they compress adjacent cardiac structures [7]. A large unruptured right coronary sinus aneurysms of Valsalva may compress the RVOT and cause obstruction. When this happens, patients may present with symptoms of right heart failure [8, 9]. In the present case, his progressive dyspnea was most likely caused by coexisting compression of the right and left atrium obstructing left and right inflow tracts, which can be seen by echocardiography imaging.

Several case reports have described other complications related to an unruptured aneurysm, including malignant arrhythmia, myocardial ischemia, and right ventricular tract obstruction [7]. Sinus of Valsalva aneurysms are commonly detected initially by two-dimensional Doppler echocardiography.

These cases are mostly seen in middle-aged or elderly patients. Sinus of Valsalva aneurysms can also rupture and result in an aorto-cardiac shunt that manifests as acute congestive heart failure [4]. Thus, it is important to make an accurate diagnosis in time.

In most cases, cross-sectional imaging modalities like CT or magnetic resonance (MR) imaging are performed to confirm the findings found on echocardiography. In recent years, CT has increasingly been used to evaluate suspected cases of SVAs, especially in the emergency care settings. High spatial resolution, faster scanning and three-dimensional reconstruction have made CT the preferred imaging modality to evaluate SVAs. The anatomic structures of the aneurysm and relation between the surrounding cardiac structures and SVA can be presented by CT excellent imaging. Computed tomography can also be used to identify suspected cases of ruptured aneurysm, which appear as a jet of contrast extending from the aneurysm to the cardiac chamber, thereby delineating any aorto-cardiac fistula [4].

Magnetic resonance imaging can also be used to assess the origin of the aneurysm and define its relationship with adjacent mediastinal structures. They have an added advantage of evaluating the hemodynamic pattern of the left ventricle, identifying any concomitant aortic regurgitation, and quantifying the amount of blood shunting across an aorto-cardiac fistula in cases of ruptured aneurysm. However, increased scan duration and cost are the limitations in MRI evaluation of suspected SVAs.

The optimal treatment of a sinus of Valsalva aneurysm has been debated, but most surgeons favor early treatment of symptomatic or large unruptured aneurysms. Operative approaches include simple plication for small aneurysm, a patch repair, aortic valve annuloplasty, or aortic root placement. The main surgical therapy is cardiopulmonary bypass surgery with closure of aneurysmal sac and repair of the defect as in our case. Percutaneous transcatheter closure can also be used for treating SVAs. In asymptomatic patients, if the aneurysmal sac is small, surgery can be deferred, but patients should receive regular follow ups; however, large aneurysms should undergo surgical repair to avoid complications.

Key Points

1. Patients with SVAs are usually asymptomatic but their aneurysms can rupture or become large enough to compress cardiac chambers.
2. The clinical presentation of patients with SVA varies from incidentally discovered cardiac murmurs to chest pain, progressive heart failure, and sudden cardiac arrest.
3. Echocardiography is the first choice to diagnose and follow up patients with SVAs; contrast-enhanced CT images can provide excellent anatomic description and prompt diagnosis, it is another important diagnosis tool.
4. Surgical repair is the mainstay of treatment with excellent prognosis. Therefore, prompt diagnosis and rapid repair are most important for patients.

References

1. Galicia-Tornell, M.M., Marin-Solis, B., Mercado-Astorga, O. et al. (2009). Sinus of Valsalva aneurysm with rupture. Case report and literature review. *Cir Cir* 77: 441–445.
2. Carita, P., Dendramis, G., Novo, G. et al. (2015). Bicuspid aortic valve and unruptured sinus of Valsalva aneurysm, a rare association. *Int J Cardiol* 202: 103–105.
3. Liu, F., Zhu, Z., Ren, J. et al. (2014). A rare case of sudden dyspnea and unexpected death in adolescence: Fistula from aortic sinus of Valsalva to right atrium. *Int J Clin Exp Med* 7: 2945–2947.
4. Bricker, A.O., Avutu, B., Mohammed, T.L. et al. (2010). Valsalva sinus aneurysms: Findings at CT and MR imaging. *Radiographics* 30: 99–110.
5. Takach, T.J., Reul, G.J., Duncan, J.M. et al. (1999). Sinus of Valsalva aneurysm or fistula: Management and outcome. Ann Thorac Surg 68: 1573–1577.
6. Barragry, T.P., Ring, W.S., Moller, J.H. et al. (1988). 15- to 30-year follow-up of patients undergoing repair of ruptured congenital aneurysms of the sinus of Valsalva. *Ann Thorac Surg* 46: 515–519.
7. Thankachen, R., Gnanamuthu, R., Doshi, H. et al. (2003). Unruptured aneurysm of the sinus of Valsalva presenting with right ventricular outflow obstruction. *Tex Heart Inst J* 30: 152–154.
8. Pastor, A., Reya, M. and Farré, J. (2011). Sinus of Valsalva aneurysm. *Rev Esp Cardiol* 64: 150.
9. Le, D.D., Orrego, C.M., Maragiannis, D. et al. (2014). An unusual case of right- sided heart failure caused by giant sinus of Valsalva aneurysm obstructing right ventricular outflow tract. *Eur Heart J* 35: 2721.

28 Isolated Pulmonary Vasculitis

Hongmei Xia[1], Yuanqing Cai[1], and Jing Ping Sun[2]

[1] Third Military Medical University, Chongqing, China
[2] The Chinese University of Hong Kong, Hong Kong

History

A 41-year-old female presented with a cough and heart murmur for half month. She had hyperthyroidism, which was well controlled.

Laboratory

Tests revealed that the function of the kidney and liver, electrolytes, and general urine were normal. The erythrocyte sedimentation rate (ESR, 32 mm/1 h, normal value < 20 mm/1 h) and C-reactive protein (CRP, 35 mg/l, normal range 0–20 mg/L) were high; hemoglobin (Hb, 122 g/L, normal value 110–160 g/l), leukocytosis (white blood cells 8.8×10^9/l, normal value $4.8–10.8 \times 10^9$/l), and thrombocytosis (299×10^9/l, normal value $100–300 \times 10^9$/l) were normal. Initial blood tests showed troponin I at 0.44 ng/mL (normal value 0–0.16 ng/mL), B-type natriuretic peptide of 1630 pg/mL (normal value 0–400 pg/mL), and creatine kinase of 6.6 ng/mL (normal value 0–4.0 ng/mL) were elevated. Immunology testing revealed negative antinuclear antibody lineage.

Chest X-ray

A chest X-ray demonstrated clear lung fields but an enlarged heart.

Electrocardiogram

An electrocardiogram showed sinus tachycardia, right axis, and signs of right atrium and right ventricle overload.

Transthoracic Echocardiography (TTE)

An apical four-chamber view with color Doppler demonstrated a giant right atrium (56 mm) and right ventricle (57 mm) with moderate to severe tricuspid regurgitation. The left ventricular (LV) size (42 mm) and systolic function (EF = 70 %) were normal (Figure 28-1A and Video 28-1). The parasternal short axis view showed the intimal of distal pulmonary artery (PA) and branches was significant thickened (Figure 28-1B). The parasternal short axis view with color Doppler flow showed turbulence color signal in the left pulmonary artery (LPA) and no flow signals within the right pulmonary artery (Figure 28-1C, and Video 28-2), The systolic pulmonary artery pressure estimated by tricuspid valve regurgitation was 95 mmHg.

Comparative Cardiac Imaging: A Case-based Guide, First Edition.
Edited by Jing Ping Sun, Xing Sheng Yang, and Bryan P. Yan.
© 2018 John Wiley & Sons Ltd. Published 2018 by John Wiley & Sons Ltd.
Companion website: www.wiley.com/sun/comparative_cardiac_imaging

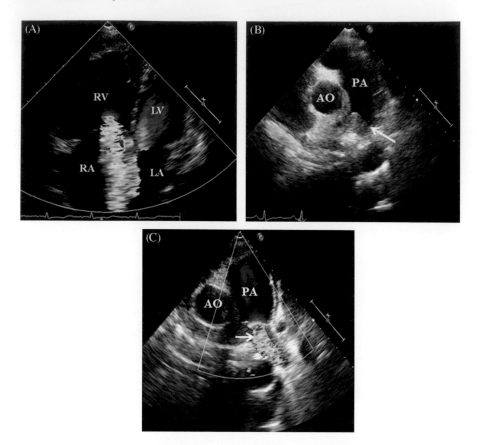

Figure 28-1 Transthoracic echocardiography. A. Transthoracic echocardiographic four-chamber view with color Doppler showed marked enlarged right atrium and ventricle with moderate to severe tricuspid regurgitation. B. Parasternal short-axis view showed significant thickening of the intimal in left and right pulmonary arteries (arrow). C. Parasternal short-axis view with color Doppler showed turbulence color signal in the left pulmonary artery (arrow) and no flow signals within the right pulmonary artery.
Notes: LA, left atrium; LV, left ventricle; RA, right atrium; RV, right ventricle; AO, aorta.

Computed Tomography

Pulmonary artery and venous angiography by 64-slice spiral computed tomography (CT) was performed. Cine imaging demonstrated right pulmonary artery occlusion and severe left PA stenosis (Figure 28-2A and D).

Exploratory surgery of pulmonary artery was performed. Intraoperative findings indicated that the right PA wall was significant thickened and solid leading to luminal obliteration, and the left PA displayed stenosis, although there were no obvious abnormalities in pulmonary veins.

Pathology

The pulmonary artery wall histological examination was performed. Microscopic examination of the tissue biopsies showed granulomatous inflammation in the endometrial tissue of the PA, with a large number of plasma cells and fiber necrosis. Immunohistochemistry staining of the tissue showed polyclonal plasma cells and

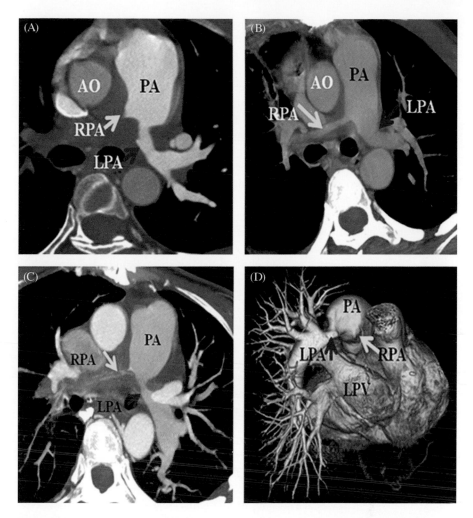

Figure 28-2 Computed tomographic pulmonary angiography and volume reconstruction images. A. Short-axis view showed the occluded right main pulmonary artery (yellow arrow) and left main pulmonary artery stenosis (red arrow). B. Short-axis view showed the right main pulmonary artery was opened with severe stenosis (yellow arrow) and left main pulmonary artery stenosis was improved (red arrow) after therapy. C. Same view showed right and left pulmonary stenosis become more severe after 2 years. D. Computed tomography reconstruction image showed left pulmonary artery stenosis (red arrow) and the occluded right main pulmonary artery (yellow arrow) at first admission.
Notes: AO, aortic; PA, pulmonary artery; LPA, left pulmonary artery; RPA, right pulmonary artery; LPV, left pulmonary vein.

lymphocyte infiltration, which was consistent with lymphomatosis, and granulomatosis. No immunoglobulin deposits were seen.

Hospital Course

The clinical and cardiac imaging findings suggested pulmonary vasculitis causing left pulmonary stenosis and right pulmonary occlusion, and this was confirmed by the histopathology. The patient was treated by the intravenous corticosteroids (20 mg of prednisone every 24 hours for 3 consecutive days) followed by prednisone 20 mg/day and low-dose aspirin. Two weeks later, her clinical symptoms were significantly improved; meanwhile, echocardiography examination showed that the pulmonary artery pressure estimated by the velocity of tricuspid regurgitation was significantly decreased (from 95 to 68 mmHg). Six weeks later, echocardiography confirmed normal size RA (35.9 mm) and RV (35.5 mm). Estimated pulmonary systolic artery pressure was 45 mmHg. The CT Cine imaging demonstrated that the right pulmonary artery was reopened with blood filling and left pulmonary artery stenosis improving (Figure 28-2B).

The clinical course of our patient confirmed the benign reactive nature of the plasma cell granuloma after treatment.

Two years later, patient experienced cough and short of breath. She was continuing to take prednisone 5 mg/day. Echocardiographic images displayed that there was severe tricuspid regurgitation and estimated systolic pulmonary artery pressure was 140 mmHg; RA and RV were significantly enlarged with dysfunction; right pulmonary artery was almost occluded and left PA stenosis was more severe, which was confirmed by CT scan (Figure 28-1C). The clinical condition of the patient was significantly declining, which might be because the dosage of prednisone was not enough to control the immunity inflammation. The patient was discharged because her family refused any further intervention.

Discussion

Vasculitis constitutes a group of heterogeneous conditions characterized by blood vessel inflammation and necrosis, leading to subsequent tissue or organ injury [1]. They are usually systemic diseases affecting multiple territories or organs with overlapping clinical and pathologic manifestations. However, there are cases in which inflammation is restricted to a single organ [2]. Isolated pulmonary vasculitis is very rare; only a few cases, mostly affecting large pulmonary vessels, have been described [3].

Although in some of these cases pulmonary vasculitis may be asymptomatic, pulmonary hypertension is a common symptom at presentation that may lead to a false-positive diagnosis of chronic thromboembolic disease [4]. When suspected, pulmonary angiogram, magnetic resonance imaging, or PET scans are useful diagnostic tools, typically showing wall thickening, narrowing, or stenosis of large vessels in these patients with isolated large-vessel pulmonary vasculitis.

In this report, we described a patient with localized pulmonary vasculitis affecting medium-sized vessels that presented as pulmonary arterial hypertension. The clinical conditions of our patient were significantly improved by treatment with intravenous corticosteroids, but did not maintain. This case is a good example of localized pulmonary vasculitis involving medium-sized vessels. Although conditions such as Behçet's syndrome or polyarteritis may share similarities with this case, our patient had no history of oral or genital ulcers, cutaneous lesions, or uveitis that are typical of Behçet's syndrome. In addition, apart from the vasculitic pulmonary involvement, there was no evidence of the involvement of other organs that is typical of cases with polyarteritis.

The nonspecific nature of the presenting symptoms, the relatively low rate of systemic symptoms and physical signs, and the variety in the pace of disease progression often resulted in delayed diagnosis of isolated pulmonary vasculitis. Early diagnosis of isolated pulmonary vasculitis is crucial as it allows early aggressive treatment, which predicts a better response and prevents irreversible stenotic and fibrotic vascular changes.

Patients with pulmonary artery hypertension due to pulmonary vasculitis had a poor prognosis and higher rates of death. Echocardiography is a useful noninvasive tool for estimating pulmonary artery systolic pressure using tricuspid regurgitation jet flow. In this case, the occlusion of the right PA and stenosis of the left PA was detected by echocardiography with careful inspection, and CT images provided more information in detail.

Key Points

1. Although the diagnosis of pulmonary vasculitis remains challenging, the identification and diagnosis of pulmonary vasculitis is critical to the care of these patients.
2. Cardiac imaging, including echocardiography and CT, is very helpful in diagnosis.
3. Effective pharmacologic therapies combined with a comprehensive, multidisciplinary approach to care for these patients may relieve the symptoms.

References

1. Atisha-Fregoso, Y., Hinojosa-Azaola, A. and Alcocer-Varela, J. (2013). Localized, single-organ vasculitis: clinical presentation and management. *Clin Rheumatol* 32 (1): 1–6.
2. Riancho-Zarrabeitia, L., Zurbano, F., Gómez-Román, J. et al. (2015). Isolated pulmonary vasculitis: case report and literature review. *Semin Arthritis Rheum* 44 (5): 514–517.
3. Hernandez-Rodriguez, J. and Hoffman, G.S. (2012). Updating single-organ vasculitis. *Curr Opin Rheumatol* 24: 38–45.
4. Hagan, G., Gopalan, D., Church, C. et al. (2011). Isolated large vessel pulmonary vasculitis as a cause of chronic obstruction of the pulmonary arteries. *Pulm Circ* 1: 425–429.

29 Giant Left Ventricular Pseudoaneurysm

Liu Chen[1], Hong Tang[1], Yuan Feng[1], and Jing Ping Sun[2]

[1] West China Hospital of Sichuan University, Chengdu, China
[2] The Chinese University of Hong Kong, Hong Kong

History

An 18-year-old male presented with fever and shortness of breath for 10 days.

Physical Examination

Body temperature was 37.5 °C. Heart rate was 120 bpm, regular. Respiration rate was 26 breaths per minute. Blood pressure was 103/62 mmHg. Bilateral jugular veins are normal. Apical impulse was downward with leftward displacement. The heart sound was distant. No murmur was noted.

Transthoracic Two- and Three-dimensional Echocardiography

The basal segment of left ventricular lateral-posterior wall ruptured and formed a large pseudoaneurysm (8×6 cm). The communication between pseudoaneurysm and left ventricular chamber was confirmed by color Doppler (Figure 29-1, Video 29-1). Three-dimensional echocardiography displayed the orifice of the ruptured left ventricular wall (Figure 29-1).

Computed Tomography

The coronal plane of the three-dimensional reconstruction cardiac CT showed that the basal segment of the left ventricular lateral-posterior wall had ruptured and formed a large pseudoaneurysm (Figure 29-2A). The front view indicates the pseudoaneurysm (8.7×7.8 cm) located beside left ventricular posterior-inferior wall (Figure 29-2B). Enhanced scanning confirmed blood filled the pseudoaneurysm.

Hospital Course

The patient was admitted into the local hospital and large pericardial effusion was detected; pericardicentesis was performed. The effusion was bloody exudates. An external drainage catheter was placed in his pericardial cavity. The patient denied any history of cardiovascular disease and chest trauma.

The patient underwent emergency surgery. Operative findings demonstrated that the pericardial wall was apparently thick, swelling, and with large amount of necrotic tissues

Comparative Cardiac Imaging: A Case-based Guide, First Edition.
Edited by Jing Ping Sun, Xing Sheng Yang, and Bryan P. Yan.
© 2018 John Wiley & Sons Ltd. Published 2018 by John Wiley & Sons Ltd.
Companion website: www.wiley.com/sun/comparative_cardiac_imaging

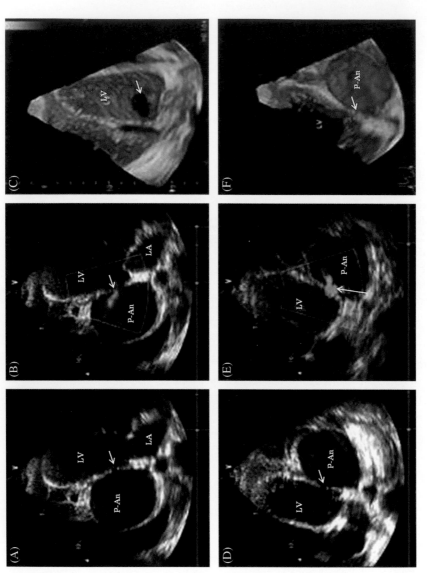

Figure 29-1 Transthoracic two- and three-dimensional echocardiography: A. Apical three-chamber view reveals the rupture (arrow) of LV lateral-posterior wall. B. Apical three-chamber view with color Doppler shows the shunt entering the pseudoaneurysm. C. Three-dimensional echocardiography displays the orifice of rupture (arrow). D. Apical four-chamber view shows the rupture hole and the pseudoaneurysm. E. Apical four-chamber view with color Doppler indicates the shunt from LV into pseudoaneurysm. F. Three-dimensional echocardiography illustrates the orifice of rupture (arrow).

Notes: RV, right ventricle; LV, left ventricle; RA, right atria; LA, left atria; P-An, pseudoaneurysm.

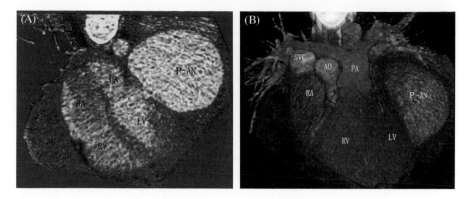

Figure 29-2 Computed tomography image: A. The coronal plane of three-dimensional reconstruction cardiac CT shows the basal segment of left ventricular lateral-posterior wall has ruptured and a large pseudoaneurysm has formed. B. The front view indicates the pseudoaneurysm (8.7 × 7.8 cm) located beside the left ventricular posterior-inferior wall.
Notes: RV, right ventricle; LV, left ventricle, RA, right atria; LA, left atria; P-AN, pseudo aneurysm; SVC, superior vena cava; AO, aorta; PA, pulmonary artery.

and organized thrombus. The lateral-posterior wall of left ventricle ruptured and connected with a giant pseudoaneurysm, the ruptured orifice was irregular, about 8 mm in diameter. The pseudoaneurysm was about 60 × 90 mm in size, with thick wall and exudates on the surface.

Discussion

According to previous study, myocardial infarction accounted for the etiology of most LV pseudoaneurysms followed by cardiac surgery, trauma, and infection.

In contrast to LV pseudoaneurysms, only about 4% of true LV aneurysms are located at the posterolateral or diaphragmatic surface [1]. One proposed explanation for the relative lack of anterior LV pseudoaneurysms is that anterior rupture may be more likely to result in hemopericardium and death than posterior rupture [2]. Because hospitalized patients usually are in the recumbent position, an inflammatory reaction of the posterior pericardium may result in pericardial adhesions and the formation of a posterior LV pseudoaneurysm rather than cardiac tamponade. Our case denied any history of cardiovascular operation or chest trauma. He has underwent pericardicentesis with drainage catheter and fever for ten days. The infection may be more likely to be the cause of a posterior LV pseudoaneurysm.

Left ventriculography may demonstrate the communication between the left ventricular cavity and the pseudoaneurysm. Because the angiography is invasive and more costly, transthoracic echocardiography is a reasonable first test. It has become the usual method for diagnosing this complication, as it may assess the exact diagnosis, anatomical relations and size [1–4]. At echocardiography, postacute myocardial infarction pseudoaneurysm may appear similar to an aneurysm, the identification of a narrow neck being crucial for a correct diagnosis. In other patients, the pseudoaneurysm may appear as an extracardiac echo-free space, and the demonstration of blood flow from left ventricular cavity to the "extracardiac" mass, apart from the proximity to an akinetic myocardial wall, plays a key role in the diagnosis in these cases. Color Doppler may be of great value in the detection of this flow [4]. Color Doppler is able to detect the blood flow in and out of the cavity. After the blood flow is detected, the subsequent use of pulsed Doppler may show a consistent "to and from" flow pattern across the myocardial defect with the characteristic. However, echocardiography may have some limitations in some cases, such as a suboptimal acoustic window and a poor visualization of the neck of the pseudoaneurysm, especially in the inferior location.

Magnetic resonance imaging (MRI) was first reported to diagnose LV pseudoaneurysm after myocardial infarction in 1991 [5]. Loss of epicardial fat at the orifice of the pseudoaneurysm is seen on MRI [6], but distinction from true aneurysms with low signal myocardium resulting from a previous infarction may be difficult [7]. Cine MRI may provide additional diagnostic capability by evaluating blood flow turbulence in the cardiac chambers, one of the hemodynamic features of the pseudoaneurysm [8].

Multidetector computed tomography (MDCT) technology with its improved spatial, contrast and temporal resolutions enables noninvasive coronary angiography as well as acquisition of accurate anatomical and functional information concerning heart chambers, myocardium and pericardium [9–12]. As demonstrated, ECG-gated MDCT was able to disclose the focal myocardial disruption, as well as to delineate the small intramural lumen and tiny neck of the left ventricular pseudoaneurysm. This is in contrast to contrast ventriculography, which demonstrated the pseudoaneurysm lumen but was unable to differentiate between left ventricular pseudoaneurysm with myocardial disruption and left ventricular diverticulum with myocardial continuity. The ECG-gated MDCT enabled not only comprehensive anatomical imaging of the coronary arteries, heart chambers and pericardium, but also offered valuable dynamic information regarding myocardial function and integrity as well. Dynamic cine evaluation demonstrated the pulsating nature of the left ventricular pseudoaneurysm, with lumen collapse during systole and expansion during diastole. Such behavior results from temporary occlusion of the pseudoaneurysm's narrow neck during systole. This is in contrast to pseudoaneurysms with larger necks, which collapse during diastole and expand during systole. Differential diagnoses of cardiac pseudoaneurysm include true aneurysm and ventricular diverticulum. The differential points are the continuity of ventricular wall and clinic manifestations [13].

Key Points

1. The myocardial infarction accounted for the etiology of most LV pseudo- aneurysms followed by cardiac surgery, trauma, and infection.
2. Transthoracic echocardiography is a reasonable first test; it may assess the exact diagnosis, anatomical relations and size of pseudoaneurysm.

References

1. Gatewood, R.P. Jr and Nanda, N.C. (1980). Differentiation of left ventricular pseudoaneurysm from true aneurysm with two-dimensional echocardiography. *Am J Cardiol* 46: 869–878.
2. Sutherland, G.R., Smyllie, J.H. and Roelandt, J.R. (1989). Advantages of colour flow imaging in the diagnosis of left ventricular pseudoaneurysm. *Br Heart J* 61: 59–64.
3. Roelandt, J.R., Sutherland, G.R., Yoshida, K. et al. (1988). Improved diagnosis and characterization of left ventricular pseudoaneurysm by Doppler color flow imaging. *J Am Coll Cardiol* 3: 807–811.
4. Weston, M.W., McKinnon, E., Donald, T. et al. (1991). Unknown extracardiac echo-free space: Diagnosis of a left ventricular pseudoaneurysm by color flow echocardiography. *Clin Cardiol* 6: 526–528.

5. Harrity, P., Patel, A., Bianco, J. et al. (1991). Improved diagnosis and characterization of postin-farction left ventricular pseudoaneurysm by cardiac magnetic resonance imaging. *Clin Cardiol* 14: 603– 606.

6. Duvernoy, O., Wikstrom, G., Mannting, F. et al. (1992). Pre- and postoperative CT and MR in pseudoaneurysms of the heart. *J Comput Assist Tomogr* 16: 401–409.

7. Kahn, J. and Fisher, M.R. (1991). MRI of cardiac pseudoaneurysm and other complications of myocardial infarction. *Magn Reson Imaging* 9: 159–164.

8. Hsu, Y.H., Chiu, I.S. and Chien, C.T. (1993). Left ventricular pseudoaneurysm diagnosed by mag-netic resonance imaging in a nine-year-old boy. *Pediatr Cardiol* 14: 187–190.

9. Ghersin, E., Lessick, J., Litmanovich, D. et al. (2004). Septal bounce in constrictive pericarditis: diagnosis and dynamic evaluation with multidetector CT. *J Comput Assist Tomogr* 28: 676–678.

10. Mollet, N.R., Cademartiri, F., Nieman, K. et al. (2004). Multislice spiral computed tomography coronary angiography in patients with stable angina pectoris. *J Am Coll Cardiol* 43: 2265–2270.

11. Ropers, D., Baum, U., Pohle, K. et al. (2003). Detection of coronary artery stenoses with thin-slice multi-detector row spiral computed tomography and multiplanar reconstruction. *Circulation* 107: 664–666.

12. Yamamuro, M., Tadamura, E., Kubo, S. et al. (2005). Cardiac functional analysis with multi-detec-tor row CT and segmental reconstruction algorithm: Comparison with echocardiography, SPECT, and MR imaging. *Radiology* 234: 381–390.

13. Ghersin, E., Kerner, A., Gruberg, L. et al. (2007). Left ventricular pseudoaneurysm or diverticu-lum: differential diagnosis and dynamic evaluation by catheter left ventriculography and ECG-gated multidetector CT. *Br J Radiol* 80 (957): e209–211.

30 Salmonela Aortitis: A Rare Cause of Fever and Back Pain in the Elderly

Jen-Li Looi, Alex Pui-Wai Lee, and Jing Ping Sun

The Chinese University of Hong Kong, Hong Kong

History

An 85-year-old man presented with fever, cough, and abdominal pain. The patient had a history of hypertension.

Laboratory

Blood cultures obtained on admission subsequently grew *Salmonella enteritidis*.
  Chest X-ray revealed right lower lobe haziness.

Transesophageal Echocardiography

A complex ulcer at the aortic arch, measuring 1.3 cm in depth was found. Small mobile strandlike densities seen in the ulcer were suggestive of vegetation (Figure 30-1, Videos 30-1, 30-2, and 30.3).

Contrast Thoracic CT Scan

The CT images confirmed an ulcerated atherosclerotic plaque measuring 1.1 cm × 1.6 cm, progressively increasing in size over 3 months despite antibiotics (Figure 30-2).

Hospital Course

The patient was initially treated for chest infection but fever and leukocytosis persisted. Computed tomography of the abdomen was unrevealing. Blood cultures obtained on admission subsequently grew *Salmonella enteritidis*. Ceftriaxone and ciprofloxacin were initiated. However he developed increasing back pain. According the findings of CT scan, a stent was deployed in view of high risk of perforation and he was placed on prolonged treatment with ceftriazone and ciprofloxacin. Post-stenting CT scan a few months later showed a patent stent with the aneurysm remained stable in size (Figure 30-2C).

Comparative Cardiac Imaging: A Case-based Guide, First Edition.
Edited by Jing Ping Sun, Xing Sheng Yang, and Bryan P. Yan.
© 2018 John Wiley & Sons Ltd. Published 2018 by John Wiley & Sons Ltd.
Companion website: www.wiley.com/sun/comparative_cardiac_imaging

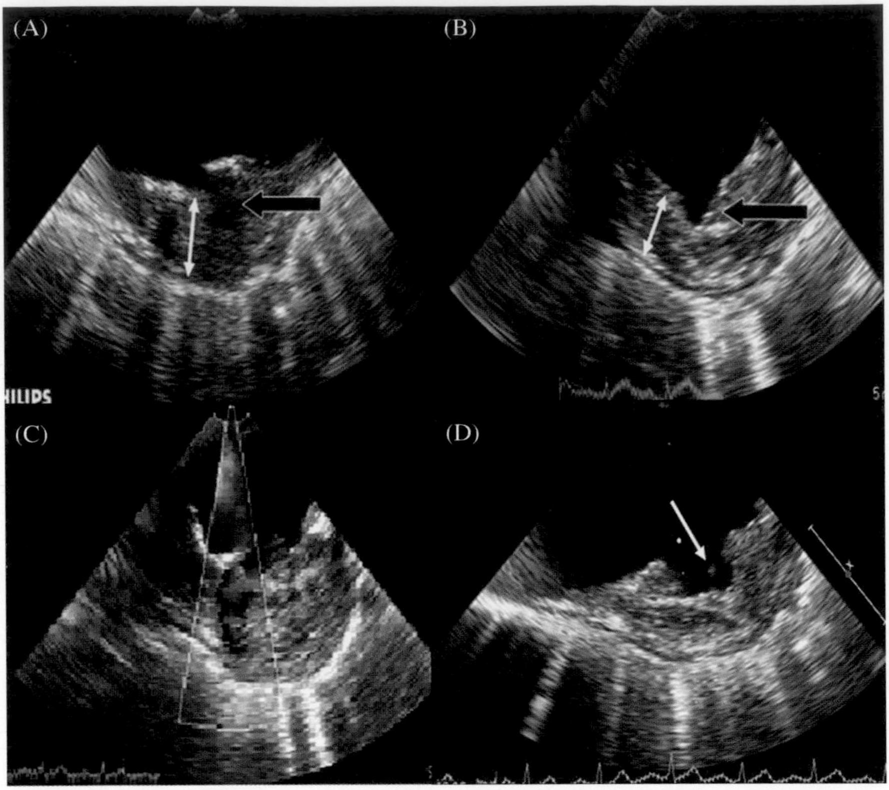

Figure 30-1 Transesophageal echocardiographic examination. A. Upper esophageal aortic arch long-axis view demonstrating moderate atheroma (white double arrow) with a complex ulcer (black arrow). B. Cross-sectional view of the aortic arch showing the ulcer (black arrow) and the atherosclerotic plaque (white double arrow). C. Color-flow Doppler image showing flow through the complex ulcer at the aortic arch. D. Small mobile strand-like densities (arrow) seen in the ulcer suggestive of vegetation along the margin of the defect.

Discussion

Cardiovascular infections develop in approximately 25% of patients with *Salmonella* bacteremia [1]. Most patients with *Salmonella* aortitis have pre-existing atherosclerosis at the site of the subsequently infected aneurysm. Our patient has hypertension and a dilated ascending aorta with moderate atherosclerosis on transesophageal echocardiography, which is a risk factor for *Salmonella* aortitis. Treatment usually requires surgical resection and a prolonged course of antibiotics. In recent years, successful treatment outcomes have been reported with the use of endovascular stent graft in selected patients [2, 3].

The diagnosis of Salmonella aortitis can be difficult because the clinical course may be indolent and the symptoms are nonspecific. A high index of suspicion is required to make the diagnosis of *Salmonella* aortitis, especially in elderly patients with risk factors for atherosclerosis who presented with Salmonella bacteremia, fever, back pain, and/or abdominal pain.

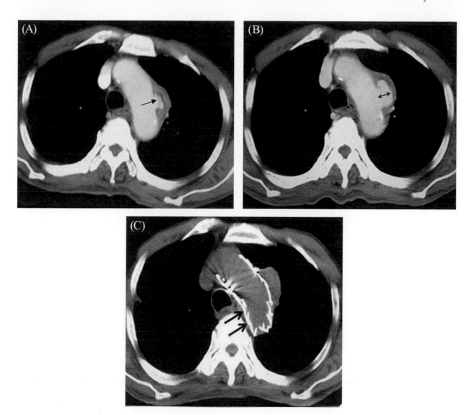

Figure 30-2   Contrast-enhanced chest CT demonstrating: A. an ulcerated atherosclerotic plaque measuring 1.1 cm × 1.6 cm affecting the aortic arch (arrow). B. The ulcer progressively increased in size (1.5 cm × 2.9 cm) over 3 months despite antibiotics (double arrow). C. Poststenting CT showed the stent deployed at the aortic arch being patent (arrows) and the aneurysm remained stable in size a few months later.

Transesophageal Echocardiography

The features of infective aortitis include a complex plaque with ulcerations, vegetation, and mycotic aneurysm formation. Almost the entire thoracic aorta can be visualized during a transesophageal examination. Thus, transesophageal echocardiography should be considered in cases of possible thoracic involvement [4].

Computed Tomography with Contrast and MRI

Tenenbaum et al. [5] used unenhanced dual-helical CT to assess calcium deposits and areas of hypoattenuation adjacent to the aortic wall in 32 patients with recent stroke or embolic events. The authors found that unenhanced dual-helical CT with thin sections appears to be useful for the rapid, noninvasive detection of a protruding aortic atheroma, especially in areas not clearly visualized with transesophageal echocardiography.

One group compared transesophageal echocardiography with MR angiography for examining protruding atheroma [6]. They found that MR angiography underestimated plaque thickness, probably because of difficulties in defining the aortic wall on the contrast-enhanced MR angiograms. Without ECG-gated cine gradient-echo images, MR imaging also provides static views of disease without assessing clinically significant mobile thrombus. However, MR imaging, like CT, can reveal the complete aorta (including the blind spots of transesophageal echocardiography) and assess great vessel disease.

Treatment

Several factors appear to be responsible for improved survival among patients with aortitis due to *Salmonella*. First, earlier diagnosis is possible because of increased awareness of this syndrome, and contrast-enhanced CT scan is usually available for use whenever the diagnosis is suspected. Second, antibacterial therapy has improved with the use of bactericidal antibiotics.

In literature review of a total of 150 patients with aortitis due to *Salmonella,* the use of bactericidal antibiotics, together with early surgical intervention and long-term suppressive antibiotic therapy, has led to improved survival. Bactericidal antibiotic therapy should be continued for at least 6 weeks after the surgical procedures. Finally, long-term suppressive therapy with daily oral antibacterial therapy seems to improve survival in patients who have undergone surgery [7] although no randomized controlled trial has formally proven this assumption. Antibiotics without surgery are not effective and are associated with a very high mortality.

In our case, a stent was deployed in view of a high risk of perforation and he was placed on prolonged treatment with ceftriazone and ciprofloxacin. Post-stenting CT scan a few months later showed a patent stent with the aneurysm remained stable in size.

Key Points

1. A high index of suspicion is required to make the early diagnosis of *Salmonella* aortitis.
2. The use of bactericidal antibiotics, together with early surgical or stent intervention and long-term suppressive antibiotic therapy, has led to improved survival.
3. The ease of performance, the detailed information obtainable, and the cost and availability of transesophageal echocardiography make this procedure as first choice for examining thoracic aortic atherosclerosis. However, MR imaging and CT can reveal the complete aorta (including the blind spots of transesophageal echocardiography) and assess great vessel disease.

References

1. Cohen, P.S., O'Brien, T.F., Schoenbaum, S.C. et al. (1978). The risk of endothelial infection in adults with salmonella bacteraemia. *Ann Intern Med* 89: 931–932.
2. Berchtold, C., Eibl, C., Seelig, M.H. et al. (2002). Endovascular treatment and complete regression of infected abdominal aortic aneurysm. *J Endovasc Ther* 9: 543–548.
3. Semba, C.P., Sakai, T. and Slonim, S.M. (1998). Mycotic aneurysms of the thoracic aorta: repair with use of endovascular stent-grafts. *J Vasc Interv Radiol* 9: 33–40.
4. Kures, P. and Soble, J. (1996). Salmonella aortitis with pseudoaneurysm formation diagnosed by tranesophageal echocardiography. *J Am Soc Echocardiogr* 9: 885–887.

5. Tenenbaum, A., Garniek, A., Shemesh, J. et al. (1998). Dualhelical CT for detecting aortic atheromas as a source of stroke: comparison with transesophageal echocardiography. *Radiology* 208: 153–158.

6. Kutz, S.M., Lee, V., Tunick, P.A. et al. (1999). Atheromas of the thoracic aorta: a comparison of transesophageal echocardiography and breath-hold gadolinium-enhanced 3-D magnetic resonance angiography. *J Am Soc Echocardiogr* 12(10): 853–858.

7. Soravia-Dunand, V.A., Loo, V.G. and Salit, I.E. (1999). Aortitis due to salmonella: Report of 10 cases and comprehensive review of the literature. *Clinical Infectious Diseases* 29: 862–868.

31 Subepicardial Aneurysm of Left Ventricle: A Rare Complication of Acute Myocardial Infarction

Ying Zheng[1], Zhiqing Qiao[1], Xuedong Shen[1], and Ben He[2]

[1] Shanghai Jiaotong University School of Medicine, Shanghai, China
[2] Tongji University School of Medicine, Shanghai, China

History

A 63-year-old, male was admitted via the emergency room because of chest pain with sweat, which he had been experiencing for 6 hours.

Physical Examination

The patient appeared pale and diaphoretic. Heart rate was 98 bpm, blood pressure was 130/80 mmHG. There was no murmur at the precordial area.

Electrocardiography

Electrocardiography (EKG) showed a complete right-bundle branch block and ST elevation on leads II, III, and aVF, V2–V6 (Figure 31-1); we therefore suspected an acute anterior and inferior wall myocardial infarction (AMI).

Coronary Angiography

Coronary angiography revealed total occlusion of the proximal left anterior descending (LAD, Figure 31-2, Video 31-1). The left circumflex and right coronary artery showed no abnormalities. The LAD was recanalized by percutaneous catheter intervention (PCI). The patient complained of chest pain the afternoon after PCI, and the EKG was unchanged.

Transthoracic Echocardiogram

An apical four-chamber view demonstrated that the apical segments of left ventricular walls were akinetic with normal thickness (Video 31-2), but apex myocardial were dyskinetic with a perforation (2 mm in diameter) connected with a small apical aneurysm (10 × 5 mm) covered by an intact epicardium, which was communicated with a left ventricular cavity demonstrated by color Doppler (Figure 31-3A, B, Video 31-3) from an

Comparative Cardiac Imaging: A Case-based Guide, First Edition.
Edited by Jing Ping Sun, Xing Sheng Yang, and Bryan P. Yan.
© 2018 John Wiley & Sons Ltd. Published 2018 by John Wiley & Sons Ltd.
Companion website: www.wiley.com/sun/comparative_cardiac_imaging

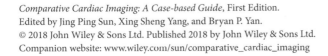

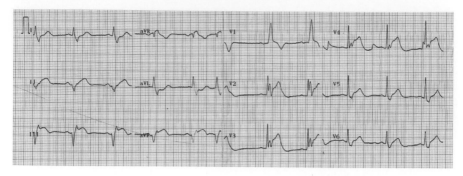

Figure 31-1 Electrocardiography showed a complete right bundle branch block, and ST elevation on leads II, III, and aVF, V2-V6.

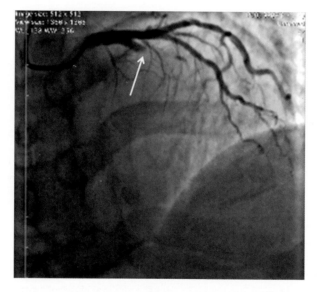

Figure 31-2 Angiogram showed the proximal segment of left anterior descending coronary was total occluded (arrow).

apical two-chamber view. This was consistent with a subepicardial aneurysm. The follow-up echocardiography was performed 8 days after infarction. There was a small thrombus at the apex and the false aneurysm could not be seen (Figure 31-3C, Video 31-4).

To confirm the diagnosis, cardiac magnetic resonance imaging (CMRI) was performed. Axial (Figure 31-4a) and short-axis (Figure 31-4b) first-pass perfusion SSFP MR images demonstrated an area of microvascular obstruction in the apical wall (filled arrows) with an small aneurysm (opened arrow) compatible with an left ventricular rupture. The magnified view (Figure 31-4C) SSFP MR image confirms an apical thrombus (arrow) at the area of the ruptured orifice (opened arrow) covered by an intact epicardium. The two-chamber view (Figure 31-4D) delayed enhancement inversion recovery MR image (SSFP-GRE) postintravenous gadolinium injection shows apical

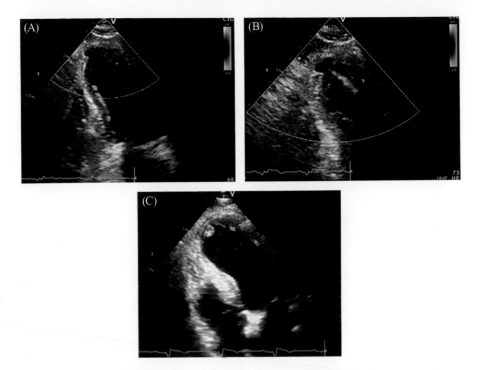

Figure 31 3 Apical two-chamber view showed apical myocardial perforation (2 mm in diameter) connected with a small apical aneurysm (10 × 5 mm) covered by an intact epicardium (A), which communicated with left ventricular cavity demonstrated by color Doppler (B). Follow-up echocardiography was performed 8 days after infarction. There was a small thrombus at apex and the false aneurysm could not be seen (C).

acute myocardial infarction with a persistent area of microvascular obstruction (filled heads), small apical thrombus, and a small aneurysm with a clot and covered by epicardia (arrow).

To prevent the epicardia rupture or sudden death, the aneurysmectomy was performed 28 days after infarction. During surgery, a small ruptured orifice filled with thrombus in the left ventricular apex was evident. Ventricular aneurysm resection and a coronary artery bypass SV-LAD side anastomosis operation were performed.

Pathological examination showed that the endocardial layer and muscle layer structure ruptured but the epicardium was integrity with fibrous tissue and a small amount of myocardial cells (Figure 31-5). The patient was discharged from hospital in good condition 10 days after surgery.

Discussion

There are several potentially life-threatening complications: arrhythmias, cardiogenic shock, and ventricular wall rupture with the formation of aneurysms. Among left-ventricular aneurysms, complete free wall ruptures account for almost 4% of patients' deaths after AMI (33% occur within the first 24 hours, 85% within the first week [1]. Complete septal ruptures account for 1–5% of all infarct-related deaths [2]. False

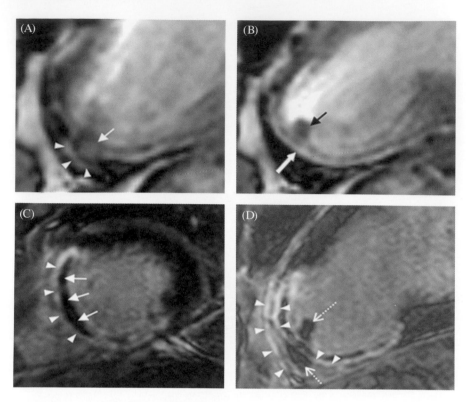

Figure 31-4 Cardiac MRI. A. Cine (SSFP) CMR imaging of a two-chamber view in the diastolic phase. A diverticulum-like cavity (arrowhead) with thrombus (white arrow) inside can be clearly observed. B. Cine imaging of a two-chamber view in the systolic phase. A diverticulum-like cavity disappeared, which indicated the formation of an aneurysm; the intact epicardia could be seen in this phase (white filled arrow), which was consistent with an subepicardial aneurysm. The thrombus (black arrow) still could be seen in LV apex. C. Late gadolinium enhancement imaging of the short axis. The scar (arrowhead) was demonstrated by enhanced myocardium, while significant microvascular obstruction (MVO) was detected as hypo-enhancement (white arrow) within the necrotic area. D. Late gadolinium enhancement imaging of the two-chamber view. Enhanced myocardium was detached in the apex. Thromboses (open arrow) can be seen in the LV and inside the aneurysm.

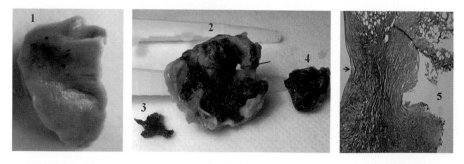

Figure 31-5 Gross pathological examination showed that the epicardium of apical surface was integrity (1*) but the endocardium and muscle-layer structure was ruptured (2, arrow) and covered by thrombus (3 and 4). Histological examination showed the epicardium was integrity (arrow) with fibrous tissue and a small amount of myocardial cells (5).

aneurysms also form. While true aneurysms typically do not require emergency treatment, false aneurysms, or pseudoaneurysms, are the result of a complete rupture of the ventricular wall with containment of the resulting hematoma by adherent pericardium and thus have a high mortality rate. Subepicardial aneurysm (SEA) is rare: of 1814 hearts examined after postmortem arteriography from autopsy subjects at the Johns Hopkins Hospital, 704 had 1140 infarcts, and only three SEAs were found (0.2% of infarcts) [3]. As SEAs are precursors to pseudoaneurysms with a high propensity to rupture, immediate treatment is often life saving. Although conservative management has been reported to be successful in asymptomatic chronic SEAs [4], surgical treatment is still considered standard care, especially for symptomatic acute SEAs, as in our case. The options include aneurysmectomy (resection) or aneurysmorrhaphy (patch repair). In addition to an elevated risk of death, patients with SEAs are initially difficult to diagnose due to a lack of specific symptoms. Although a transthoracic echocardiogram demonstrates the abnormality, sometimes the features are not distinct enough to differentiate aneurysm subtypes; MRI or CT may be helpful for accurate diagnosis. Due to the fact that subepicardial aneurysms have high risk of rupture, cardiac surgery should be performed as soon as diagnosis is confirmed in patients with a history of AMI or signs of coronary artery disease.

In a patient with continued chest pain post-AMI, subendocardial left-ventricular aneurysm / impending rupture should be considered as an uncommon life-threatening differential diagnosis. In our case, the SEA was found by transthoracic echocardiography and confirmed with a dedicated cardiac MRI. Emergency surgery guided by these imaging findings most likely saved the patient's life.

Key Points

1. Subepicardial aneurysm is a rare complication of acute myocardial infarction.
2. Due to the fact that subepicardial aneurysms have high risk of rupture, cardiac surgery should be performed as soon as diagnosis is confirmed.
3. Echocardiography is the first choice to detect this lesion in patients with acute myocardial infarction; MRI or CT may be needed for accurate diagnosis.

Reference

1. Pollak, H., Nobis, H. and Mlczoch, J. (1994). Frequency of left ventricular free wall rupture complicating acute myocardial infarction since the advent of thrombolysis. *Am J Cardiol* 74: 184–186.
2. Fox, A.C., Glassman, E. and Isom, O.W. (1979). Surgically remediable complications of myocardial infarction. *Prog Cardiovasc Dis* 21: 461–484.
3. Epstein, J.I. and Hutchins, G.M. (1983). Subepicardial aneurysms: A rare complication of myocardial infarction. *Am J Med* 75: 639–644.
4. Yang, H.S. (2008). Subepicardial aneurysm evaluated by Multiplane 2D and real-time 3D volumetric transesophageal echocardiography. *Circulation: Cardiovascular Imaging* 1: 171–172.

32 Coronary Artery Disease and Systemic Vasculitis

Ligang Fang[1], Jing Ping Sun[2], and Yining Wang[1]

[1] Affiliated Hospital of Peking Union Medical College, Beijing, China
[2] The Chinese University of Hong Kong, Hong Kong

History

A 32-year-old male presented with right lower limb intermittent claudication and left-limb dysfunction, which he had for 4 years. The left upper limb disability occurred recently. There was no history of chest pain. The patient had been smoking for more than 10 years, 20–30 cigarettes/day.

Physical Examination

Temperature was 37.1 °C; heart rate was 82 BPM, respiration rate was 18 times/min, BP: upper right 125/74 mmHg, upper left 131/80 mmHg, lower right 00/00 mmHg, lower left 49/24 mmHg. There were no remarkable findings from a heart examination. The pulse of the right femoral, popliteal, tibial, and dorsalis pedis arteries was not palpated; the left femoral artery could be felt but was weak.

Artery Ultrasound

The bilateral carotid artery, vertebral artery and subclavian artery were normal; the proximal segments of bilateral common iliac and external iliac artery embolization was detected. The distal segment of superior mesenteric artery could not be seen well. The resistance of the left renal artery increased; the velocity of bilateral femoral artery blood flow was reduced; and the popliteal artery embolization was detected.

Transthoracic Echocardiography

Transthoracic two-dimensional echocardiography parasternal short-axis and apical four-chamber view showed that the apical myocardium displayed echodensity and was akinetic. There is a mobile thrombus in LV apex (Figure 32-1A–C, Videos 32-1 to 32-3).

Magnetic Resonance Imaging

Cine cardiovascular magnetic resonance delineates the apical thrombus; late gadolinium enhancement imaging clearly confirms the avascular nonenhancing thrombus (Figure 32-1D-F small arrow) close to the transmural infarcted myocardium (bright

Comparative Cardiac Imaging: A Case-based Guide, First Edition.
Edited by Jing Ping Sun, Xing Sheng Yang, and Bryan P. Yan.
© 2018 John Wiley & Sons Ltd. Published 2018 by John Wiley & Sons Ltd.
Companion website: www.wiley.com/sun/comparative_cardiac_imaging

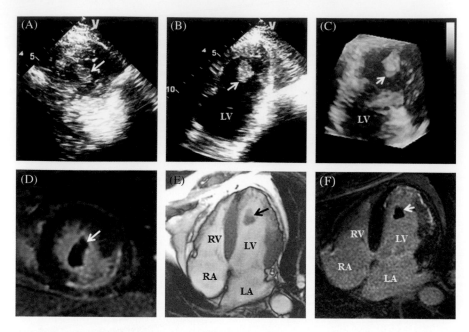

Figure 32-1   Transthoracic echocardiography. A mass was seen in the apex of the parasternal short-axis view (A), the apical four-chamber view (B), and in the three-dimensional four-chamber real-time image (C). Cine cardiovascular magnetic resonance imaging delineates the apical thrombus; late gadolinium enhancement imaging clearly confirms the avascular nonenhancing thrombus (D–F small arrow) close to the transmural infarcted myocardium (bright hyper enhanced, longer arrows).

hyperenhanced, longer arrows). Cranial magnetic resonance angiography showed the middle cerebral artery stenosis. The right side of the brain artery presented as arteritis.

Computed Tomography

Cranial CT showed cerebral infarction. Cardiac CT showed left anterior descending coronary artery stenosis.

Hospital Course

The cardiac thrombus was moved by surgery. The mass was 2.5 cm × 1.8 cm × 1 cm, and the characteristics of histology were in line with focal organizing thrombosis. This was a young patient with multiple artery lesion, so the diagnosis of systemic vasculitis was considered. The patient was given glucocorticoid, cyclophosphamide and anticoagulant therapy; the symptoms quickly improved, and the patient underwent lower extremity artery bypass surgery. The patient was doing well 2 years after operation.

Discussion

Primary systemic vasculitis (PSV) refers to a group of autoimmune conditions characterized by occlusion, stenosis, or aneurysmal dilatation of blood vessels secondary to intramural inflammation. Numerous classifications of vasculitis have been proposed. The American College of Rheumatology has classified seven forms of primary vasculitis: polyarthritis nodosa, Churg–Strauss syndrome, Wegener granulomatosis, hypersensitivity vasculitis, Henoch–Schönlein purpura, giant-cell arteritis, and Takayasu arteritis [1]. Microscopic polyangiitis is not included in the classification criteria. The American College of Rheumatology criteria were designed for research studies, but are often used for diagnosis, and do not include antineutrophil cytoplasmic antibody (ANCA) testing for the diagnosis of small vessel vasculitis or require biopsy or angiography for vasculitis classification. The criteria have poor reliability when applied for diagnosis [2].

In 1994, the Chapel Hill Consensus Conference proposed a nomenclature defining 10 forms of primary vasculitis based on vessel size (large, medium, and small) [3]. There is no recommended diagnostic standard for vasculitis. In the absence of validated diagnostic criteria, the American College of Rheumatology classification criteria and the Chapel Hill Consensus Conference nomenclature are most widely used in clinical practice to distinguish different forms of vasculitis.

Pathogenesis

The pathogenesis of vasculitis is poorly understood. Three possible mechanisms of vascular damage are immune complex deposition, ANCAs (humoral response), and T-lymphocyte response with granuloma formation (cell-mediated) [4, 5]. The end result of these various pathways is endothelial cell activation, with subsequent vessel obstruction and ischemia of dependent tissue. This may cause hemorrhage in the surrounding tissues and, in some cases, weakening of the vessel wall, which leads to the formation of aneurysms. For almost all forms of vasculitis, the triggering event initiating and driving this inflammatory response is unknown.

Clinical Appearance

Patients with vasculitis typically have prodromal symptoms, constitutional disturbances, and organ-specific manifestations. Patients can present with nonspecific signs or symptoms (e.g., fever, rash, myalgia, arthralgia, malaise, weight loss) or to the emergency department with life-threatening features (e.g., massive hemoptysis, renal failure). Manifestations vary, depending on the size, site, and extent of vessels involved. Our patient presented with lower limb intermittent claudication and left-limb dysfunction caused by multiple small and medium-sized arteritis.

Diagnostic Approach

Primary systemic vasculitis is difficult to diagnose because of the clinical manifestations. The patient's age, sex, and demographic or ethnic origin are also important. Finally, type and extent of organ involvement and the size of the vessels involved should be determined. Certain organ-specific symptoms, not otherwise explained, may be clues leading to a more specific diagnosis. A definitive diagnosis of systemic vasculitis should be made by the presence of characteristic symptoms and signs of vasculitis and at least one of the following: histologic evidence of vasculitis; or specific indirect evidence of vasculitis [6–8]. It is important to ascertain that no other diagnosis accounts for the presenting symptoms and signs.

Imaging
Chest Radiography
Nonspecific abnormalities that can be seen on chest radiography include infiltrates, nodules, patchy consolidation, pleural effusion, and cardiomegaly. These findings can occur in many settings but if unexplained may raise the suspicion of vasculitis.

Angiography
Angiography can show vascular occlusion and aneurysm. A diagnosis of polyarthritis nodosa can be confirmed by detection of aneurysms in the mesenteric and renal arteries. Although conventional angiography is still accepted as the recommended diagnostic modality, computed tomography angiography and magnetic resonance angiography may be superior because they can provide valuable information regarding intraluminal pathology and thickening of the vessel wall.

Echocardiography
Transthoracic echocardiography is useful to detect cardiac abnormalities caused by coronary arteritis. For example, apical myocardial dysfunction and a thrombus were found by transthoracic echocardiography in our case.

Magnetic Resonance Imaging
Magnetic resonance angiography imaging may be superior because it can provide valuable information regarding intraluminal pathology and thickening of the vessel wall; cardiac MRI can also provide the information of coronary arteritis, as in our case.

Computed Tomography
Computed tomography angiography is very useful to detect the abnormalities of multiple arteritis in the whole body. Cranial CT showed cerebral infarction. Cardiac CT showed left anterior descending coronary artery stenosis in our case.

Management
High-dose glucocorticoid therapy has a definite role in inducing remission in systemic multiple arteritis. Low-dose aspirin should be considered in all patients to reduce the risk of developing cardiovascular and cerebrovascular events [9, 10].

Management of systemic vasculitis is complicated. Educating patients about signs and symptoms, and monitoring typical adverse effects are helpful. Many patients will have a relatively benign, self-limited course, especially if the disease is limited to the skin; however, for patients with aggressive disease, it is imperative to begin treatment without delay. Multisystem involvement in systemic vasculitis necessitates a multidisciplinary team approach to patient care. Recent advances in therapy have led to considerably better outcomes in patients with vasculitis.

Monitoring and Follow Up
All patients with systemic arteritis may have a higher risk of cardiovascular events than the general population. They should be monitored in the long term due to the risk of relapse, cardiovascular events, and iatrogenic complications. Blood pressure monitoring

is recommended for all patients at each follow-up visit. Hypertension may be iatrogenic due to glucocorticoid therapy or nephrotoxic drugs, or as a result of the disease.

Key Points

1. Primary systemic vasculitis (PSV) is a group of autoimmune conditions characterized by occlusion, stenosis, or aneurysmal dilatation of blood vessels secondary to intramural inflammation.
2. Primary systemic vasculitis is difficult to diagnose because of the clinical manifestations.
3. It is crucial to keep knowledge of systemic multiple arteritis in mind in diagnosis.

References

1. Bloch, D.A., Michel, B.A., Hunder, G.G. et al. (1990). The American College of Rheumatology 1990 criteria for the classification of vasculitis. Patients and methods. *Arthritis Rheum* 33 (8): 1068–1073.
2. Rao, J.K., Allen, N.B., and Pincus, T. (1998). Limitations of the 1990 American College of Rheumatology classification criteria in the diagnosis of vasculitis. *Ann Intern Med* 129 (5): 345–352.
3. Jennette, J.C., Falk, R.J., Andrassy, K. et al. (1994). Nomenclature of systemic vasculitides. Proposal of an international consensus conference. *Arthritis Rheum* 37 (2): 187–192.
4. Sneller, M.C. and Fauci, A.S. (1997). Pathogenesis of vasculitis syndromes. *Med Clin North Am* 81 (1): 221–242.
5. Danila, M.I. and Bridges, S.L. Jr. (2008). Update on pathogenic mechanisms of systemic necrotizing vasculitis. *Curr Rheumatol Rep* 10 (6): 430–435.
6. Merkel, P.A., Polisson, R.P., Chang, Y. et al. (1997). Prevalence of anti-neutrophil cytoplasmic antibodies in a large inception cohort of patients with connective tissue disease. *Ann Intern Med* 126 (11): 866–873.
7. Roggenbuck, D., Buettner, T., Hoffmann, L. et al. (2009). High-sensitivity detection of autoantibodies against proteinase-3 by a novel third-generation enzyme-linked immunosorbent assay. *Ann N Y Acad Sci* 1173: 41–46.
8. Savige, J., Pollock, W. and Trevisin, M. (2005). What do antineutrophil cytoplasmic antibodies (ANCA) tell us? *Best Pract Res Clin Rheumatol* 19 (2): 263–276.
9. Hogan, S.L., Falk, R.J., Chin, H. et al. (2005). Predictors of relapse and treatment resistance in antineutrophil cytoplasmic antibody-associated small-vessel vasculitis. *Ann Intern Med* 143 (9): 621–631.
10. Pagnoux, C., Hogan, S.L., Chin, H. et al. (2008). Predictors of treatment resistance and relapse in antineutrophil cytoplasmic antibody-associated small-vessel vasculitis: comparison of two independent cohorts. *Arthritis Rheum* 58 (9): 2908–2918.

Part III
Cardiac Mass

33 Primary Cardiac Angiosarcoma in Left Atrium

Hongjun Wang[1], Junli Hu[1], Shaochun Wang[1], and Jing Ping Sun[2]

[1] Affiliated Hospital of Jining Medical University, Jining, China
[2] The Chinese University of Hong Kong, Hong Kong

History

A 22-year-old male presented with palpitations and chest tightness on exertion.

Physical Examination

Heart rate was regular at 80 bpm. Blood pressure was 105/78 mm Hg. On auscultation, there was a diastolic murmur at the left parasternal border of the fourth intercostal space. There were no signs of heart failure.

Echocardiogram

Transthoracic echocardiography showed a mural mass (16×53 mm) (Figure 33-1A) attached to the left atrial posterior wall, which protruded across the mitral valve during diastole. A second mass (15×30 mm) was seen infiltrating the anterior mitral leaflet (Figure 33-1B, supplemental Video 33-1); The two masses caused dynamic obstruction of mitral inflow with high color Doppler velocity during cardiac diastole; M-mode echo-cardiography of the mitral valve of this case showed the masses obstructed the mitral inflow tract (Figure 33-1C and D, Videos 33-1 and 33-2) and the left atrium was dilated. Moderate pericardial effusion was detected. Malignant cardiac tumor was suspected and the patient was referred for surgery.

Operation

During operation, the surgeon found lobulated masses with wide bases attached to the left atrial posterior wall infiltrating into the orifice of the left pulmonary vein, the mitral annulus, and leaflets. The tumors were excised and the left atrium was repaired with the pericardium.

Pathology

Histology and the immunohistochemical staining of the masses was diagnosed as undifferentiated angiosarcoma (Figure 33-2).

Comparative Cardiac Imaging: A Case-based Guide, First Edition.
Edited by Jing Ping Sun, Xing Sheng Yang, and Bryan P. Yan.
© 2018 John Wiley & Sons Ltd. Published 2018 by John Wiley & Sons Ltd.
Companion website: www.wiley.com/sun/comparative_cardiac_imaging

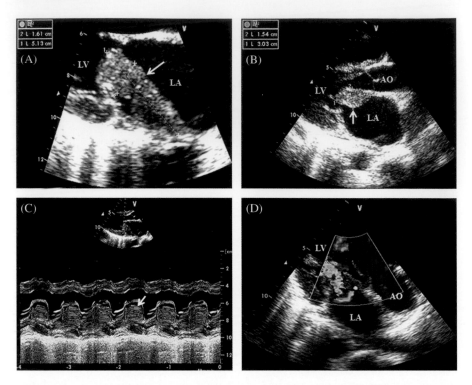

Figure 33-1 Transthoracic echocardiography showed a mural mass (16 × 53 mm) (A) attached to the left atrial posterior wall, which protruded across the mitral valve during diastole. Another mass (15 × 30 mm) was seen infiltrating the anterior mitral leaflet (B). M-mode echocardiography of mitral valve of this case showed the mass filled in the mitral inflow tract. The two masses caused dynamic obstruction of the mitral inflow with high-color Doppler velocity (C and D).

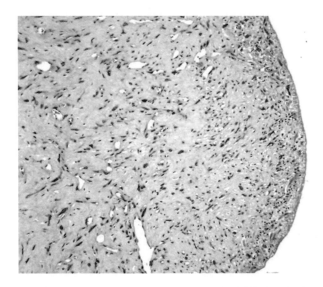

Figure 33-2 Histologic photomicrograph. The tumor consists of spindle-shaped cells with pleomorphic nuclei lining anastomosing vascular spaces. Mitotic figures and areas of hemorrhage and necrosis can also be found. These findings support the diagnosis of angiosarcoma.

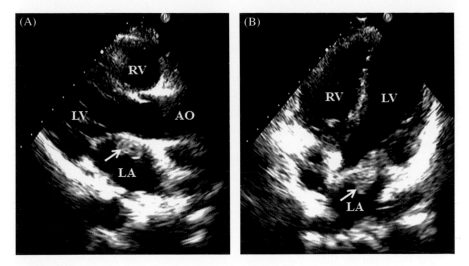

Figure 33-3 The follow-up echocardiography found a recurrence of tumor attached to the anterior mitral leaflet.

Follow Up

Three months after operation, the patient was doing well. However, follow-up echocardiography found a recurrence of the tumor attached to the anterior mitral leaflet (Figure 33-3; Video 33-3).

Discussion

Primary cardiac sarcoma is a rare clinical entity, with an incidence of 0.0001% in collected autopsy series [1]. Several subtypes of primary cardiac sarcoma exist (e.g., angiosarcoma [2], rhabdomyosarcoma, mesothelioma, fibrosarcoma, and malignant schwannoma), which occur in decreasing order of frequency in adults [3, 4]. Nearly 80% of cardiac angiosarcomas arise as mural masses in the right atrium. Typically, they completely replace the atrial wall and fill the entire cardiac chamber. They may invade adjacent structures (e.g., the vena cava; tricuspid valve).

The low incidence of primary cardiac sarcomas reflects the overall low incidence of sarcomas in the general population and the small percentage of body weight of the heart (0.5%) compared with muscle (40%). Angiosarcomas are the commonest cardiac sarcomas and make up 33% of cases. We describe a case of undifferentiated angiosarcoma infiltrating the left atrium and mitral valve.

Primary cardiac sarcoma seldom causes symptoms until late in the course. The most common symptoms include dyspnea, chest pain, heart failure, palpitation, fever, and myalgia. Case reports in the literature describe a variety of clinical manifestations, which included arrhythmia, vena cava obstruction, pericardial effusion with or without features of tamponade, and conduction disturbances. In contrast with benign tumors, which are usually located in the left atrium, malignant tumors are found almost exclusively in the right heart, particularly in the right atrium. Our case is particularly rare. The angiosarcoma was in the left atrium, and swung into the mitral inflow tract during the cardiac diastole leading to dynamic mitral inflow obstruction, which caused the symptoms of palpitations and chest tightness.

Despite the availability of modern imagine techniques, the diagnosis of cardiac sarcoma is usually late. According to a large single-center case series (33 cases) report, transthoracic echocardiography (TTE) as the initial diagnostic test had 75% sensitivity for visualizing primary cardiac angiosarcoma (9/12 patients); computed tomographic (CT) angiography was initially performed in four patients to evaluate the possibility of pulmonary embolus and correctly identified cardiac angiosarcoma in three (75%). Pericardial effusion was a common finding but pericardial fluid cytology was invariably negative. Thus, a normal pericardial fluid analysis does not exclude a potentially malignant cause. The absence of a tumor stalk was a universal TTE finding that may help to distinguish angiosarcoma from benign, primarily pedunculated tumors such as myxoma and papillary fibroelastoma [5].

The prognosis of cardiac angiosarcoma is poor with a median survival ranging from 6 to 11 months. The therapy for primary cardiac tumors is still controversial but surgery remained the therapy of choice in the cases of localized disease. However, complete resection of cardiac sarcoma can be difficult depending on the location and extent of involvement. Often tumors are so large at the time of the operation that complete resection cannot be done. Furthermore, metastases and local invasion are often present at time of diagnosis. There are some reported cases of patients with metastatic angiosarcoma treated with partial resection followed by chemotherapy and radiotherapy who survived from 34 to 53 months [6]. Based on these case reports, we might consider chemotherapy and/or radiotherapy as adjuvant therapy after radical or debulking surgery, in order to improve overall survival. Unfortunately, the patient did not receive chemotherapy or radiotherapy and the tumor recurred 3 months after surgery.

In conclusion, primary cardiac angiosarcoma is associated with a poor prognosis, with life expectancy between 6–11 months. In general, recommendations for the treatment of nonmetastatic cardiac sarcoma include surgical removal of the primary tumor to relieve obstructive symptoms.

Key Points

1. Primary cardiac angiosarcoma is a rare but highly aggressive tumor with a poor prognosis.
2. The absence of a tumor stalk was a universal finding on TTE that may help distinguish angiosarcoma from benign, primarily pedunculated tumors such as myxoma and papillary fibroelastoma.
3. Partial resection followed by chemotherapy and radiotherapy may have a survival benefit.

References

1. Look Hong, N.J., Pandalai, P.K., Hornick, J.L. et al. (2012). Cardiac angiosarcoma management and outcomes: 20-year single-institution experience. *Ann Surg Oncol* 19 (8): 2707–2715.
2. Simpson, L., Kumar, S.K., Okuno, S.H. et al. (2008). Malignant primary cardiac tumors: Review of a single institution experience. *Cancer* 12 (11): 2440–2446.

3. Zhang, P.J., Brooks, J.S., Goldblum, J.R. et al. (2008). Primary cardiac sarcomas: A clinicopathologic analysis of a series with follow-up information in 17 patients and emphasis on long-term survival. *Hum Pathol* 39 (9): 1385–1395.

4. Talbot, S.M., Taub, R.N., Keohan, M.L. et al. (2002). Combined heart and lung transplantation for unresectable primary cardiac sarcoma. *J Thor Cardiovasc Surg* 124 (6): 1145–1148.

5. Kupsky, D.F., Newman, D.B., Kumar, G. et al. (2016). Echocardiographic features of cardiac angiosarcomas: The Mayo Clinic experience (1976–2013). *Echocardiography* 33: 186–192.

6. Nakamichi, T., Fukuda, T., Suzuki, T. et al. (1997). Primary cardiac angiosarcoma: 53 months' survival after multidisciplinary therapy. *Ann Thor Surg* 63 (4): 1160–1161.

34 Atypical Left-Atrial Papillary Fibroelastoma

Kevin Ka-Ho Kam, Alex Pui-Wai Lee, and Jing Ping Sun

The Chinese University of Hong Kong, Hong Kong

History

A 55-year-old lady was referred because of a suspicious left-atrial mass. She was known to have hypertension and chronic headache. She was well, without any fever, limb weakness, chest pain, or symptoms of heart failure.

Physical Examination

The blood pressure and pulse were normal. The jugular venous pressure was within normal range. There was grade 2 over 6 pansystolic murmur over the apex with no radiation. The lung field was clear. An ECG showed normal sinus rhythm.

- Transthoracic echocardiography. A subcostal four-chamber view showed a suspicious left atrial tumor (Figure 34-1). There were no significant valvular lesions. Transesophageal echocardiography illustrated a 1 cm highly mobile anemone-like echogenic mass attaching to the left atrium (Figure 34-2A and B). Provisional diagnosis of left atrial papillary fibroelastoma was made.
- High-slice multidetector row computed tomography (MDCT) of the heart was performed but it did not reveal any mass (Figure 34-3A).
- Cardiac magnetic resonance (CMR) imaging only showed mild left-atrial enlargement without identifiable abnormal structure or mass within the left atrium (Figure 34-3B). The radiologist suggested that the abnormality previously seen on an echocardiogram may represent an artifact.

Hospital Course

Surgical excision was carried out and it confirmed the diagnosis pathologically. It was a 6 mm frond-like tumor with a pedicle attached to the posterior wall of the left atrium below the entrance of the inferior pulmonary vein.

Discussion

Papillary fibroelastoma is the second most common cardiac tumor, which ranks just after the myxoma. It accounts for 10% of all primary cardiac tumors [1]. Most of the time, fibroelastoma is less than 1 cm in size and usually attached to mitral or aortic

Comparative Cardiac Imaging: A Case-based Guide, First Edition.
Edited by Jing Ping Sun, Xing Sheng Yang, and Bryan P. Yan.
© 2018 John Wiley & Sons Ltd. Published 2018 by John Wiley & Sons Ltd.
Companion website: www.wiley.com/sun/comparative_cardiac_imaging

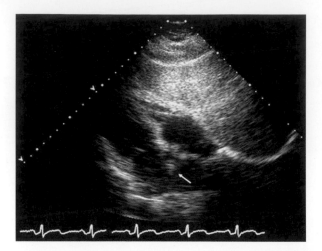

Figure 34-1 The subxiphoid window of transthoracic echocardiography showed a suspicious mass (indicated by a white arrow) moving within the left atrium.

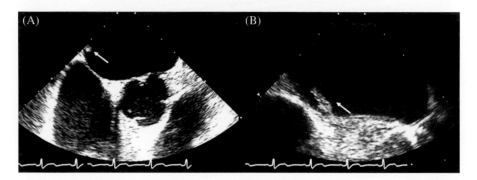

Figure 34-2 The transesophageal echocardiography: A. View at 45° showed a 1 cm echogenic mass (indicated by a white arrow) attached to left atrial wall. B. The transesophageal echocardiography at the bicaval view clearly demonstrated a frond-like mass with a stalk (indicated by a white arrow) attached to the left atrial wall. The features were compatible to papillary fibroelastoma.

valves [2]. On rare occasions it may be found within the heart chambers. The majority of patients are asymptomatic and diagnosed incidentally by echocardiography. Clinical examination, ECG, and plain chest radiography are unhelpful in establishing the diagnosis. Clinical manifestations including embolic events such as stroke, transient ischemic attack, myocardial infarction, heart failure or sudden cardiac death may occur in some patients [2, 3]. Owing to its mobile nature, small fibroelastomas are not well visualized by MDCT or CMR. Thus, echocardiography, especially transesophageal echocardiography, is the gold standard for diagnosis, as in our case. Surgery is generally recommended if the mass is more than 1 cm or highly mobile [2, 4]. Excision should also be performed for patients who have had embolic events or complications related to tumor mobility [2, 4, 5], for example coronary ostial occlusion. Recurrence of fibroelastoma after operation has not been reported [5].

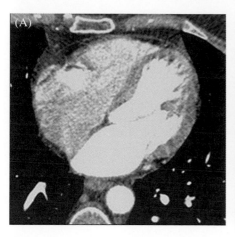
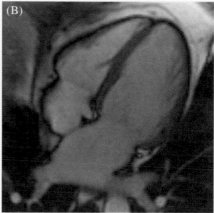

Figure 34-3 Computed tomography image. A. The four-chamber view from multidetector computed-tomography could not identify any suspicious mass in the left atrium. B. The four-chamber view from cardiac magnetic resonance imaging should be more sensitive in detecting small cardiac structure but could not visualize any mass in the left atrium in our case.

Prognosis is generally good for patients with papillary fibroelastoma. The perioperative mortality rate is low. Prognosis becomes worse if complications like embolic events occurred. Thus the patient should be operated on as soon as possible if the mass is significant in size or highly mobile.

Key Points

1. Papillary fibroelastoma is the second most common cardiac tumor, which ranks just after the myxoma. It accounts for 10% of all primary cardiac tumors.
2. Echocardiography, especially transesophageal echocardiography, is the most useful tool for diagnosing this highly mobile cardiac mass.
3. Surgical excision is recommended if the papillary fibroelastoma is larger than 1 cm or mobile. It should also be done if there has been an embolic complication.

References

1. Palecek, T., Lindner, J., Vitkova, I. et al. (2008). Papillary fibroelastoma arising from the left ventricular apex associated with nonspecific systemic symptoms. *Echocardiography* 25: 526–528.
2. Gowda, R.M., Khan, I.A., Nair, C.K. et al. (2003). Cardiac papillary fibroelastoma: A comprehensive analysis of 725 cases. *Am Heart J* 146 (3): 404.
3. Liebeskind, D.S., Buljubasic, N. and Saver, J.L. (2001). Cardioembolic stroke due to papillary fibroelastoma. *J Stroke Cerebrovasc Dis* 10 (2): 94–95.
4. Sun, J.P., Asher, C.R., Yang, X.S. et al. (2001). Clinical and echocardiographic characteristics of papillary fibroelastomas: a retrospective and prospective study in 162 patients. *Circulation* 103 (22): 2687.
5. Grinda, J.M., Couetil, J.P., Chauvaud, S. et al. (1999). Cardiac valve papillary fibroelastoma: Surgical excision for revealed or potential embolization. *J Thoracic Cardiovasc Surg* 117 (1): 106.

35 Cardiac Lipoma with Ventricular Arrhythmias

Litong Qi[1], Ying Yang[1], Yong Huo[1], and Jing Ping Sun[2]

[1] Beijing Medical School, Beijing, China
[2] The Chinese University of Hong Kong, Hong Kong

History

A 24-year-old female was admitted to the hospital because of intermittent episodes of palpitation for 2 years, and increased episodes with syncope for 6 months.

Physical Examination

Temperature was 37 °C. Heart rate was 68 bpm with ventricular premature beats (VPBs). Respiration rate was 16 /min. Blood pressure was 110/60 mmHg. A grade 2/6 systolic heart murmur was heard in the apical area.

Electrocardiogram

Electrocardiogram showed ST elevation 0.1–0.2 mv with T-wave bidirection on I, II, III, AVL, V2-V6 leads with paroxysmal ventricular tachycardia (VT) (Figure 35-1). Holter recording indicated frequent VPBs (2458 beats/24 h) and paroxysmal VT.

Echocardiography There was a large mass at the left ventricular posterior-lateral wall within the pericardium (Figure 35-2A, and Videos 35 1, 35-2, and 35-3). There was no pericardial effusion. Both left and right ventricles and atriums were normal in size. The left ventricular posterior wall displayed mild hypokinesis; the left ventricular eject fraction was 56%. There was mild to moderate mitral regurgitation.

Computed Tomography There was a large fat density lesion with the size of 10.0×9.5×5.2 cm in the left ventricular lateral-posterior wall, CT value of about −81 HU. The adjacent myocardium was thin and there were moderate density radial cord tissue extended into the lesion (Figure 35-2B). The large lesion in the heart suggested the diagnosis of cardiac lipoma.

Magnetic Resonance Imaging A cardiac MRI scan showed a large lesion with the size of 8.5×8.3×5.9 cm in the pericardium connected with left ventricular and left atrial wall. The outer boundary of the lesion was smooth and clear. There were several low radial cord signals from the myocardial of the LV wall extending to the lesion (Figure 35-2C). The lateral-posterior wall of left ventricle was mildly hypokinetic.

Comparative Cardiac Imaging: A Case-based Guide, First Edition.
Edited by Jing Ping Sun, Xing Sheng Yang, and Bryan P. Yan.
© 2018 John Wiley & Sons Ltd. Published 2018 by John Wiley & Sons Ltd.
Companion website: www.wiley.com/sun/comparative_cardiac_imaging

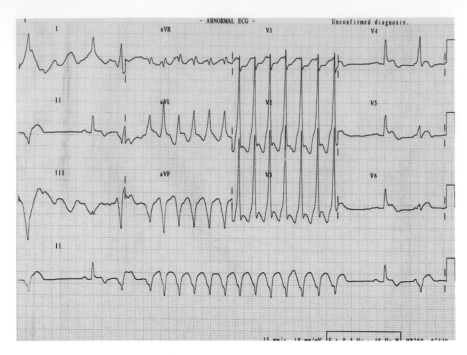

Figure 35-1 An electrocardiogram showed ST elevation 0.1–0.2 mv with T-wave bidirection on I, Ii, III, AVL, V2-V6 leads with paroxysmal ventricular tachycardia (VT).

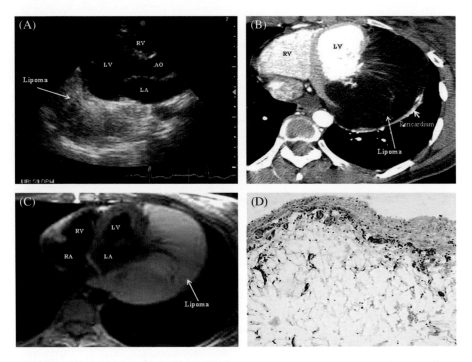

Figure 35-2 Echocardiography: A. There was a large mass at left ventricular posterior-lateral wall within pericardium. B. Computed tomography. There was a large fat density lesion with a size of 10.0×9.5×5.2 cm in the left ventricular lateral-posterior wall. C. A cardiac MRI scan showed a large lesion with the size of 8.5×8.3×5.9 cm in the pericardium connected with the left ventricular and left atrial wall. D. Histological section shows mature adipose tissue intermixed with myocardium, and thinning fibrous connective tissue surrounding it.

The signals within the lesion were homogeneous in Double IR T1 and T2 images. The T1 weighted image revealed homogenous signal intensity as well as a loss of signal due to fat tissue. Diffusion-weighted MRI imaging revealed that the signals of lesion was low. The characteristics of a mass revealed by MRI are consistent with the diagnosis of a large cardiac lipoma derived from myocardial tissue.

Hospital Course

An 8×5 cm mass was found in the posterior wall of left ventricle, commencing from the myocardium and partially embedded LAD, LCX coronary arteries, which could not be fully removed. Partially excision was performed during open heart surgery. The patient recovered well and was discharged from hospital.

Pathological Findings

Histological section shows mature adipose tissue intermixed with myocardium, and thinning fibrous connective tissue surrounding it (Figure 35-2D). The pathological diagnosis was lipoma of the left ventricular wall.

Discussion

Cardiac lipomas are rare, benign tumors composed of adipose tissue. These tumors are usually found in adults but can affect patients of all ages. Most of them cause no symptoms but a few can have a detrimental effect on myocardial function as well as displacing and encasing the coronary arteries [1].

Cardiac lipomas have been associated with a variety of arrhythmias, including atrial fibrillation [2], ventricular tachycardia [3], and atrioventricular block [4]. There were episodes of ventricular tachycardia in our case.

Echocardiography is the primary modality for imaging intracardiac disease. It provides high-resolution, real-time images, the quality of which has further improved with the introduction of new ultrasonographic imaging techniques such as tissue harmonics [5]. However, as image acquisition with CT and MR imaging has steadily become faster, these modalities have played an increasingly important role in the evaluation of cardiac neoplasms. Although spatial and temporal resolution are far lower with these modalities than with echocardiography, the soft-tissue contrast of both CT and MR imaging is superior to that of echocardiography, and both modalities allow imaging of the entire mediastinum and evaluation of the extracardiac extent of disease.

Cardiac lipomas manifest on CT as homogeneous, low-attenuation masses either in a cardiac chamber or in the pericardial space. Both CT and MR imaging can help identify fat with a high degree of specificity and can therefore be used to diagnose cardiac lipomas without equivocation. For this reason, reports of cardiac lipomas over the past 10–15 years have tended to emphasize the role of CT and MR imaging and go into detail about the imaging features of these tumors [1]. With MR imaging, lipomas have homogeneous increased signal intensity on T1-weighted images, which decreases with fat-saturated sequences. They may have a few thin septations but no soft-tissue component. Like soft-tissue lipomas, cardiac lipomas do not enhance with the administration of contrast material.

Unlike MR imaging, CT is capable of helping detect calcification, which is an important variable in the differential diagnosis of cardiac neoplasms. In addition, CT is faster, easier to perform, and generally has more reliable image quality. Magnetic resonance imaging has better soft-tissue contrast than CT and allows much greater flexibility in the selection of imaging planes.

Key Points

1. Cardiac lipomas are rare, benign tumors composed of adipose tissue.
2. Most of cases with cardiac lipomas have no symptom; some of them may have a variety of arrhythmias. Including atrial fibrillation, ventricular tachycardia and atrioventricular block.
3. Cardiac imaging modalities are the most important diagnosis tools.

References

1. Araoz, P.A., Mulvaqh, S.L., Tazelaar, H.D. et al. (2000). CT and MR Imaging of benign primary cardiac neoplasms with echocardiographic correlation. *RadioGraphics* 20: 1303–1319.
2. Grande, A.M., Minzioni, G., Pederzolli, C. et al. (1998) Cardiac lipoma description of three cases. *J Cardiovasc Surg* 39: 813–815.
3. Conces, D.J., Jr, Vix, V.A. and Tarver, R.D. (1989). Diagnosis of a myocardial lipoma by using CT. *Am J Roentgenol* 153: 725–726.
4. Vanderheyden, M., De Sutter, J., Wellens, F. et al. (1998). Left atrial lipoma: Case report and review of the literature. *Acta Cardiol* 53: 31–32.
5. Thomas, J.D. and Rubin, D.N. (1998). Tissue harmonic imaging: why does it work? *Am Soc Echocardiogr* 11: 803–808.

36 Primary Cardiac Pheochromocytoma

Ligang Fang[1], Jing Ping Sun[2], and Yining Wang[1]

[1] Affiliated Hospital of Peking Union Medical College, Beijing, China
[2] The Chinese University of Hong Kong, Hong Kong

History

A 51-year-old man presented with intermittent hypertension, palpitation, and excessive sweating.

Physical Examination

Supine blood pressure was 130/90 mmHg. Orthostatic blood pressure was 90/60 mmHg. Heart rate was 62 bpm. There were no pathological heart murmurs.

Laboratory

Both plasma and urinary catecholamine levels were significantly elevated. 131-I-Metaiodobenzylguanidine scintigraphy was positive.

Echocardiography

A mass was noted between the right and left atriums (Figure 36-1A) in the subcostal short-axis view.

Computed Tomography

The computed tomography scan of bilateral adrenal glands was normal. The contrast enhanced CT showed the tumor located at the root of the aorta, between the left atrium and right atrium (Figure 36-1B).

Coronary angiography showed that the majority of the blood supply to the mass was from the branch of the RCA and a minority from the branch of the LCX (Figure 36-1C).

Hospital Course

Cardiac surgery was performed in accordance with the clinical and laboratory findings. The mass was a cardiac paraganglioma between left and right atrium, which was completely resected.

Pathology

The immunohistochemical staining of lesion showed chromogranin A (CgA) staining positive.

Comparative Cardiac Imaging: A Case-based Guide, First Edition.
Edited by Jing Ping Sun, Xing Sheng Yang, and Bryan P. Yan.
© 2018 John Wiley & Sons Ltd. Published 2018 by John Wiley & Sons Ltd.
Companion website: www.wiley.com/sun/comparative_cardiac_imaging

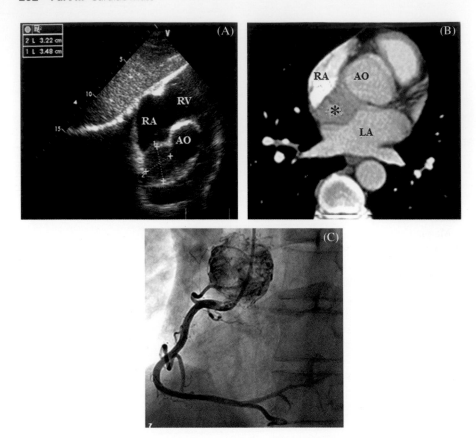

Figure 36-1   A. Two-dimensional echocardiography. A subcostal short axis view showed a mass between the right atrium and the left atrium. B. Contrast-enhanced computed tomography showed a tumor located between the left atrium and right atrium. C. The coronary angiography showed the majority of the blood supply to the mass was from the branch of the right coronary artery.

At follow-up 12 months after operation, the patient was symptom free, the blood pressure was normal, and the 24 hours urine catecholamine levels were within the normal range.

Discussion

Pheochromocytomas are tumors of the sympathetic nervous system arising from chromaffin cells. In adults the majority of these masses are located in the adrenal medulla, where chromaffin cells are concentrated. Small amounts of these cells can exist in the walls of blood vessels, mainly the aorta, and scattered through organs like the ovaries, prostate, and heart [1]. Cardiac pheochromocytomas produce large amounts of catecholamine, particularly norepinephrine [2]. These tumors occur in less than 0.1% of hypertensive patients [3].

Clinical Features

Pheochromocytoma present with a variety of symptoms. In a review of 30 cases [2], the most common presentation of pheochromocytoma was hypertension, and dyspnea accounted for only three cases. Our patient displayed intermittent hypertension, palpitations, and excessive sweating at the time of presentation, which are common symptoms of this disease.

Diagnosis

The diagnostic tests includes two-dimensional and transesophageal echocardiographic studies [4], coronary angiography, magnetic resonance imaging, CT, and 131-I-metaiodobenzylguanidine scintigraphy. Ultrasound can have a variable appearance ranging from solid to mixed cystic and solid to cystic [5].

Computed tomography is the first imaging modality to be used, with an overall sensitivity of 89%. This is on account of 98% of tumors being located within the abdomen and 90% limited to the adrenal glands [6]. They are usually large, heterogeneous masses with areas of necrosis and cystic change.

Magnetic resonance imaging is the most sensitive modality for identification of pheochromocytoma and is particularly useful in cases of extra-adrenal location. The overall sensitivity is said to be 98% [6].

In the heart, most of the tumors reported are intimally associated with the left atrial wall originating from the visceral autonomic paraganglia of the atrium. The tumor described in our case was between left and right atrium, which was cardiac paraganglioma confirmed by histology.

Treatment and Prognosis

The definitive treatment is surgical, and if complete resection is achieved, without metastases, then surgery is curative, and hypertension usually resolves.

Preoperative medical management is essential in reducing the risk of intraoperative hypertensive crises and typically consists of a noncompetitive alpha adrenergic blockade (e.g. phenoxybenzamine). Later, but never before 7–10 days of alpha blockade, a beta-blocker may need to be added to control tachycardia or some arrhythmias [6]. Adequate preoperative preparation with adrenergic blockers might not prevent serious intraoperative hypertension or high peripheral vascular resistance during cardiopulmonary bypass. Fortunately, our patient underwent the surgery smoothly after adequate preoperative preparation with phenoxybenzamine.

In our case, coronary angiography was performed to determine the blood supply of the tumor, which is important to guide the surgical procedures.

Key Points

1. One of the more unusual benign tumours affecting the heart is pheochromocytoma
2. Surgical excision during cardiopulmonary bypass is the treatment of choice, and cure is the usual result.

References

1. Shapiro, B., Sisson, J., Kalff, V. et al. (1984). The location of middle mediastinal pheochromocytomas. *J Thorac Cardiovasc Surg* 87: 814–820.
2. Jebara, V.A., Uva, M.A., Farge, A. et al. (1992). Cardiac pheochromocytomas. *Ann Thorac Surg* 53: 356–361.

3. Lee, H.H., Brenner, W.I., Vardhan, I. et al. (1990). Cardiac pheochromocytoma originating in the interatrial septum. *Chest* 97: 760–762.

4. David, T.E., Lenkei, S.C., Marquez Julio, A. et al. (1986). Pheochromocytoma of the heart. *Ann Throrac Surg* 41: 98–100.

5. Leung, K., Stamm, M., Raja, A. et al. (2013). Pheochromocytoma: The range of appearances on ultrasound, CT, MRI, and functional imaging. *Am J Roentgenol* 200 (2): 370–378.

6. Blake1, M.A., Cronin, C.G.. and Boland, G W. (2010). Adrenal imaging. *Am J Roentgenol* 194 (6): 1450–1460.

37 Cardiac Rhabdomyosarcoma of the Left Atrium

Lan Ma[1], Ming Chen[2], and Jing Ping Sun[3]

[1] Jiaotong University, Shanghai, China
[2] Tongji University School of Medicine, Shanghai, China
[3] The Chinese University of Hong Kong, Hong Kong

History

A 27-year-old man complained of frequent chest pain and recurrent syncope for three months.

Physical Examination

He was in mild respiratory distress with a respiratory rate of 20/min, and a heart rate of 94 bpm, regular in rhythm. His blood pressure was 120/70 mm Hg. Cardiac auscultation revealed a distinct early diastolic click followed by a grade 2/5 diastolic decrescendo murmur at the apex that was variable in character with postural changes. A grade 2/6 systolic ejection murmur was heard at the left lower sternal border.

Transthoracic Echocardiography

Transthoracic echocardiography showed a large mass with blood flow within the left atrial chamber, protruding into the left ventricular cavity and obstructing mitral inflow during diastole (Figure 37-1A and B, Videos 37-1 and 37-2).

Hospital Course

In view of severe mitral valve obstruction by the atrial mass, surgical removal of the tumor was recommended. During operation, the patient was found to have pericardial effusion; an irregular tumor mass measuring $5 \times 6 \times 6$ cm was found attached to the roof of left atrium, with adhesions to the left atrial posterior and lateral walls. The tumor almost filled the entire left atrium and extended across the mitral valve orifice. The mass was removed by clean dissection along the atrial wall; the mitral valve appeared normal without gross evidence of tumor invasion. On surgical inspection, the surface of the posterior atrial wall where the tumor attached appeared to be slightly roughened; no tumor permeation of the atrium wall was evident. There was also no evidence of intramyocardial or pericardial spread of the tumor mass.

Comparative Cardiac Imaging: A Case-based Guide, First Edition.
Edited by Jing Ping Sun, Xing Sheng Yang, and Bryan P. Yan.
© 2018 John Wiley & Sons Ltd. Published 2018 by John Wiley & Sons Ltd.
Companion website: www.wiley.com/sun/comparative_cardiac_imaging

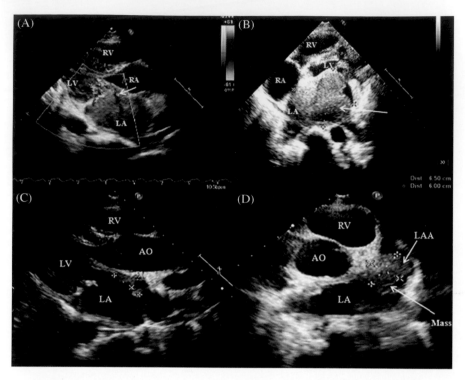

Figure 37-1   Echocardiography: A. Parasternal long-axis view showed a huge mass occupying most of the left atrium, with blood flow within the tumor on color-Doppler examination. B. Modified four-chamber view showed the mass protruding into the left ventricle during diastole. C. On postoperative day 38, a parasternal long-axis view of echocardiography revealed a small mass attached to the atrial septum. D. A modified parasternal short-axis view showed another mass in the left atrial appendage.

Pathology

Gross appearance of the excised tumor showing hemorrhagic and necrotic areas. Histology revealed roundish tumor cells with pleomorphic nuclei and large eosinophilic cytoplasm that are typical of rhabdomyosarcoma. (Figure 37-2).

Predischarge echocardiography showed normal ventricular function, no significant dysfunction of the cardiac valves, and the left atrium appeared to be clean without residual tumor. The patient was symptom free and discharged 10 days after the operation.

The patient did well after discharge and returned for a follow up 38 days post operation. At this time, echocardiography revealed a recurrent small echodense mass attached to atrial septum and another bigger mass in the left atrial appendage (Figure 37-1C; Video 37-3). These two masses were progressively enlarged in size on echocardiography performed 54 days postoperatively (Figure 37-1C and D, Video 37-4). There are several soft tissue masses in the left atrium demonstrated by CT 60 days after operation, which suggested recurrence of the tumor. A. A CTA four-chamber view showed three masses in the left atrium. B. A CTA short-axis view showed several masses in the left atrium. (Figure 37-3).

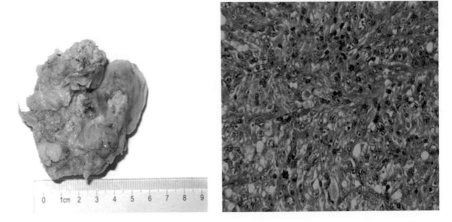

Figure 37-2 Left. Gross appearance of the excised tumor showing hemorrhagic and necrotic areas. Right. Histology revealed roundish tumor cells with pleomorphic nuclei and large eosinophilic cytoplasm that are typical of rhabdomyosarcoma. Histological examination of the excised tumor mass revealed typical features of a rhabdomyosarcoma.

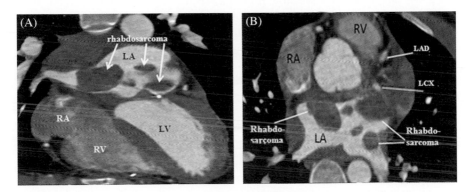

Figure 37-3 There are several soft tissue masses in the left atrium demonstrated by CT 60 days after operation, which suggested recurrence of the tumor. A. A CTA four-chamber view showed three masses in the left atrium. B. A CTA short-axis view showed several masses in the left atrium.

Discussion

Primary malignant cardiac rhabdomyosarcoma is a rare neoplasm that has been reported in all age groups and occurs with similar frequency in both males and females [1]. The usual location of this tumor in order of frequency is right atrium, left atrium and both ventricles [2]. Rhabdomyosarcomas usually originate intramurally, sometimes protruding into cardiac chambers, causing obstruction [3]. The mass in our patient originated in the left atrium and protruded through the mitral valve, causing mechanical obstruction to the left ventricular inflow, clinically mimicking mitral stenosis with a low-pitched diastolic murmur, manifested clinically as recurrent syncope that was indicative of intermittent cardiac and brain ischemia. Tumor invasion to the right side of the heart can mimic tricuspid or pulmonary valve diseases with clinical presentation of right heart failure. Tumor metastases are usually found in the lung, liver, thoracic lymph nodes, and pancreas. Occasionally, cardiac rhabdomyosarcoma can present with cerebral embolism [4].

Echocardiographic (ECHO) findings can provide diagnosis, while electrocardiography and X-ray findings can be nonspecific [5]. Echocardiography is very useful in revealing the location of the tumor mass, and confirming the normal structure of mitral valve.

Cardiac magnetic resonance imaging (MRI) and computed tomography (CT) are used for diagnostic purposes. Signal intensity characteristics at MR imaging are variable. Isointensity relative to the myocardium [6] as well as heterogeneous signal intensity and contrast material enhancement have been reported [7]. In one study, necrotic areas appeared at MR imaging as a large defect in communication with the pericardial space [7]. Computed tomography may show a smooth [8] or irregular [9] low-attenuation mass in a cardiac chamber. Extracardiac extension is clearly depicted at CT and MR imaging. Extension into the pulmonary arteries has been demonstrated at CT [6], and MR imaging has been used to delineate invasion of the pulmonary artery [10], descending aorta [11], and pulmonary valve [6].

Before surgery, differentiation between benign and malignant tumors is important but sometimes difficult. The most common benign cardiac tumor is the atrial myxoma, which may be accompanied by systemic embolization mimicking the metastasis of malignant tumors. In our case, atrial myxoma was initially suspected. However, atrial myxoma are typically more mobile because of its attachment to the atrial septum through a stalk, as compared to a malignant tumor that may have a more broad-based adhesion to the chamber walls which may be at multiple sites. Moreover, the highly vascular nature demonstrated by color-Doppler flows within the tumor mass is more suggestive of a vascularized malignant tumor rather than a myxoma. This case illustrated the role of echocardiography in differentiating malignant tumor mass from benign atrial tumor before surgery. Echocardiographic contrast perfusion imaging aids in the differentiation of cardiac masses. Compared with the adjacent myocardium, malignant and vascular tumors hyper-enhanced, whereas stromal tumors and thrombi hypo-enhanced [12].

Surgical resection, when possible, is the treatment of choice for all primary cardiac tumors in which effective palliation is possible with resection of malignant tumors. There is no consensus on adjuvant chemotherapy or radiotherapy. Case reports indicate that certain histological subtypes may benefit from adjuvant therapy, although there is no standard chemotherapy regimen recommended.

In our case, the mass was surgically resected. The patient was symptom free after the operation; unfortunately, this malignant tumor recurred after a short period.

Key Points

1. Primary malignant cardiac rhabdomyosarcoma is a rare neoplasm that has been reported in all age groups.
2. Echocardiographic (ECHO) findings can provide diagnosis; extracardiac extension can be clearly depicted with CT and MR imaging.

References

1. Kramer, S., Meadows, A. T., Jarrett, P. et al. (1983). Incidence of childhood cancer: experience of a decade in a population-based registry. *J Natl Cancer Inst* 70: 49–55.
2. McAllister, H.A. (1979). Primary tumors and cysts of the heart and pericardium. *Curr Probl Cardiol* 4 (2): 350–352.

3. Chaudron, J.M.S., Saint Remy, J.M., Schmitz, A. et al (1977). Right atrium rhabdomyosarcoma. *Acta Cardiol* 32: 75–81.
4. Mata, M., Wharton, M., Geisinger, K. et al. (1981). Myocardial rhabdomyosarcoma in multiple neurofibromatosis. *Neurology* 31: 1549–1551.
5. Chen, H.Z., Jiang, L., Rong, W.H. et al. (1992). Tumors of the heart. An analysis of 79 cases. *Chin Med J (Engl)* 105: 153–158.
6. Wantanabe, A.T., Teitelbaum, G.P., Henderson, R.W. et al. (1989). Magnetic resonance imaging of cardiac sarcomas. *J Thorac Imaging* 4: 90–92.
7. Siripornpitak, S. and Higgins, C.B. (1997). MRI of primary malignant cardiovascular tumors. *J Comput Assist Tomogr* 21: 462–466.
8. Rheeder, P., Simson, I.W., Mentis, H. et al. (1995) Cardiac rhabdomyosarcoma in a renal transplant patient. *Transplantation* 60: 204–205.
9. Jack, C.M., Cleland, J. and Geddes, J.S. (1986). Left atrial rhabdomyosarcoma and the use of digital gated computed tomography in its diagnosis. *Br Heart J* 55: 305–307.
10. Satoh, M., Horimoto, M., Sakurai, K. et al. (1990). Primary cardiac rhabdomyosarcoma exhibiting transient and pronounced regression with chemotherapy. *Am Heart J* 120:1458–1460.
11. Szucs, R.A., Reher, R.B., Yanovich, S. et al. (1991). Magnetic resonance imaging of cardiac rhabdomyosarcoma: quantifying the response to therapy. *Cancer* 67: 2066–2070.
12. Kirkpatrick, J.N., Wong, T., Bednarz, J.E. et al. (2004). Differential diagnosis of cardiac masses using contrast echocardiographic perfusion imaging. *J Am Coll Cardiol* 43 (8): 1412–1419.

38 Unusual Cardiac Fibroelastoma

Fanxia Meng[1], Ming Chen[1], and Jing Ping Sun[2]

[1] Tongji University School of Medicine, Shanghai, China
[2] The Chinese University of Hong Kong, Hong Kong

History

A 12-year-old boy presented with paroxysmal chest pain for 2 months, and a sudden onset of syncope, which lasted about 2 minutes.

Physical Examination

The patient was well developed. There was a diastloic murmur at the left fourth intercostal space.

Echocardiography

The parasternal long-axis view showed an echo-dense mass attached to the left ventricular anterior papillary muscle, extending to the anterior mitral valvular chordae, the left ventricular outflow tract (LVOT), and the aortic root (Figure 38-1A; Video 38-1). The apical five-chamber view demonstrated the mass in the LVOT extending into aortic root through the aortic valves (Figure 38-1B). The apical four-chamber view illustrated that the mass was on the mitral valvular chordae and papillary muscle (Figure 38-1C, D; Video 38-2). The series of parasternal long-axis views showed the mass in the aortic root was close to the orifice of the right coronary artery (RCA) and swung into the RCA dur- ing the cardiac circle (Figure 38-2; Video 38-1). The left ventricular function was normal with an ejection fraction of 61%.

Cardiac Computed Tomography (CT)

A coronal view showed that a big mass with a long tail extended from left mid-ventricle via the LVOT into the ascending aorta through the aortic valve (Figure 38-3A, white and black arrows). The CT cardiac long axis view clearly illustrated that the mass on the papillary muscle extended to the mitral valvular chordae, and appeared in the aortic root, invading into the right Valsalva sinus (Figure 38-3B). The CT short-axis view showed that the mass was on the papillary muscle and mitral valvular chordae (Figure 38-3C).

Comparative Cardiac Imaging: A Case-based Guide, First Edition.
Edited by Jing Ping Sun, Xing Sheng Yang, and Bryan P. Yan.
© 2018 John Wiley & Sons Ltd. Published 2018 by John Wiley & Sons Ltd.
Companion website: www.wiley.com/sun/comparative_cardiac_imaging

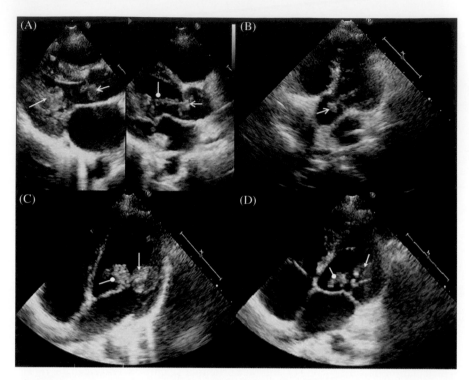

Figure 38-1 A. The parasternal long-axis view showed an echo-dense mass attached to the left ventricular anterior papillary muscle (arrows), extended to the anterior mitral valvular chordae (oval arrows), LVOT, and aortic root (open arrows). B. The apical five-chamber view demonstrated the mass in the LVOT extended into the aortic root through the aortic valves. C and D. The apical four-chamber view illustrated that the mass was on the mitral valvular chordae and papillary muscle.

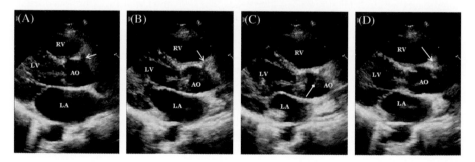

Figure 38-2 The series of parasternal long axis views (A, B, C, D) illustrated the mass (diamond arrows) in aortic root was closed to the orifice of RCA (open arrows) and swung into the RCA during cardiac circle.

Surgery

During operation, the surgeon found one large frond-like appearance, resembling a sea anemone mass on the papillary muscle with a long tail, which extended to the anterior mitral valvular chordae, LVOT, to the aortic root through the aortic valve (Figure 38-4 and Figure 38-5). Part of the mass in the aortic root invaded into the RCA.

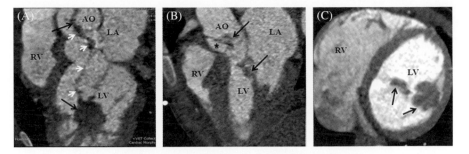

Figure 38-3 A. Cardiac CT coronal view showed a big mass with a long tail (white arrows) extended from left mid-ventricular via LVOT into the ascending aorta through the aortic valve. B. The CT cardiac long axis view clearly illustrated the mass on the papillary muscle, extended to the mitral valvular chordae, and appeared in the aortic root, invaded into right Valsalva sinus (*). C. The CT short-axis view showed the mass was on the papillary muscle and mitral valvular chordae.

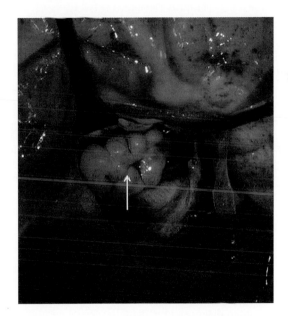

Figure 38-4 The appearance of the cardiac mass (arrow) during operation.

Pathology

The histological diagnosis of the mass was cardiac papillary fibroelastoma (CPF).

Discussion

Cardiac papillary fibroelastoma (CPF) is a rare primary cardiac neoplasm of unknown prevalence [1]. Since the introduction of echocardiography, the diagnosis of these tumors in living patients has been reported sporadically. The largest report of a pathologically confirmed CPF includes 162 patients [2]. The echocardiographic characteristics include the following: (i) the tumor is round, oval, or irregular in appearance, with

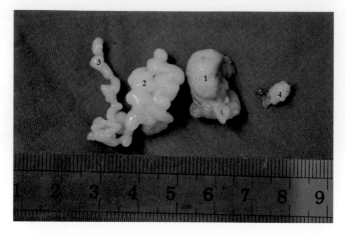

Figure 38-5 The gross appearance of the mass. Part 1 was on the papillary muscle. Part 2 was on the mitral valvular chordae. Part 3 was in the LVOT. Part 4 was in the aortic root.

well-demarcated borders and a homogeneous texture; (ii) most CPFs are small (99% were < 20 mm in the largest dimension); (iii) nearly half of CPFs had small stalks, and those with stalks were mobile; (iv) CPFs may be single or multiple lesions and are most often associated with cardiac valvular disease [2].

Approximately 90% of the CPFs reported in the literature were attached to valves [2–4] and the majority were on the aortic valve [2, 3]. For the aortic valve, no predilection for the tumor to appear on the aortic or the ventricular side has been reported [4]. In the largest study, 49 of the 110 CPFs (44.5%) were attached to the aortic valve, predominantly on the aortic side. This common location of the tumor suggests a potential for dynamic coronary ostial obstruction leading to myocardial ischemia [2]. The mitral valve was the next most common location of involvement in published data, with tumors occurring on the anterior or posterior leaflets, the chordae, and the papillary muscles [2]. Tumors arising from the right atrium are described in only three cases [3, 5]. It is readily apparent that the lower rate of right-sided detection is likely due to a lack of symptoms from right-sided embolization and under-reporting due to uncommon excision of right-sided valves or entry to the right heart.

Although CPFs are often diagnosed incidentally, neurological events, sudden death, angina, acute myocardial infarction, pulmonary emboli, and retinal artery embolism related to CPF have been reported [6–8]. With the increased use of 2D TTE, CPF are detected during life and are occasionally found in patients without symptoms.

Echocardiography is a convenient and noninvasive diagnostic technique and should be the first choice of tests to search for CPFs. Transesophageal echocardiography (TEE) is an important tool for delineating the extent and anatomic attachment of these small tumors because only this technique allows optimal high-resolution imaging. However, many CPFs go undetected by echocardiography. The reasons echocardiography may fail to diagnose tumors include the following: (i) the tumor was masked by an associated lesion; (ii) the tumor was too small to be seen; (iii) the examination was not done carefully with a sufficient index of suspicion; or (iv) there were no significant characteristics to differentiate the CPF from the degenerative valve disease [2].

Computed tomography imaging has the advantage to show a complete picture and the relation with the surrounding strictures. In our case, CT imaging showed a big mass with a long tail extended from left mid-ventricular via LVOT into the ascending aorta through the aortic valve, which indicates that this is one mass.

Management

On the basis of our previous findings and a review of the literature, we recommend the following guidelines for the assessment and management of patients with CPF. Patients with events that may be embolic in nature and are not explained by other cardiovascular or neurological diseases should undergo TTE and TEE if necessary to exclude cardiac sources of emboli, including CPF. A mass seen by echocardiography should be characterized by size, shape, location of attachment, mobility, presence of a stalk, and multiplicity. Although the differential diagnosis may still include vegetation (infective or noninfective), thrombi, degenerative valve tissue, and other benign tumors, these lesions can often be differentiated by clinical information, blood cultures, and laboratory tests. Because the presence of a stalk and associated mobility is a significant predictor of embolic risk, patients with presumed CPF, especially if left-sided, should undergo TEE to determine if a stalk is present.

Decisions regarding the primary surgical excision of CPF depend on the size, location, mobility, and potential or strength of association of the tumor with symptoms. Excision of isolated right-sided CPFs is indicated only for large mobile tumors, including those that result in obstruction or embolization that is hemodynamically significant. The presence of a patent foramen ovale with a sizeable right-to-left shunt is an additional consideration for management of right-sided CPF. Asymptomatic patients with small, left-sided, nonmobile (no stalk) CPFs are usually observed. However, larger (≥1 cm) CPFs, especially if mobile, should be considered for excision, especially if other cardiovascular disease is detected or the patient is young, with low risk of surgery and a high cumulative risk for embolization. Patients with residual tumors who have had an embolic event should similarly be considered for excision, depending on the risks of surgery and other cardiovascular indications. Isolated CPF excision of aortic or mitral valve lesions can often be performed through a minimally invasive approach, with no damage to the valve. Incidentally detected CPFs in patients undergoing cardiac surgery should generally be removed unless they add substantial time and risk to the operation that cannot be justified based on size, location, and mobility.

In this case, a CPF presented as a large tumor that extended into multiple structures in the heart, which is very rare. This irregular tumor was well demarcated and homogenous on echocardiography, and its characteristics could be differentiated from malignant tumors, which are rich in blood vessels. This teenage boy had angina, which could be due to a temporary obstruction of RCA by the mass in aortic root. The surgery was performed successfully without any complications.

Key Points

1. Although symptoms related to fibroelastomas are uncommon, there is a potential for serious morbidity, particularly among patients with large, mobile, left-sided lesions.

2. The presence of tumors should be determined in patients with symptomatic unexplained cardiac or neurological events. Consideration for surgical excision should be given to those patients, whether asymptomatic or symptomatic – especially those with a high cumulative risk of embolization and a low risk for surgery.
3. Although a CPF is a histologically benign tumor, it may result in life-threatening complications, such as stroke, myocardial infarction, pulmonary embolism and sudden death, although the frequency with which that occurs is not well established.

References

1. Burke, A. and Virmani, R. (1996). Tumors of the heart and great vessels. In: *Atlas of Tumor Pathology*, Third Series, 47–54. Washington DC: Armed Forces Institute of Pathology.
2. Sun, J.P., Asher, C.R., Yang, X.S. et al. (2001). Clinical and echocardiographic characteristics of papillary fibroelastomas: A retrospective and prospective study in 162 patients. Circulation 103: 2687–2693.
3. McAllister, H.A. Jr. and Fengolio, J.J. Jr. (1978). Papillary fibroelastoma. In: *Tumors of the Cardiovascular System* (ed. B.H. Landing), 20–25. Washington DC: Armed Forces Institute of Pathology.
4. Edward, F.H., Hale, D., Cohen, A., et al. (1991). Primary cardiac valve tumors. *Ann Thorac Surg* 52: 1127–1131.
5. Gallas, M.T., Reardon, M.J., Reardon, P.R., et al. (1993). Papillary fibroelastoma: A right atrial presentation. Texas Heart Inst J 20: 293–295.
6. Gowda, R.M., Khan, I.A., Nair, C.K. et al. (2003). Cardiac papillary fibroelastoma: A comprehensive analysis of 725 cases. *American Heart Journal* 146 (3): 404–410.
7. Boone, S., Higginson Lyall, A.J., Walley, V.M. (1992). Endothelial papillary fibroelastomas arising in and around the aortic sinus, filling the ostium of the right coronary artery. *Arch Pathol Lab Med* 116: 135–137.
8. Zamora, R.L., Adelberg, D.A., Berger, A.S. et al. (1995). Branch retinal artery occlusion caused by a mitral valve papillary. fibroelastoma. *Ophthalmology* 119: 325–329.

39 Pulmonary and Cardiac Inflammatory Myofibroblastic Tumor

Yong Jiang[1], Hao Wang[1], and Jing Ping Sun[2]

[1] Fuwai Hospital, Beijing, China
[2] The Chinese University of Hong Kong, Hong Kong

History

A 9-year-old girl was admitted to hospital because of exertional dyspnea.

Physical Examination

She was in mild respiratory distress with a respiratory rate of 34/minute, and a heart rate of 100 bpm, regular in rhythm. Her blood pressure was 94/62 mm Hg. Cardiac auscultation revealed a distinct early diastolic click followed by a grade 2/5 diastolic decrescendo murmur at the apex, which was variable in character with postural changes.

Electrocardiogram

The ECG showed sinus rhythm, left atrium enlargement demonstrated by bifid P wave with >40 ms between the two peaks and a total P-wave duration of >110 ms in lead II. A biphasic P wave was seen with a terminal negative portion that was >40 ms in duration and >1 mm deep in V_1.

Chest X-ray

This showed an irregular shadow seen at the lower left of the parahilar. Pulmonary texture was significant; the aortic node was widened; the pulmonary artery segment straight; the cardiothoracic ratio was increased (Figure 39-1).

Transthoracic Echocardiography

The parasternal long-axis view revealed a large mass with clear boundary in the left atrial chamber, protruding into the left ventricular cavity through the mitral annulus during diastole, and obstructing the mitral inflow (Figure 39-2A; Video 39-1). An atypical four-chamber view showed a mass in the left atrium and connected with mass in the dilated left lower pulmonary vein (Figure 39-2B; Video 39-2).

Magnetic Resonance Imaging (MRI) Magnetic resonance imaging four-chamber view showed the mass was smooth and lobulated, one part located in the left atrium, which was connected with another part in the left lung through the left lower pulmonary

---

Comparative Cardiac Imaging: A Case-based Guide, First Edition.
Edited by Jing Ping Sun, Xing Sheng Yang, and Bryan P. Yan.
© 2018 John Wiley & Sons Ltd. Published 2018 by John Wiley & Sons Ltd.
Companion website: www.wiley.com/sun/comparative_cardiac_imaging

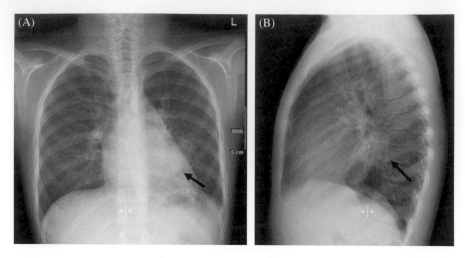

Figure 39-1 Chest X-ray. A. Posterior-anterior view showed that the cardiothoracic ratio was increased, and a high density was noted behind the heart (arrow). B. A left lateral view showed an enlarged left atrium and an abnormally high density (arrow) at the region of the lower left pulmonary hilar.

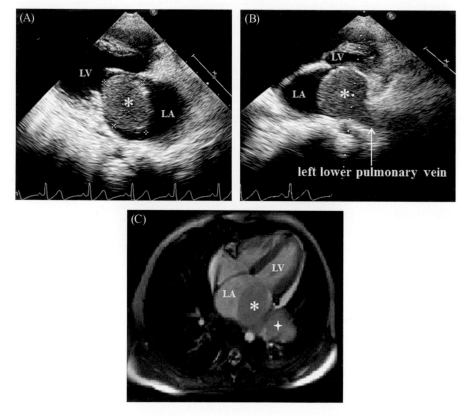

Figure 39-2 A. An echocardiographic parasternal long-axis view showed a mass (*) in the left atrium and a blocked left ventricular inflow tract. B. An atypical four-chamber view showed a mass (*) in the left atrium connected with mass in the left lower pulmonary vein. C. MRI 4-chamber imaging showed a mass (*) in the left atrium and connected with mass in the left lung.

vein (Figure 39-2C; Video 39-3). The precontrast T1WI showed that the tumor was substantially uniform and significantly enhanced by early and late contrast infusion.

Operation

According to the examination results, the primary diagnosis was cardiac malignant tumor, and a surgical resection of the tumor was performed.

Pathology

The pathology gross examination revealed that the left lung lower lobe and left atrial tumor were in a dumb-bell shape with a smooth surface, and clear boundary but no capsule; the larger part was in the left atrium, its size was 3.5 cm × 2.5 cm, the small part was in the lung, its size was 1.0 cm × 1.0 cm × 0.5 cm. The tumor sections were homogeneous solid, gray white, and hard (Figure 39-3, left and middle). Histologic examination revealed that the tumor consisted of spindle-shaped cells and myxoid stroma with infiltration of lymphocytes, plasma cells, and monocyte inflammatory cells (Figure 39-3, right). The results of pathology examination were consistent with inflammatory myofibroblastic tumor.

After the operation, the patient recovered smoothly. She was in good condition including normal echocardiographic examination at the follow up visit after one year.

Discussion

An inflammatory myofibroblastic tumor (IMT) of the heart is rare, with fewer than 60 cases being reported in the literature under various designations, including IMT, plasma cell granuloma, inflammatory pseudotumor, and inflammatory fibrosarcoma [1]. An IMT is considered a low-grade neoplasm. The recent classification of the World Health Organization recognized the uncertainty of its biological nature – that is, its clinical features might resemble malignant neoplasia. Up to now, the recurrence rate of pulmonary IMT has been low. However, the local recurrence rate of extrapulmonary IMT is up to

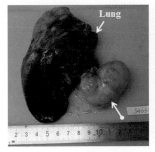 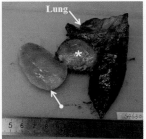 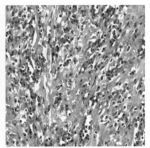

Figure 39-3 Pathology: Left. Gross examination: left lung lower lobe and left atrial tumor with smooth surface, size of 3.5 cm × 2.5 cm. Middle: Gross examination: the left inferior pulmonary vein and left lower lung hilum, and mass with dumbbell shape and clear boundary but no capsule; the larger part was in the left atrium, the small part was in the lung, its size was 1.0 cm × 1.0 cm × 0.5 cm. The tumor sections were homogeneous solid, gray white, and hard. Right: Histologic examination revealed the tumor consisted of spindle-shaped cells and myxoid stroma with infiltration of lymphocytes, plasma cells, and monocyte inflammatory cells.

25 % [2]. Although the majority of cardiac tumors followed a benign course after surgical resection, sudden unexpected death due to cardiac IMT has been reported in five cases, including two cases as a results of a tumor occluding coronary artery [3, 4]. The possibility of recurrence and the long-term prognosis after cardiac surgery have not been determined due to the rarity of these lesions. The recurrence of inflammatory myofibroblastic tumors in the left atrium was reported in a case who received cardiac surgery for complete resection of inflammatory myofibroblastic but died suddenly due to a left atrial tumor that protruded into the left ventricle through the mitral annulus during diastole 5 months after surgery [5].

As cardiac IMT may be potentially fatal if a cardiac valve or the coronary arteries are involved, whenever feasible, a complete surgical resection of the tumor remains the mainstay of treatment and seems to have a satisfactory outcome. The patients should be closely followed up including regular echocardiography, even if they were asymptomatic after surgical resection of cardiac IMT.

We report a very rare case of a patient with exertional dyspnea caused by obstruction of the mitral inflow by a large IMT in the left atrium. The echocardiographic image indicated that the tumor extended to the lung via its connection at the dilated left lower pulmonary vein, which was confirmed by cardiac magnetic resonance imaging. In fact, the operative finding indicated that the tumor originated from the pulmonary vein, which extended into the left atrium. The diagnosis of IMT was confirmed by histopathology. The tumor was successfully removed by surgery, and the patient was in good condition at the 1 year follow up. To the best of our knowledge, this is the first case of a cardiac IMT connected to another part of the tumor in the left lower lung.

Our case indicates that the cardiac imaging is very useful for the diagnosis of cardiac tumors. Echocardiography is readily available and relatively inexpensive, and cardiac magnetic resonance imaging or CT can be used as complementary imaging.

Key Points

1. Inflammatory myofibroblastic tumor (IMT) of the heart is rare but might have potentially catastrophic consequences such as sudden death or acute heart failure.
2. Complete surgical resection of the tumor remains the mainstay of treatment for inflammatory myofibroblastic tumor.
3. To prevent the recurrence of the tumor, patients should be closely followed up including with echocardiography after surgery.

Reference

1. Sunbul, M., Cagac, O. and Birkan, Y. (2013). A rare case of inflammatory pseudotumor with both involvement of lung and heart. *Thorac Cardiovasc Surg* 61 (7): 646–648.
2. Coffin, C.M., Watterson, J., Priest, J.R. et al. (1995). Extrapulmonary inflammatory myofibroblastic tumor (inflammatory pseudotumor). A clinicopathologic and immunohistochemical study of 84 cases. *Am J Surg Pathol* 19: 859–872.
3. Li, L., Burke, A., He, J. et al. (2011). Sudden unexpected death due to inflammatory myofibroblastic tumor of the heart: A case report and review of the literature. *Int J Legal Med* 125 (1): 81–85.
4. Burke, A., Li, L., Kling, E. (2007). Cardiac inflammatory myofibroblastic tumor: A "benign" neoplasm that may result in syncope, myocardial infarction, and sudden death. *Am J Surg Pathol* 31: 1115–1122.
5. Hartyanszky, I.L., Kadar, K., Hubay, M. (2000). Rapid recurrence of an inflammatory myofibroblastic tumor in the right ventricular outflow tract. *Cardiol Young* 10: 271–274.

40 Intravenous Leiomyomatosis with Cardiac Metastases

Ligang Fang[1], Jing Ping Sun[2], and Yining Wang[1]

[1] Affiliated Hospital of Peking Union Medical College, Beijing, China
[2] The Chinese University of Hong Kong, Hong Kong

History

The patient is a 44-year-old female with intermittent exertional dyspnea for more than 1 week. She underwent a hysterectomy 2 years earlier due to a multiple myoma of the uterus.

Physical Examination

Blood pressure 120/80 mmHg. A diastolic murmur was heard the fourth intercostal space at the right parasternal. The ECG was normal.

Abdomen Ultrasound

A mass was observed in the front of left iliac vein, and multiple masses were seen in the pelvic cavity.

Transthoracic Echocardiography

Parasternal short and apical four-chamber views showed A 5.5 × 3.4 cm free-flowing echogenic mass in the right atrium and extending into right ventricle to the right out flow tract (Figure 40-1A, D; Videos 40-1 and 40-2) during diastole, obstructing the right inflow tract. A long strip mass was seen in the inferior vena cava and extending into the right atrium (Figure 40-1C and Video 40-3). The right atrium was significantly enlarged. Left and right ventricular systolic function was normal. The aortic valve right cups were mild thickened; there was no pericardial effusion, and tricuspid valve blood flow velocity was slightly increased. Mild tricuspid regurgitation was detected. The estimated pulmonary artery systolic blood pressure was 32 mmHg.

Computed Tomography

A cardiac CT scan showed a big mass in right atrium (Figure 40-2A, *) extending into the right ventricle through the tricuspid valve (Figure 40-2B, *). An abdominal CT scan showed a long strip mass in the inferior vena cava extending into the right atrium (Figure 40-2C, arrows).

Comparative Cardiac Imaging: A Case-based Guide, First Edition.
Edited by Jing Ping Sun, Xing Sheng Yang, and Bryan P. Yan.
© 2018 John Wiley & Sons Ltd. Published 2018 by John Wiley & Sons Ltd.
Companion website: www.wiley.com/sun/comparative_cardiac_imaging

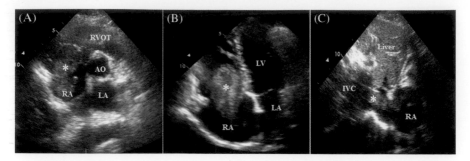

Figure 40-1 Transthoracic echocardiography: A. A parasternal short-axis view shows a soft echogenic mass in the right atrium and extending into the right ventricle to the right outflow tract. B. Apical four-chamber views during diastole; the right inflow tract was obstructed by a mass. The right atrium was significantly enlarged. C. A long strip mass was seen in the inferior vena cava and extended into the right atrium.

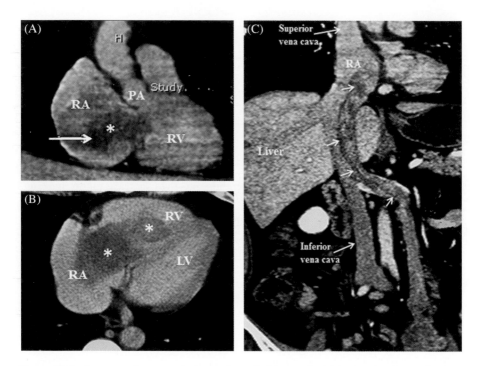

Figure 40-2 A computed tomography image showed a big mass in right atrium (A, *) extending into the right ventricle through the tricuspid valve (B, *). An abdominal CT scan showed a long strip mass in the inferior vena cava extending into the right atrium (C, arrows).

Hospital Course

The patient underwent an operation, which was performed by the cooperation of cardiac and vascular surgeons and a gynecologist. All of the tumors in the heart, IVC, and pelvic cavity were removed, and a bilateral adnexectomy was performed.

Pathology

The left ovarian tissue, tumors in right atrium and inferior vena cava were in line with vascular vein leiomyoma.

Discussion

Intravenous leiomyomatosis was first described by Durl and Horman in 1907 [1]. The exact etiology of this neoplasm is not entirely known. Two contrasting theories have been presented, both of which have supporting evidence [2] The first one suggests that the neoplasm arises from estrogen-induced smooth muscle cell proliferation in the venous wall of the uterine veins, while the second one suggests that the neoplasm arises from uterine leiomyomas that invaded the venous system [3]. The extension of the tumor is mostly through the uterine veins and it can progress along the veins into the inferior vena cava. Further extension into the right-sided cardiac chambers will lead to intracardiac leiomyomatosis. Since 1900, only 73 cases of cardiac leiomyomatosis have been reported [2] and 60% of the reports were within the last 15 years. However, it is believed that diagnosis is still significantly underestimated [4] because it is easily missed, particularly at early stages when the tumor's extension remains inside the small vessels of myometrium and cannot be detected easily.

Clinical Presentation

Clinical onset of these tumors usually reflects the extension of the lesions. The majority of the patients present with numerous nonspecific symptoms that include vaginal bleeding, pelvic pain, dyspnea, syncope, and congestive heart failure [3]. Predominant cardiac symptoms have been reported in 10% of the patients; our case presented with exertional dyspnea due to the tricuspid valve obstructed by the mass. However, patients may be completely asymptomatic [2], and correct diagnosis relies on a higher index of suspicion.

Imaging

Echocardiography In patients with intracardiac leiomyomatosis, transthoracic echocardiography can show the presence of a free-flowing echogenic intracardiac mass in the right cavities or in the pulmonary arteries, as in our case. Transesophageal echocardiography usually reveals an elongated, mobile, serpentlike polypoid mass proceeding from the inferior vena cava into the right atrium and ventricle, passing through the tricuspid valve.

Computed Tomography and Magnetic Resonance Magnetic resonance and multidetector computed tomographic angiography are the most sensitive methods to reveal IVL even in early stages without intracardial leiomyomatosis. A heterogeneous uterine mass that can be seen unilaterally or bilaterally into the iliac veins and in the inferior vena cava is the most common finding. Masses in the subhepatic region, extending down to the pelvis, and tumor masses within the ovarian veins or the renal veins have also been reported [4].

Treatment

Surgical resection is the treatment of choice [2, 3, 5]. Attempts must be made to remove the entire neoplasm, which usually involves hysterectomy [1]. Incomplete excision can result in recurrence of the neoplasm. A recurrence rate of 30% from 7 months to 17 years follow up has been reported [1, 3]. It has been suggested that recurrence may show the same pattern even after hysterectomy and bilateral adnexectomy. This shows that the tumor growth is independent of the presence of the uterus and, although histologically benign, might be considered clinically malignant [5]. When recurrence is seen, reintervention is universally recommended to achieve long-term disease-free survival [5].

Key Points

1. Cardiac leiomyomatosis is a rare metastasis lesion but it might be underdiagnosed.
2. The correct diagnosis relies on a higher index of suspicion.
3. Since cardiac metastasis may be long delayed, prolonged clinical follow up is recommended.

References

1. Kocica, M.J., Vranes, M.R., Kostic, D. et al. (2005). Intravenous leiomyomatosis with extension to the heart: Rare or underestimated? *J Thorac Cardiovasc Surg* 130: 1724–1726.
2. Butany, J., Singh, G., Henry, J. et al. (2006). Vascular smooth muscle tumors: 13 cases and a review of the literature. *Int J Angiol* 15: 43–50.
3. Ling, F.T., David, T.E., Merchant, N. et al. (2000). Intracardiac extension of intravenous leiomyomatosis in a pregnant woman: a case report and review of the literature. *Can J Cardiol* 16: 73–79.
4. Lam, P.M., Lo, K.W., Yu, M.Y. et al. (2004). Intravenous leiomyomatosis: Two cases with different routes of tumor extension. *J Vasc Surg* 39: 465–469.
5. Castelli, P., Caronno, R., Piffaretti, G. et al. (2006). Intravenous leiomyomatosis with right heart extension: successful two-stage surgical removal. *Ann Vasc Surg* 20: 405–407.

41 Intramural Left Atrial Hematoma Complicating Catheter Ablation for Atrial Fibrillation

Jen-Li Looi, Alex Pui-Wai Lee, and Jing Ping Sun

The Chinese University of Hong Kong, Hong Kong

History and Hospital Course

A 52-year-old woman with drug refractory paroxysmal atrial fibrillation was referred for radiofrequency catheter ablation. Trans-septal puncture was performed under fluoroscopy guidance. During the procedure, the patient suddenly became hypotensive. Focused transthoracic echocardiography with a handheld device revealed a moderate amount of pericardial effusion in the posterolateral region and a mass in the left atrium, which gave rise to suspicions of a thrombus. Activated coagulation time was 270 s during the procedure. Emergency pericardiocentesis was performed with removal of blood stained pericardial fluid, resulting in rapid improvement in systemic hemodynamics.

Cardiac computed tomography (CT) performed subsequently showed a homogenous, hyperdense, nonenhancing mass at the postero-inferior aspect of the left atrium consistent with a hematoma, which was thought to be extracardiac and compressing on the left atrium (Figure 41-1). However, the patient remained hemodynamically stable and therefore was managed conservatively. Anticoagulation was stopped and a comprehensive transthoracic echo study 3 days after the procedure revealed a well-circumscribed mass in the posterior wall of the left atrium (Figure 41-2A, 2B and 2C; Video 41-1 and Video 41-2). Contrast echocardiography was performed to exclude communication between the intramural cavity and the left atrium (Figure 41-3, Video 41-3). The results of echocardiography were strongly suggestive of an intramural hematoma. There was no obstruction of the mitral valve or pulmonary veins by the mass, and no pericardial effusion. Two weeks later, a follow-up echo demonstrated that the intramural hematoma had evolved into a cyst-like structure (Figure 41-4A, B and C; Videos 41-4, 41-5, and 41-6). The echocardiograph strongly suggested a partially resolved intramural left-atrial hematoma, rendering the dissection flap in the left atrial wall more clearly visible by echocardiography. The patient remained well clinically, thus no further intervention was taken. Anticoagulation was resumed, and echocardiography repeated 2 months later (Figure 41-3) demonstrated significant reduction in the size of the intramural cavity.

Comparative Cardiac Imaging: A Case-based Guide, First Edition.
Edited by Jing Ping Sun, Xing Sheng Yang, and Bryan P. Yan.
© 2018 John Wiley & Sons Ltd. Published 2018 by John Wiley & Sons Ltd.
Companion website: www.wiley.com/sun/comparative_cardiac_imaging

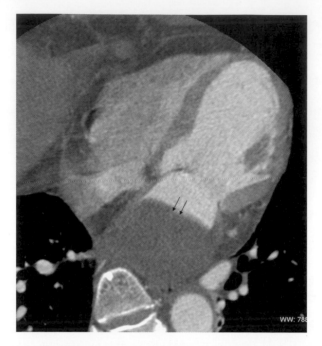

Figure 41-1   Cardiac CT showed a large hematoma (arrows) measuring 5.5 cm × 3.5 cm × 3.3 cm at the posteroinferior aspect of the left atrium, which was thought to be extracardiac.

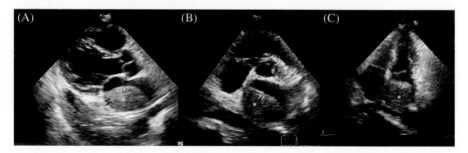

Figure 41-2   Transthoracic echocardiography. A parasternal long-axis view (A), parasternal short-axis view (B) and apical four-chamber view (C) showed a smoothly contoured echogenic mass (*) measuring 3.0 cm × 4.2 cm in the posterior left atrial wall. The left atrial wall was clearly delineated (arrows), raising the possibility of left-atrial haematoma. The outer cardiac border (black arrows) could be clearly delineated on the parasternal short-axis view, making the diagnosis of extracardiac mass unlikely.

Discussion

Transcatheter radiofrequency ablation is increasingly used for treatment of drug refractory atrial fibrillation. Intramural left-atrial hematomas are rare complications, but they have been described as occurring either spontaneously [1] or iatrogenically [2, 3]. We report a case of intramural left-atrial hematoma during catheter ablation for atrial fibrillation, which was managed conservatively with a good outcome. Damage to the left atrial wall during transeptal puncture with continued anticoagulation or laceration of

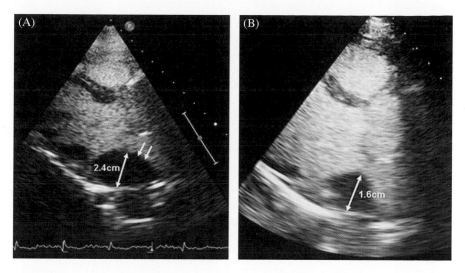

Figure 41-3   A. Contrast echocardiography. A parasternal long-axis view showed a nonenhancing mass in the posterior left atrial wall (arrows) and excluded the diagnosis of pseudoaneurysm of the left atrium. The mass measured 2.4 cm (double arrow). B. Contrast echocardiography. A parasternal long-axis view demonstrated that a nonenhancing mass had reduced in size significantly. The mass measured 1.6 cm (double arrow).

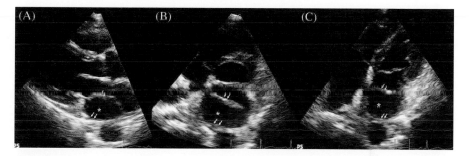

Figure 41-4   Transthoracic echocardiography. A parasternal long-axis view (A), parasternal short-axis view (B) and modified apical 4-chamber view (C) showed a cystlike structure (*) measuring 2.3 cm × 3.9 cm. The dissection flap in the left atrial wall (arrows) was clearly visualized. Again, the outer cardiac border (white arrows) could be clearly visualized, excluding the diagnosis of extracardiac mass.

the right inferior pulmonary vein [4] have been hypothesized to cause this complication. However, in our case, transseptal puncture was performed smoothly and there was no distinct intimal tear identified on 2D, color-Doppler and contrast echocardiography. A partially resolved left atrial wall hematoma may give a misleading appearance of a cystic mass inside the atrial cavity, and therefore it should be included in the differential diagnosis of cystic left-atrial masses. This case also highlights the importance of echocardiography in the diagnosis of intramural left-atrial hematoma. The atrial wall is highly echogenic and can therefore be visualized clearly by echocardiography. Contrast echocardiography can exclude the presence of persistent communication between the intramural and intravascular spaces of the left atrium, which might be useful to identify cases that can be managed conservatively.

Key Points

1. Transcatheter radiofrequency ablation is increasingly used for the treatment of drug-refractory atrial fibrillation. Complications should be noted in time.
2. Echocardiography is an important modality in the diagnosis of intramural left atrial hematoma and other complications of transcatheter radiofrequency ablation.

References

1. Shaikh, N., Rehman, N.U., Salazar, M.F. et al. (1999). Spontaneous intramural atrial haematoma presenting as a left atrial mass. *J Am Soc Echocardiogr* 12: 1101–1110.
2. Kelly, S., Bickneel, S.G. and Sharma, S. (2006). Left atrial wall hematoma after radiofrequency ablation for atrial fibrillation. *Am J Roentgenol* 186: 1317–1319.
3. Sah, R., Epstein, L.M. and Kwong, R.Y. (2007). Intramural atrial hematoma after catheter ablation for atrial tachyarrhythmias. *Circulation* 115: e446–e447.
4. Echahidi, N., Philippon, F., O'Hara, G. et al. (2008). Life-threatening left atrial wall haematoma secondary to a pulmonary vein laceration: an unusual complication of catheter ablation for atrial fibrillation. *J Cardiovasc Electrophysiol* 19: 556–558.

42 Primary Cardiac Lymphoma: Two Rare Cases

Yi Liu[1], Min Xu[1], Bo Zhang[1], and Jing Ping Sun[2]

[1] Tongji University School of Medicine, Shanghai, China
[2] The Chinese University of Hong Kong, Hong Kong

History
- Case 1: A 61-year-old female with palpitation and dyspnea for 10 days.
- Case 2: A 74-year-old man who presented with dyspnea for 2 months.

Physical Examination
- Case 1. There was a systolic and diastolic murmur at the third intercostal of left sternal border.
- Case 2. The patient's jugular veins were distended.

Electrocardiography (EKG)
- Case 1. Electrocardiography showed low voltages on all limb leads and sinus tachycardia.
- Case 2. Electrocardiography showed atrial fibrillation.

Chest X-ray
- Case 1. Chest X-ray revealed cardiomegaly.
- Case 2. Chest X-ray showed blunted costophrenic angles on both sides.

Laboratory Test
In Case 1, tumor markers showed cancer antigen 125 was elevated (167.9 U/ml; normal range: 0 to 35 U/ml).

Transthoracic Echocardiogram (TTE)
The TTE showed:
- Case 1. A large mass, almost completely filling the right atrium (RA), penetrated the right atrial free wall, the tricuspid annulus, and the right ventricular free wall, resulting in functional tricuspid stenosis. There was a large amount of pericardial effusion. The left ventricular ejection fraction (LVEF) was normal (Figure 42-1A and Video 42-1). Contrast-enhanced echocardiography showed a lobulated mass with plenty of blood in the right atrium and a thickened right ventricular wall (Figure 42-1B and Video 42-2).

Comparative Cardiac Imaging: A Case-based Guide, First Edition.
Edited by Jing Ping Sun, Xing Sheng Yang, and Bryan P. Yan.
© 2018 John Wiley & Sons Ltd. Published 2018 by John Wiley & Sons Ltd.
Companion website: www.wiley.com/sun/comparative_cardiac_imaging

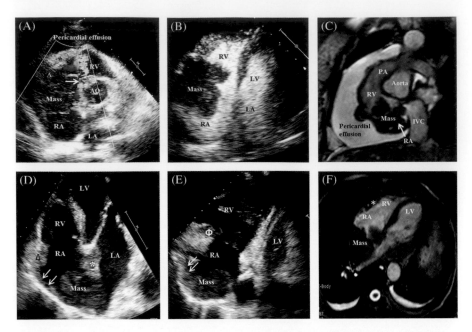

Figure 42-1   Case 1. Transthoracic echocardiogram. A. Parasternal short-axis view at great-vessel level showed a large mass almost completely filling right atrium, penetrated into right atrial free wall, tricuspid annulus (Δ) and ventricular free wall (*), resulting in functional tricuspid stenosis (arrow). There was large amount of pericardial effusion. B. Contrast-enhanced echocardiography of four-chamber view showed a lobulated mass in right atrium and thickened right ventricular free wall (red *). C. The bright blood SSFP sequence MRI showed a large, lobulated mass fill in the right atrium, invading right ventricular free wall and tricuspid annulus. Case 2. Transthoracic echocardiogram. D. Four-chamber view showed a large mass in the right atrium, penetrating the interatrial septum (*), right atrial lateral wall (arrow), and tricuspid annulus (Δ). E. The atypical four-chamber view showed the mass in the right atrial cavity and extended into the RA roof, the lateral wall and part of tricuspid annulus (Φ). F. The bright blood SSFP sequence MRI imaging showed a large mass in the right atrium, penetrating interatrial septum and tricuspid annulus. A small amount of pleural effusion was seen. *Notes:* LV, left ventricle; RV, right ventricle; LA, left atrium; RA, right atrium; AO, aortic valve; PA, pulmonary artery; IVC, inferior vena cava.

- Case 2. The TTE revealed a large mass in the roof of the right atrium, which had invaded into the atrial septum, the right atrial lateral wall, and the tricuspid annulus (Figure 42-1C, D and Video 42-3). The LVEF was normal.

Magnetic Resonance Imaging (MRI)

- Case 1. The MRI showed a large, lobulated mass fill in the right atrium, invading the pericardium and part of the right ventricular free wall (Figure 42-1E, Videos 42-4).
- Case 2. The bright blood SSFP sequence MRI imaging showed a large mass in the right atrium, penetrating the interatrial septum and tricuspid annulus. A small amount of pleural effusion was seen on both sides (Figure 42-1E). Contrast-enhanced magnetic resonance imaging (MRI) showed the mass invading tricuspid annulus, inferior vena cava, atrial septum, and part of the right atrial wall (Figure 42-1 F, Video 42-5).

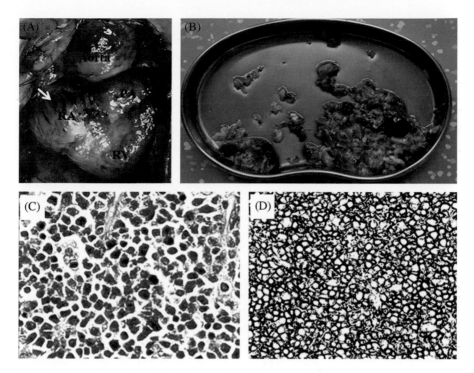

Figure 42-2   Case 1. A. The surface of RA was dark red appearance (white arrow), which resulted from malignant tumor infiltration. B. The gross appearance of gelatinous, friable fragments in the kidney basin were cleared from right atrium. C. Histological examination confirmed that the mass was diffuse lymphoma (hematoxylin–eosin stain, original magnification × 400). D. Histological examination using immunochemical staining showed cytoplasmic expression of CD79a (original magnification × 200). *Notes:* RV, right ventricle; PA, pulmonary artery; RA, right atrium.

Operation

- Case 1. According to the imaging information, malignancy cardiac mass was considered, cardiac surgery was performed to relieve the symptoms and for diagnosis. The surgeon found a large amount pericardial effusion in light yellow color. The surface of the right atrium and the ventricular free wall was infiltrated by a crisp texture tumor tissue with numerous vessels (Figure 42-2A). There was a huge, opaque, jellylike, mass (4 × 5 × 6 cm) with a crisp texture in the right atrium. The tumor infiltrated into the tricuspid annulus. There was no capsule and clear border, so it was hard to remove the whole mass. The surgeon cleared the tumor from the right atrium as far as possible. For the content see Figure 42-2B. As the result, the right ventricular inflow tract was cleared. The patient died due to heart failure 2 weeks later.
- Case 2. The patient underwent a transjugular intracardiac mass biopsy under ultrasound guidance. The patient died suddenly 1 week after biopsy.

Pathology

- Case 1. The histopathologic diagnosis was a diffuse large B cell lymphoma (Figure 42-2C, D).

- Case 2. The pathologic diagnosis was a diffuse large B cell lymphoma. Immunoperoxidase stains were strongly positive for CD20, CD79a and negative for CD3, CD5, CD10 and CD38.

Both of these patients were negative for HIV. An extracardiac tumor was excluded by Computed tomography (CT) scan through the body in these cases.

Discussion

Primary cardiac lymphoma (PCL) with no evidence of extracardiac involvement is a very rare cardiac malignancy. The incidence of PCL was 1.3% of all primary cardiac tumors, and 0.5% of all lymphomas. It is especially rare in immunocompetent patients [1]. We reported two cases with isolated primary cardiac lymphomas in the right atrium; the extra-cardiac tumor was excluded by CT scan.

More than 80% of PCLs are diffuse B-cell non-Hodgkin's lymphomas, and B-cell lymphomas should be positive for CD 20 [2]. Primary cardiac lymphomas are mainly seen in the right atrium, followed by the right ventricle, left ventricle, left atrium, atrial septum, and ventricular septum, but rarely invading the tricuspid valve. The clinical features of PCLs vary. They can include intractable, rapidly progressive heart failure, arrhythmia, atrioventricular heart block, chest pain, syncope, pulmonary embolism, myocardial infarction, superior vena cava syndrome, pleural effusion, and cardiac tamponade [3].

Among the diagnostic tools, TTE should be considered as a first approach. Transesophageal echocardiography is the more sensitive imaging technique, and can provide a higher quality of image of the cardiac structure than TTE. Contrast-enhanced echocardiography can show the blood supply of the tumor [3]. A CT scan is more sensitive in distinguishing pericardial and extracardial masses, but MRI can demonstrate poorly marginated and heterogeneous lesions. Although imaging techniques are of great value, a definite diagnosis of PCL must be made on the basis of histology, which can guide appropriate therapy. Besides surgical biopsy, an histology of the mass can also be obtained by a transvenous intracardiac biopsy with transesophageal ultrasound guidance, or transthoracic guide needle biopsy. Both methods are associated with the risk of a tumor embolism and cardiac tamponade [4]. In patients who have pericardial effusion, cytological specimens can also be obtained from the pericardial fluid [5]. An operation can relieve obstruction and chemotherapy might be to prolong the median survival time [6]. Unfortunately, more than half of patients died before chemotherapy, as in our cases. Usual causes of sudden death include refractory heart failure, massive pulmonary embolism, and cardiac rupture due to rapid intramural tumor lysis during chemotherapy.

Our two cases did not have any specific clinical signs. The primary impressions were made by echocardiography, and confirmed by MRI. An extracardiac tumor was excluded by CT scan through the body in both cases. The final diagnosis was made by pathology.

The characteristics of the tumor from imaging studies are: irregular shape, no capsule, and penetration into the cardiac chamber walls and the tricuspid annulus.

Key Points

1. Primary cardiac lymphoma with no evidence of extracardiac involvement is very rare cardiac malignancy tumor.

2. Primary cardiac lymphomas are mainly seen in the right atrium, followed by the right ventricle and other cardiac chambers.

3. The prognosis is poor. Mean survival of patients with sarcoma is 9 to 11 months depending on the stage of the disease at the time of diagnosis.

Reference

1. Antoniades, L., Eftychiou, C., Petrou, P.M. et al. (2009). Primary cardiac lymphoma: Case report and brief review of the literature. *Echocardiography* 26 (2): 214–219.
2. Hsueh, S.C., Chung, M.T., Fang, R. et al. (2006). Primary cardiac lymphoma. *J Chin Med Assoc* 69: 169–174.
3. Gowda, R.M. and Khan, I.A. (2003). Clinical perspectives of primary cardiac lymphoma. *Angiology* 54: 599–603.
4. Kang, S.M., Rim, S.J., Chang, H.J., et al. (2003). Primary cardiac lymphoma diagnosed by transvenous biopsy under transesophageal echocardiographic guidance and treated with systemic chemotherapy. *Echocardiography* 20: 100–101.
5. Faganello, G., Belham, M., Thaman, R. et al. (2007). A case of primary cardiac lymphoma: Analysis of the role of echocardiography in early diagnosis. *Echocardiography* 24: 889–892.
6. Kosugi, M., Ono, T., Yamaguchi, H. et al. (2006). Successful treatment of primary cardiac lymphoma and pulmonary tumor embolism with chemotherapy. *Int J Cardiol* 111: 172–173.

43 Mass in Left Atrium and Appendage

Jing Ping Sun[1], Fanxia Meng[2], Xing Sheng Yang[1], Alex Pui-Wai Lee[1], and Bo Zhang[2]

[1] The Chinese University of Hong Kong, Hong Kong
[2] Tongji University School of Medicine, Shanghai, China

History
Case 1
A 75-year-old, male, visited cardiology clinic because of atrial fibrillation. Transesophageal echocardiography indicated:

- Significant expansion of the left atrial appendage ($4.7 \times 2.6\,cm^2$) with spontaneous echo contrast.
- A pedunculated mass ($3.6 \times 1.8\,cm^2$) in left atrium appendage (Figure 43-1 and Video 43-1).
- After thrombolytic therapy, the size of mass was shrinking gradually and almost dissolved (Figure 43-1, Videos 43-1, 43-2, and 43-3).

Case 2
A 72-year-old female visited the cardiology clinic because of palpitations. Transthoracic echocardiography indicated:

- Mitral stenosis with significantly dilated left atrium (LA) and a subtle echo density (*) in the top of the LA closing to atrial septum (Figure 43-2, Video 43-4).
- A definite mass in the LA could be seen in the subcostal view (Figure 43-2).

A cardiac CT scan demonstrated:

- Coronary artery disease proximal left anterior descending artery mix multiple spots, mild luminal stenosis. Middle of the right coronary artery myocardial bridge.
- Cardic CT image showed: There is a mass in the enlarged left atrium (Figure 43-3).

Cases 3 and 4 and Several Other Cases from our Laboratory
A 56-year-old woman and a 60-year-old male were referred to our hospital for further cardiovascular examination because of a mild stroke. Physical examinations, electrocardiogram, and routing transthoracic echocardiography were normal. Findings from transesophageal echocardiography were as follows:

- Images were obtained from several cases. They showed the atrial pouch on the left (Figure 43-4A, B, arrows) and right sides (Figure 43-4D arrows). An image with contrast (Figure 43-4C) showed that there are no microbubbles through the atrial septum pouch. There was also an image of a patent foramen oval (PFO) (Figure 43-4E) with color flow, and a contrast echo image showing microbubbles through the PFO (Figure 43-4F, arrow).

Comparative Cardiac Imaging: A Case-based Guide, First Edition.
Edited by Jing Ping Sun, Xing Sheng Yang, and Bryan P. Yan.
© 2018 John Wiley & Sons Ltd. Published 2018 by John Wiley & Sons Ltd.
Companion website: www.wiley.com/sun/comparative_cardiac_imaging

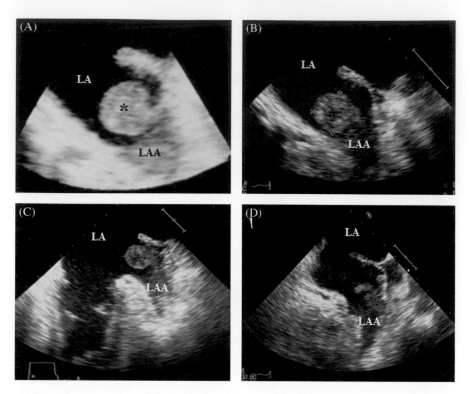

Figure 43-1 Case 1. Transesophageal echocardiography showed significant expansion of the left atrial appendage (4.7×2.6 cm²) with spontaneous echo contrast, and a pedunculated mass (3.6×1.8 cm²). After thrombolytic therapy, the mass was shrinking gradually and almost dissolved (A–D).

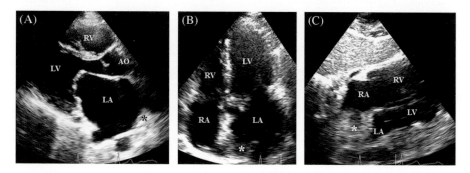

Figure 43-2 Case 2. Transthoracic echocardiography indicated mitral stenosis with significantly dilated left atrium (LA) and a subtle echo density in the top of the LA closing to the atrial septum in the parasternal and apical four-chamber views (A and B*); a definite mass in the LA could be seen in subcostal view (C*).

- An image was obtained from Case 3, which showed a thrombus within the left atrial (LA) septal pouch (Figure 43-5A, arrow, Video 43-5).
- An image (Case 4) showed a tiny thrombus arising from right atrial (RA) septal pouch (Figure 43-5B, arrow, Video 43-6).

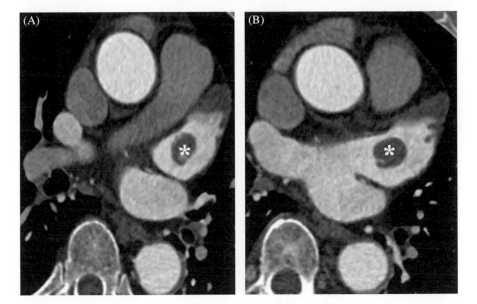

Figure 43-3 Cardiac CT scan demonstrated a left atrial mass and left atrial enlargement.

Discussion

Cardiac masses are common findings in clinical practice. Myxomas are the most benign primary tumors of the heart. On echocardiography, myxomas appear as mobile masses attached to the endocardial surface by a stalk, usually arising from fossa ovals [1]. A left atrial mass can be diagnosed as a thrombus if it is associated with atrial fibrillation, a dilated left atrium, mitral or tricuspid stenosis, low ejection fraction, prosthetic mitral or tricuspid valves, spontaneous atrial contrast echoes, hypertrophic cardiomyopathy, or infective endocarditis. Atrial fibrillation is almost always a finding that accompanies other findings; the etiology in cases without atrial fibrillation or additional cardiac disorders is not clear.

The differential diagnosis between thrombi and myxoma is sometimes difficult but is critical in making the right therapeutic decision. When the thrombus moves freely in the cardiac cavity the diagnosis is relatively simple. In some patients, atrial thrombi may have a stalk and may be mistaken as myxoma or other tumor, which can lead to unnecessary and potential harmful surgery. The pathophysiology may be growth from the thrombus in the left atrium, taking on the shape of the cavity and then becoming a pedunculated mobile mass [2, 3].

The authors presented a case of a 75-year-old male with a history of atrial fibrillation. Transesophageal echocardiography showed significant expansion of the left atrial appendage with spontaneous echo contrast, and a pedunculated mass. This pedunculated mass was confusing but an attempt was made to begin thrombolytic therapy for this case. The mass shrank gradually and almost dissolved after thrombolytic therapy; this result confirmed the diagnosis of mass as thrombus.

In clinical practice, we should careful to view several different plains in an echocardiography study. We presented Case 2 with mitral valve stenosis and a dilated left atrium as an example; the left atrial mass was not clear, and could be missed easily but a clear mass could be seen in subcostal view.

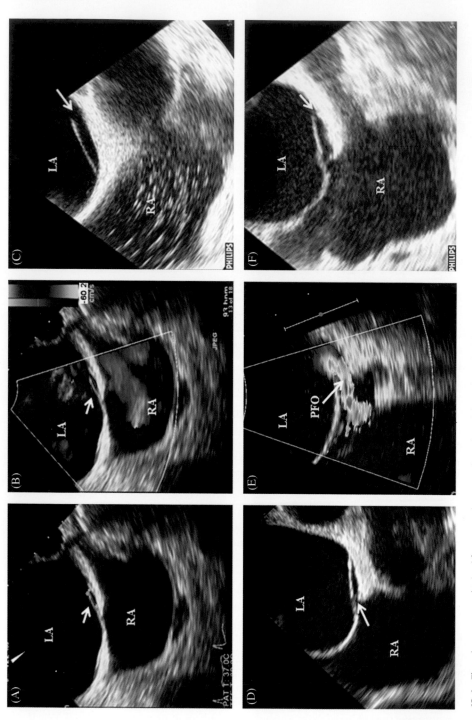

Figure 43-4 These images were obtained from several cases to show the atrial pouch on the left side (A and B, arrows) and right side (D, arrows). An image with contrast (C) shows there are no microbubbles through the atrial septum pouch. A patent foramen ovale with color flow (E). A contrast echo image showing microbubbles through PFO (F, arrow).

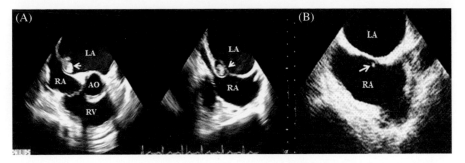

Figure 43-5 This image was obtained from Case 3. It shows a thrombus (arrow) within the left atrial (LA) septal pouch (A, arrow). An image (Case 4) shows a tiny thrombus arising from the right atrial (RA) septal pouch (B, arrow).

The diagnosis of cryptogenic stroke remains presumptive in a vast majority of patients. Recently, a new anatomical entity, the atrial septal pouch (ASP), has been defined in a pathology study. It was described as an incomplete fusion in the cranial segment of the overlap between the septum primum (SP) and septum secundum (SS), resulting in a recess that opens into the left (LASP) or right atrium (RASP), with no interatrial shunting [4]. The LASP might serve as a nidus for thrombus formation in the presence of low flow states, and therefore predispose to embolic events. There are a number of case reports demonstrating a thrombus arising from the cavity of LASP [5, 6] but the association between LASP and cryptogenic strokes from several retrospective studies is controversial. We studied 324 patients with TEE studies; the risk of ischemic stroke was twice more among patients with LASP than cases without LASP. We also found thrombus arising from ASP. Our findings suggest that LASP might be the source of emboli contributing to ischemic stroke [7].

We also presented several cases in this report, to show the characteristics of ASP, PFO in echocardiography, and the thrombus arising from ASP.

Echocardiography has been the mainstay for thrombus detection but its prevalence varies considerably among echocardiographic studies because of modest image reproducibility and poorer spatial and soft-tissue resolution than cardiac MRI. Magnetic resonance imaging allow useful differentiation between tumor and thrombus [8, 9]. Thrombus in T2-weighted sequences and in TrueFISP (true fast imaging with steady-state precession) sequence appears significantly homogeneously hypointensive / dark. The vascular supply of myocardial thrombi is poor so that the thrombus do not enhance after the administration of gadolinium contrast material. The most typical feature of myxoma is an increase in the signal after application of contrast medium during perfusion examination [10].

Key Points

1. The mass in the left atrium is common, the differential diagnosis is important.
2. The thrombus is mostly sessile and immobile but can be pedunculated and mobile.
3. In particular case, magnetic resonance imaging of the heart is helpful in differential diagnosis between tumow and thrombus.

References

1. Burke, A., Jeudy, J. Jr and Virmani, R. (2008). Cardiac tumours: An update: Cardiac tumours. *Heart* 94: 117–123.
2. Yoshida, K., Fujii, G., Suzuki, S. et al. (2002). A report of a surgical case of left atrial free floating ball thrombus in the absence of mitral valve disease. *Ann Thorac Cardiovasc Surg* 8: 316–318.
3. O'Donnell, D.H., Abbara, S., Chaithiraphan, V. et al. (2009). Cardiac tumors: Optimal cardiac MR sequences and spectrum of imaging appearances. *Am J Roentgenol* 193 (2): 377–387.
4. Krishnan, S.C. and Salazar, M. (2010). Septal pouch in the left atrium: A new anatomical entity with potential for embolic complications. *J Am Coll Cardiol Intv* 3: 98–104.
5. Shimamoto, K., Kawagoe, T., Dai, K. et al. (2014). Thrombus in the left atrial septal pouch mimicking myxoma. *J Clin Ultrasound* 42 (3): 185–188.
6. Wong, J.M., Lombardo, D., Handwerker, J. et al. (2014). Cryptogenic stroke and the left atrial septal pouch: A case report. *J Stroke Cerebrovasc Dis* 23 564–565.
7. Sun, J.P., Meng, F., Yang, X.S. et al. (2016). Prevalence of atrial septal pouch and risk of ischemic stroke. *Int J Cardiology* 214: 37–40.
8. Lima J.A. and Desai M.Y. Cardiovascular magnetic resonance imaging: Current and emerging applications. *J Am Coll Cardiol.* 2004; 44: 1164–1171.
9. Hendel, R.C., Patel, M.R., Kramer, C.M. et al. (2006). ACCF/ACR/SCCT/SCMR/ASNC/ NASCI/ SCAI/SIR 2006 appropriateness criteria for cardiac computed tomography and cardiac magnetic resonance imaging. *J Am Coll Cardiol* 48: 1475–1497.
10. Larose, E., Rodes-Cabau, J., Delarochelliere, R. et al. (2007). Cardiovascular magnetic resonance for the clinical cardiologist. *Can J Cardiol* 23(Suppl B): 84B–88B.

44 Metastatic Cardiac Lymphoma

Jing Ping Sun, Xing Sheng Yang, and Alex Pui-Wai Lee

The Chinese University of Hong Kong, Hong Kong

History
A 49-year-old female was admitted due to exertion dyspnea.

Physical Examination
Blood pressure was 114/75 mmHg. Heart rate was 112 bpm. Physical examination showed tachypnea.

Echocardiography
The left ventricle and atrium were normal in size and systolic function. The right ventricle was normal in size and systolic function. A huge heterogeneous mass (5.7 × 5.1 cm) was in the right atrium; the right atrial cavity was significantly occupied by the mass with impaired filling (Figure 44-1, Videos 44-1 to 44-4). The right ventricular inflow was obstructed by the mass without evidence of tumor infiltration. Inflow velocity was >2 m/s. There was a positive agitated saline test with contrast filling in the right and left sides of the heart (Video 44-2).

Computed Tomography
There was a large (8 cm deep × 7 cm wide × 11 cm long) irregular mixed hypodense anterior mediastinal mass with fat density or cystic change. The mass invades and protrudes into the right atrium. The right atrium is distended and largely filled by the tumor (Figure 44-2). This leads to engorgement of the superior vena cava and inferior vena cava. The mass also encases the right coronary artery, which is patent. The root of the aorta, pulmonary trunk and right ventricle is abutted by the mass. This may represent an aggressive tumor such as a mediastinum malignant lymphoma with metastatic cardiac lymphoma.

Hospital Course
The patient underwent biopsy. The diagnosis of metastatic cardiac lymphoma was confirmed by histology.

Comparative Cardiac Imaging: A Case-based Guide, First Edition.
Edited by Jing Ping Sun, Xing Sheng Yang, and Bryan P. Yan.
© 2018 John Wiley & Sons Ltd. Published 2018 by John Wiley & Sons Ltd.
Companion website: www.wiley.com/sun/comparative_cardiac_imaging

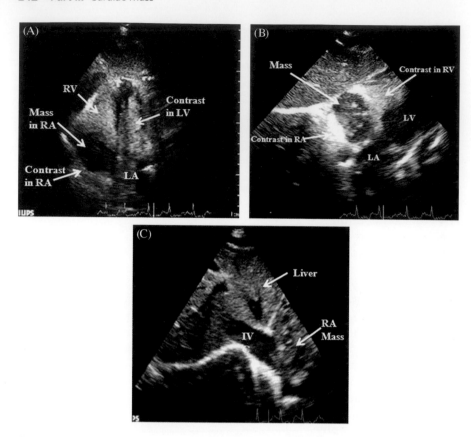

Figure 44-1 Echocardiography: A. Apical four-chamber view showed a huge heterogeneous mass (5.7 × 5.1 cm) filling the right atrium, and a positive agitated saline test with right to left shunting. B. Subcostal four-chamber view with agitated saline contrast showed a huge mass in the right atrium. C. Subcostal view showed dilated inferior vena cava and hepatic vein.

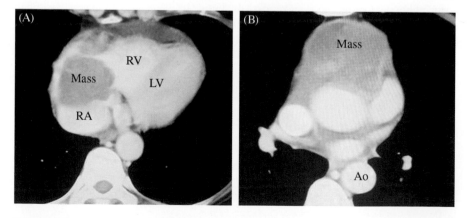

Figure 44-2 Computed tomography images showed there is a large (8 cm deep × 7 cm wide × 11 cm long) irregular mixed hypodence anterior mediastinal mass with fat density or cystic change. The mass invades and protrudes into the right atrium.

Discussion

On clinical observation of an intracavitary cardiac mass, the differential diagnosis may include mural thrombus, benign primary cardiac tumor (myxoma, lipoma), malignant primary cardiac tumor (sarcoma, lymphoma), or secondary involvement from extracardiac tumors [1]. Left atrial thrombi are most often associated with atrial fibrillation and/or rheumatic mitral stenosis, which accounts for over 45% of cardiogenic thromboemboli [2]. Cardiac myxoma, usually involving the left atrium, is another possible diagnosis [1, 3].

In our patient, a normal cardiac history and normal cardiac structures by echocardiography and ECG findings may help in distinguishing an intracardiac tumor from a mural thrombus. The differentiation of a mass in the right atrium as primary or cancer metastasis is challenging with our echocardiographic images. Computed tomography provides a more complete picture. It found that the mediastinal mass invaded and protruded into the right atrium.

The mediastinum is divided into three compartments: anterior, middle, and posterior. Masses can be found in all three compartments.

The most common mediastinal masses are neurogenic tumors (20% of mediastinal tumors), usually found in the posterior mediastinum, followed by a thymoma (15–20%) located in the anterior mediastinum [4].

Masses in the anterior portion of the mediastinum can include thymoma, lymphoma, pheochromocytoma, germ-cell tumors including teratoma, thyroid tissue, and parathyroid lesions. Masses in this area are more likely to be malignant than those in other compartments [5].

Malignant lymphoma initially presenting as an intracardiac mass is very rare [6]. Most patients remain clinically undetected and are diagnosed from autopsy findings [6, 7]. When the heart is involved, patients often present with impaired ventricular function caused by ventricular invasion, and the prognosis is poor. Differentiation between primary cardiac lymphoma and secondary heart invasion by lymphoma is challenging. The two conditions share similar and nonspecific symptoms (fever, chills, night sweats, weight loss, fatigue, and occasionally chest discomfort due to pleural or pericardial effusion or external compression). Primary cardiac lymphoma mainly involves the right side of the heart in 69 to 72% of cases, with rare extracardiac involvement [1, 2]. Chest CT with contrast enhancement and cardiac magnetic resonance may offer the best methods to distinguish a primary cardiac tumor from a direct extension from adjacent mediastinal structures [1]. However, histological evaluation is necessary for a definitive diagnosis.

Key Points

1. The differential diagnosis of an intracavitary cardiac mass may include mural thrombus, benign primary cardiac tumor (myxoma, lipoma), malignant primary cardiac tumor (sarcoma, lymphoma), or secondary involvement from extracardiac tumors.
2. Chest CT with contrast enhancement and cardiac magnetic resonance may offer the best methods to distinguish primary cardiac tumor from direct extension from adjacent mediastinal structures.
3. Histological evaluation is necessary for a definitive diagnosis.

References

1. McManus, B. (2011). Primary tumors of the heart. In: *Braunwald's Heart Disease: A Textbook of Cardiovascular Medicine*, 9th edn. (eds. R.O. Bonow, D.L. Mann, D.P. Zipes and P. Libby), 1638–1648. Philadelphia, PA: Elsevier Saunders.
2. Ban-Hoefen, M., Zeglin, M.A. and Bisognano, J.D. (2008). Diffuse large B cell lymphoma presenting as a cardiac mass and odynophagia. *Cardiol J* 15: 471–474.
3. Nguyen, D.T., Meier, C.R. and Schneider, D. (2008). Primary cardiac lymphoma mimicking left atrial myxoma in an immunocompetent patient. *J Clin Oncol* 26:150–152.
4. Macchiarini, P. and Ostertag, H. (2004). Uncommon primary mediastinal tumours. *Lancet Oncol* 5 (2): 107–118.
5. Davis, R.D., Oldham, H.N. and Sabiston, D.C. (1987). Primary cysts and neoplasms of the mediastinum: recent changes in clinical presentation, methods of diagnosis, management, and results. *Ann Thorac Surg* 44 (3): 229–237.
6. Tanaka,T., Sato, T., Akifuji, Y. et al. (1996). Aggressive non-Hodgkin's lymphoma with massive involvement of the right ventricle. *Intern Med* 35: 826–830.
7. O'Mahony, D., Peikarz, R.L., Bandettini, W.P. et al. (2008). Cardiac involvement with lymphoma: a review of the literature. *Clin Lymphoma Myeloma* 8: 249–252.

45 Metastatic Renal Carcinoma in Inferior Vena Cava

Jing Ping Sun and Jen-Li Looi

The Chinese University of Hong Kong, Hong Kong

History
A 67-year-old female presented with 5 months' history of anemia and recurrent fever.

Physical Examination
Heart rate was regular at 90 bpm. Blood pressure was 105/78 mm Hg. Cardiovascular examination was unremarkable. There was a big mass palpable on the left side of the abdomen. No ankle edema was present.

Laboratory
Hemoglobin: 6.9 g/100 ml.

Echocardiogram
Both atria and ventricles were normal in size. The systolic function of the left and right ventricles was normal. There was a large, long linear thrombus in the inferior vena cava (IVC) extending into the right atrium and ventricle (Figure 45-1A, B, and Videos 45-1 to 45-3).

Abdomen Ultrasonography
A large irregular heterogeneous mass over the left kidney, which suggests renal cell carcinoma.

Computed Tomography
There was a large left renal cell carcinoma with a thrombus in the kidney (Figure 45-2), which was extending into the hepatic vein, IVC, right atrium and crossing tricuspid valve into right ventricle. Retroperitoneal nodal masses were seen at the pancreatic tail and upper retrocaval region.

Magnetic Resonance Imaging
A long linear filling defect was seen in the left renal vein, extending into the inferior vena cava, the right atrium and possibly to the tricuspid valve level (Figure 45-3).

Comparative Cardiac Imaging: A Case-based Guide, First Edition.
Edited by Jing Ping Sun, Xing Sheng Yang, and Bryan P. Yan.
© 2018 John Wiley & Sons Ltd. Published 2018 by John Wiley & Sons Ltd.
Companion website: www.wiley.com/sun/comparative_cardiac_imaging

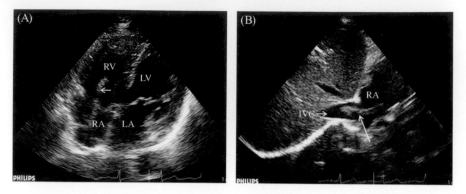

Figure 45-1   Echocardiography. A. Apical four-chamber view demonstrates a long strip in the right atrium extending into ventricle. B. A subcostal view shows a long strip in the inferior vena cava extending into RA.

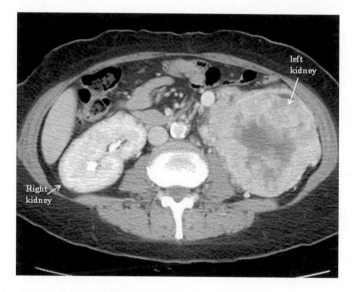

Figure 45-2   Computed tomography image showed a large left renal cell carcinoma.

Hospital Course

Biopsy confirmed the diagnosis of renal cell carcinoma. Because of metastatic disease, local control and facilitated laser targeted therapy were given.

Discussion

The detection of inferior vena cava (IVC) masses has important clinical implications for the management of patients with retroperitoneal or metastatic tumors and migratory thrombi. Due to the direct connection between the renal vein and the inferior vena cava, renal cell carcinoma is a well-recognized cause of an IVC mass. Surgical resection may be curative for many patients with renal cell carcinoma without metastases, so IVC involvement should be assessed preoperatively. Inferior vena cavography and magnetic

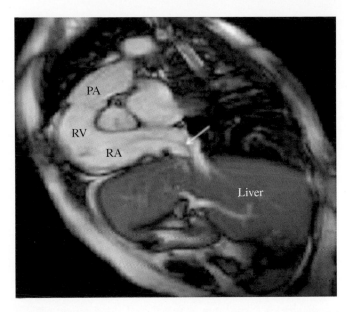

Figure 45-3 Magnetic resonance image showed a long linear filling defect inside the left renal vein to the confluence of the left renal vein with the inferior vena cava, along the retro hepatic segment of IVC and extending into the right atrium and possibly to the tricuspid valve level.

resonance imaging (MRI) are reliable and established methods to identify the presence of an IVC thrombus and to define the location and extent of invasion [1–3]. Other modalities for diagnosis of IVC masses include transabdominal ultrasonography, computerized tomography (CT), and echocardiography. We have previously reported the usefulness of echocardiography in the evaluation of IVC before surgical resection of solid organ tumors in 62 patients [4].

Previous studies have reported the most common causes of IVC masses include hypernephroma, hepatoma, Wilm's tumor, lymphosarcoma, and leiomyosarcoma [5]. Our study found a similar distribution of etiologies with renal cell carcinoma being by far the most prevalent tumor in this setting. Generally, these tumors invade the inferior vena cava through direct hematogenous extension, which explains the high proportion of abdominal and retroperitoneal sources. Although an IVC mass may result in partial or total obstruction of the inferior vena cava, the most common manifestation is pulmonary embolization [6]. Often, these emboli may not be clinically apparent and may be detected only by ventilation and/or perfusion scanning, pulmonary angiography, or occasionally by directly visualizing their passage through the inferior vena cava, right heart chambers, and pulmonary artery by echocardiography.

Preoperative imaging studies are essential to determine the presence and distal limits of an IVC mass. This provides important information with regards to the surgical approach for their removal.

Removal of an IVC mass from a patient with renal cell carcinoma is most likely to be curative when there is no lymph node or distant metastatic disease [7].

Contrast inferior vena cavography, although considered the gold standard, is invasive and associated with complications, such as contrast-induced renal dysfunction. Transthoracic echocardiography is a reliable and convenient diagnostic tool for evaluation of cardiac sources of embolism, cardiac tumors, valvular heart disease, and cardiac function and is, therefore, often used during preoperative testing. The subcostal view is part of a routine transthoracic echocardiographic study. It enables accurate evaluation of the proximal inferior vena cava as it extends into the right atrium. This view is useful for screening of IVC masses and assessment of right atrial pressure. Transthoracic echocardiography is able to detect and localize IVC masses with a diagnostic accuracy of 90% compared with operative findings, supporting the use of transthoracic echocardiography as an effective screening modality instead of the more time-consuming and expensive MRI or CT scanning. The additional advantages of transesophageal echocardiography compared with transthoracic echocardiography have been previously described, including the opportunity to use higher frequency transducers with less obstructed views [8].

Computed tomography (CT) provides a detailed cross-sectional image of the body. A CT scan provides precise information about the size, shape, and position of a tumor. It is also useful for the assessment of metastatic disease, which will help in the management of the patient, as described in our case.

Magnetic resonance imaging is used less often than CT scans in patients with kidney cancer. It may be indicated in cases where CT is contraindicated, for example if the patient is allergic to the CT contrast. Magnetic resonance imaging is useful in the assessment of metastatic disease to the brain or spinal cord, if the patient has symptoms suggestive of neurological involvement.

Key Points

1. Tumors may travel up to the inferior vena cava into the right side of the heart and also into the left heart through a patent foramen oval.
2. These tumors may cause obstruction of the tricuspid valve.
3. These masses may be the source of pulmonary embolization. Echocardiography is a useful tool for detection of intracardiac masses and CT provides a detailed assessment of the tumor.

References

1. Siminovitch, J.M.P., Montie, J.E. and Straffon, R.A. (1982). Inferior venacavography in the preoperative assessment of renal adenocarcinoma. *J Urol* 128: 908 –909.
2. Abrams, H.L. (1982). Renal venography. In: *Abrams Angiography: Vascular and Interventional Radiology*, 3rd edn (ed. S. Brown), 1339–1342. Boston, MA: Little, Brown & Co.
3. Glazer, A. and Novick, A.C. (1997). Preoperative transesophageal echocardiography for assessment of vena caval tumor thrombi: A comparative study with venacavography and magnetic resonance imaging. *Urology* 49: 32–34.
4. Sun, J.P., Asher, C.R., Xu, Y. et al. (1999). Inferior vena caval masses identified by echocardiography. *Am J Cardiol* 1;84 (5): 613–615.
5. Weyman, A.E. (1994). *Principle and Practice of Echocardiography*, 2nd edn. Philadelphia, PA: Lee & Febiger.
6. Van Kuyk, M., Mols, P. and Englert, M. (1984). Right atrial thrombus leading to pulmonary embolism. *Br Heart J* 51: 462– 464.
7. Marshall, V.F., Middleton, R.G., Holswade, G.R. et al. (1970). Surgery for renal cell carcinoma in the vena cava. *J Urol* 103: 414–420.
8. DeVille, J.B., Corley, D., Jin, B.S. et al. (1995). Assessment of intracardiac masses by transesophageal echocardiography. *Tex Heart Inst J* 22: 134–137.

46 Pericardial Metastasis Mass from Thyroid Carcinoma

Changchun Hao[1] and Jing Ping Sun[2]

[1] Qinglong Country Hospital, Hebei Province, China
[2] The Chinese University of Hong Kong, Hong Kong

History

A 74-year-old female presented with progressive shortness of breath over the previous 2 years. She had a total thyroidectomy for thyroid adenocarcinoma 6 years ago and had pericardial metastasis from her thyroid cancer diagnosed by echocardiogram and confirmed by cytological examination of pericardial fluid 5 years ago. She was treated conservatively with a yearly echocardiogram follow up in a rural hospital, since then, visiting the country hospital almost once a year.

Physical Examination

A physical examination revealed that her general condition was stable. Blood pressure was normal. On auscultation, a 3/6 systolic murmur was heard at the right sternal edge.

Echocardiography

A series of transthoracic echocardiography images obtained over 5 years was reviewed. Five years ago, a pericardial mass (1.0 × 1.2 cm) and moderate effusion were seen in a parasternal short-axis view. Four years ago, the mass had grown bigger (2 × 2 cm), partially compressing the right ventricle (RV). Two years ago the mass with a plentiful blood supply had grown in size pressing on the RV more. One year ago, the parasternal long-axis view showed severe external compression of the RV by the pericardial mass. After 5 years, the RV was almost completely pressed by a huge pericardial mass with a plentiful blood supply (5.8 cm × 8 cm) (Figure 46-1; Videos 46-1, 46-2, and 46-3).

The mass was clearly seen within the pericardial space without penetrating into the right ventricular wall (Figure 46-2; Video 46-4). Apical four-chamber view with color Doppler showed moderate tricuspid regurgitation (Figure 46-2; Video 46-4). The Doppler recording showed the peak velocity of tricuspid regurgitation is mild elevated (Figure 46-2).

Comparative Cardiac Imaging: A Case-based Guide, First Edition.
Edited by Jing Ping Sun, Xing Sheng Yang, and Bryan P. Yan.
© 2018 John Wiley & Sons Ltd. Published 2018 by John Wiley & Sons Ltd.
Companion website: www.wiley.com/sun/comparative_cardiac_imaging

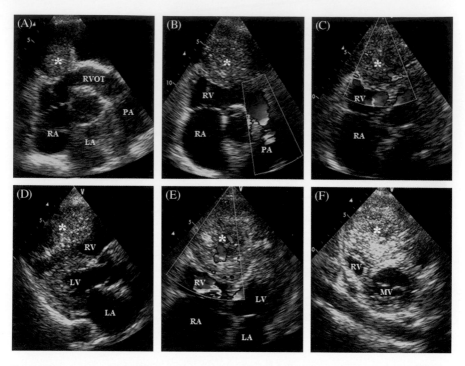

Figure 46-1 A series of transthoracic echocardiography images obtained over 5 years was reviewed. A. Five years ago, a pericardial mass (1.0 × 1.2 cm) and moderate effusion were seen in parasternal short-axis view. B. Four years ago, the mass had grown bigger (2 × 2 cm), partially compressing the right ventricle (RV). C. Two years ago, the mass had grown in size compressing the RV more, with a plentiful blood supply. D. One year ago, the parasternal long-axis view showed the RV was severely pressed by the pericardial mass. E and F. After 5 years, the RV was almost completely compressed by the huge vascular pericardial mass (5.8 cm × 8 cm).

Discussion

Metastasis pericarditis represents approximately 5%–7% of the cases with acute pericarditis [1–4]. Theoretically, any malignant tumor may cause a pericardial effusion or a mass [1, 2] through direct extension or metastasis via lymphatic or blood vessels into the pericardium [3, 5]. The most common malignancy causing pericardial effusion is lung cancer, followed by breast cancer, lymphomas, leukemia, and esophageal cancer. Only a few cases of neoplastic pericarditis in patients with thyroid cancer have been reported in the literature. Here, we present a case of thyroid carcinoma that metastasized into the pericardium causing moderate pericardial effusion and a mass initially, and then the effusion absorbed but the mass gradually grew and pressed the right ventricle.

Neoplastic pericarditis [6], massive pericardial effusion [7], or cardiac tamponade [7–12] have been reported as the first manifestation of a thyroid cancer. Although the best treatment for metastatic pericardial mass has not been established, most would advocate surgical removal at time of diagnosis. For reasons unknown to us, the patient did not undergo surgery 5 years ago. As a result, we were able to observe longitudinally the natural progression of the mass, which became vascular and grew in size causing progressive compression on the right ventricle without the evidence of other metastasis. This case might indicate that if patient get surgical therapy early, she might have better outcome.

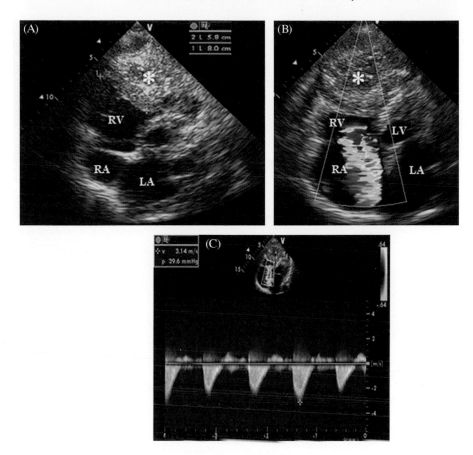

Figure 46-2 Echocardiography. A. Atypical short axis view showed the size of the mass was 5.8×8 cm. B. The mass was clearly seen within the pericardial space without penetrating into the right ventricular wall. Apical four-chamber view with color Doppler showed moderate tricuspid regurgitation. C. The Doppler recording showed the peak velocity of tricuspid regurgitation is mildly elevated.

Key Points

1. Massive pericardial metastatic mass caused by thyroid cancer is rare.
2. Metastatic thyroid carcinoma to the pericardium can be slow growing but can cause pressing on adjacent cardiac structures.

References

1. Imazio, M., Brucato, A., Derosa, F.G. et al. (2009). Aetiological diagnosis in acute and recurrent pericarditis: When and how. *J Cardiovasc Med (Hagerstown)* 10: 217–30.
2. Imazio, M., Spodick, D.H., Brucato, A. et al. (2010). Diagnostic issues in the clinical management of pericarditis. *Int J Clin Pract* 64: 1384–1392.
3. Imazio, M., Brucato, A, Mayosi, B.M. et al. (2010). Medical therapy of pericardial diseases: Part II: Noninfectious pericarditis, pericardial effusion and constrictive pericarditis. *J Cardiovasc Med (Hagerstown)* 11: 785–794.
4. Azam, S. and Hoit, B.D. (2011). Treatment of pericardial disease. *Cardiovasc Ther* 29: 308–314.
5. Refaat, M.M. and Katz, W.E. (2011). Neoplastic pericardial effusion. *Clin Cardiol* 34: 593–598.

6. Nissimov, R., Machtey, I. and Salomon, M. (1973). Thyroid carcinoma with pericardial involvement simulating rheumatic heart disease. *Harefuah* 84: 83–87.

7. Chiewvit, S., Pusuwan, P., Chiewvit, P. et al. (1998). Metastatic follicular carcinoma of thyroid to pericardium. *J Med Assoc Thai* 81: 799–802.

8. Jancić-Zguricas, M. and Janković, R. (1986). Occult papillary carcinoma of the thyroid gland revealed by cancer pericarditis. *Pathol Res Pract* 181: 761–766.

9. Kovacs, C.S., Nguyen, G.K., Mullen, J.C. et al. (1994). Cardiac tamponade as the initial presentation of papillary thyroid carcinoma. *Can J Cardiol* 10: 279–281.

10. de la Gándara, I., Espinosa, E., Gómez Cerezo, J. et al. (1997). Pericardial tamponade as the first manifestation of adenocarcinoma. *Acta Oncol* 36: 429–431.

11. Fukuda, A., Saito, T., Imai, M. et al. (2000). Metastatic cardiac papillary originating from the thyroid in both ventricles with a mobile right ventricular pedunculated tumor. *Jpn Circ J* 64: 890–892.

12. González Valverde, F.M., Gómez Ramos, M.J., Moltó Aguado, M. et al. (2005). Pericardial tamponade as initial presentation of papillary thyroid carcinoma. *Eur J Surg Oncol* 31: 205–207.

47 Spindle Cell Sarcoma: A Rare Case of Multicardiac Chamber Mass

Chengzheng Zhang[1], Junli Hu[1], Shaochun Wang[1], and Jing Ping Sun[2]

[1] Affiliated Hospital of Jining Medical University, Jining, China
[2] The Chinese University of Hong Kong, Hong Kong

History

A 49-year-old Chinese female admitted to our hospital due to worsening shortness of breath and palpitations for a few months. She was previously well and has no significant past history.

Physical Examination

On examination, she was hemodynamically stable. Cardiovascular and respiratory examination was unremarkable except for bilateral pleural effusions, which were confirmed on a chest X-ray. Incidentally, a palpable soft nontender mass was noted on the left buttock.

Echocardiography

Transthoracic echocardiography revealed a large mobile mass in the left atrium obstructing into the mitral valve and three smaller round mobile masses within the right atrium, and right and left ventricles. (Figure 47-1, Videos 47-1, 47-2, and 47-3). The size and function of both ventricles were normal. There was a small amount of pericardial effusion and massive pleural effusion.

Hospital Course

A core biopsy of the left buttock mass was performed. Thoracentesis was performed.

Pathology

The characteristic of histology examination from left buttock mass biopsy is consistent with undifferentiated spindle-cell sarcoma (Figure 47-2). The immunohistochemistry included cancer cell Vimentin (+),CR(−), EMA (−), SMMHC(−), MyoD1 (−), Myogenin (−), CD 31 vascular (+),CD 34 vascular (+), Ki-67 (+30–40%).

A preliminary diagnosis of undifferentiated spindle-cell sarcoma of the left-buttock mass was made. Cytology of the pleural effusion did not find evidence for a spindle-cell sarcoma.

Comparative Cardiac Imaging: A Case-based Guide, First Edition.
Edited by Jing Ping Sun, Xing Sheng Yang, and Bryan P. Yan.
© 2018 John Wiley & Sons Ltd. Published 2018 by John Wiley & Sons Ltd.
Companion website: www.wiley.com/sun/comparative_cardiac_imaging

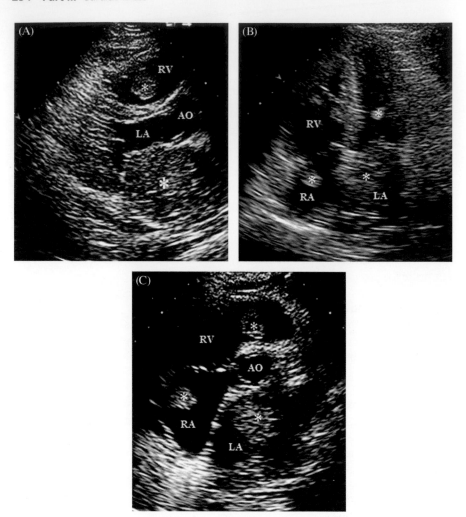

Figure 47-1 Transthoracic 2-D echocardiography examination revealed: A. The parasternal long-axis view showed a large mass (*) in the left atria, obstructing into the mitral inflow tract and a small mass (*) in the right ventricle. The systolic function of the left and right ventricles was normal. B. An apical four-chamber view showed a large mobile mass (*) obstructing into the mitral valve. A small round (*) mobile mass was seen in the left ventricle and the right atrium. C. A parasternal short-axis view showed three mobile masses (*) within the left atrium, right ventricle and atrium separately. *Notes:* LA, left atrium; LV, left ventricle; RA, right atrium; RV, right ventricle; AO, aorta.

Diagnosis

The presumptive diagnosis was metastasis pleural effusion and multiple cardiac masses.

Discussion

Metastatic cardiac tumors are 20-40 times more common than primary cardiac tumors [1]. The most common primary cardiac tumors are angiosarcoma and rhabdomyosarcoma [1]. Fibrosarcoma, primary osteogenic cardiac sarcoma, leiomyosarcoma,

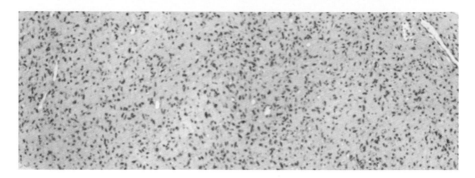

Figure 47-2 The characteristic of histology examination from left buttock mass biopsy is consistent with undifferentiated spindle-cell sarcoma.

liposarcoma, and primary cardiac lymphomas are less common. Undifferentiated sarcomas usually occur in the left atrium. Advances in cardiac imaging have enabled earlier detection of these rare malignant tumors [2].

Mayer et al. [1] described a series of 14 patients with sarcomas arising from the heart or the great vessels. We reported a case of spindle-cell sarcoma presenting with multiple cardiac chamber masses, which is seldom seen in the literature.

Transthoracic echocardiography (TTE) is the primary imaging modality for the initial diagnosis of intracardiac masses. It is noninvasive and inexpensive, and it provides functional information in addition to morphological details in multiple planes, it should be used as the first choice for detecting cardiac tumors.

Key Points

1. Spindle-cell sarcoma of soft tissue is a rare cause of cardiac masses.
2. Metastasis multiple cardiac chamber masses are very rare.

References

1. Meyer, F., Aebert, H., Rudert, M. et al. (2007). Primary malignant sarcomas of the heart and great vessels in adult patients – a single-center experience. *The Oncologist* 12: 1134–1142.
2. Araoz, P.A., Eklund, H.E., Welch, T.J. et al. (1999). CT and MR imaging of primary cardiac malignancies *Radiographics* 19: 1421–1434.

Part IV
Cardiomyopathy and Myocarditis

48 Fulminant Myocarditis

Lei Zhang¹, Jingjin Wang², and Jing Ping Sun³

¹ Tongji University School of Medicine, Shanghai, China
² Fuwai Hospital, Beijing, China
³ The Chinese University of Hong Kong, Hong Kong

History

A 48-year-old male was admitted because of severe shortness of breath. He had influenza about 2 weeks earlier.

Physical Examination

Patient was apyretic and presented severe dyspnea at rest. His respirations were 25/min, the pulse was 120, and the blood pressure was 90/60 mmHg. At the cardiac examination a grade 3 systolic murmur and a third tone were audible along the left sternal border. Crackles and wet rales were heard in lungs. The abdomen was normal.

Laboratory

The laboratory evaluations showed increased myocardia and liver enzymes (aspartate aminotransferase128 IU/L, alanine aminotransferase 194 IU/ L, lactate dehydrogenase 808 IU/ L, creatine kinase 988 IU/ L, MB fraction 76 IU/ L, alkaline phosphatase 307 IU/L, c glutam yltransferase101 IU/L) and high in ammatory parameters (C-reactive protein 76 mg/ L).

Electrocardiogram

An electrocardiogram showed sinus tachycardia with nonspecific ST segment changes (Figure 48-1).

Chest X-ray

Anteroposterior chest radiograph shows interstitial and alveolar pulmonary edema (Figure 48-2).

Echocardiography Examination

Transthoracic echocardiography showed that the left ventricle (LV) and atrium were mild enlarged with diffuse enhanced echo genesis of ventricular wall, and severe LV systolic dysfunction (LVEF 20 %). The right ventricle was in normal size with systolic dysfunction. There was a small amount of pericardial effusion (Video 48-1). The cardiac

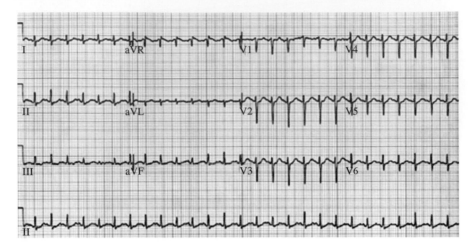

Figure 48-1 Electrocardiogram showing sinus tachycardia with nonspecific ST segment changes.

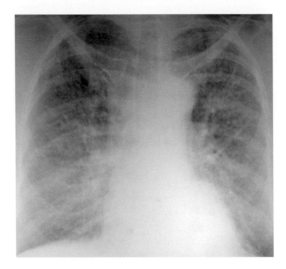

Figure 48-2 Chest X-ray anteroposterior chest radiograph showed interstitial and alveolar pulmonary edema.

strain image was analyzed; the LV global longitudinal (Figure 48-3A), circumferential and radial strains were significantly decreased.

Cardiac Magnetic Resonance Imaging

T2-weighted short tau inversion recovery (STIR) imaging showed myocardial edema in the intraventricular septum, and the anterior and lateral walls of the left ventricle (red arrow). Pericardial effusion is detected as hyperintense (Figure 48-4A). Early T1-weighted (early gadolinium enhancement [EGE]) images showed patch hyperintense in myocardia in the washout phase (Figure 48-4B). Late gadolinium enhanced areas were detected in the subepicardial layers of the LV inferolateral wall and in the

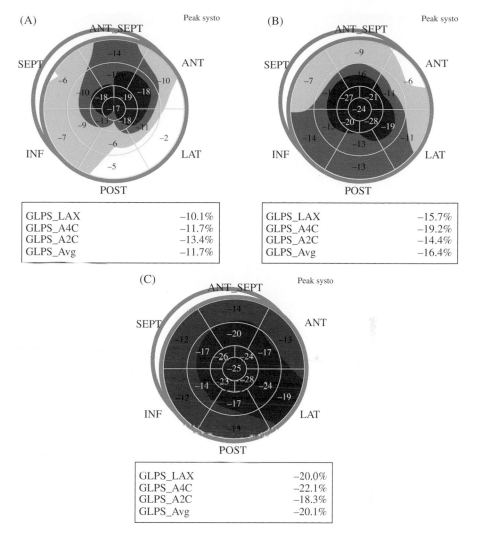

Figure 48-3 The results of cardiac longitudinal strain showed that the LV global longitudinal strain was significantly impaired excepting apex (A); it partially recovered after 2 weeks (B) and totally recovered three month later (C).

intraventricular septum of short-axis image (Figure 48-4C) and in LV lateral wall of four-chamber image (Figure 48-4D).

Hospital Course

According to the clinical characteristics above, the diagnosis of fulminant myocarditis was made. Prednisone at 30 mg/day, low doses of β-blocker and angiotensin-converting enzyme inhibitor were initiated. The patient's condition became stable and recovered smoothly. At 2-week follow-up, his LVEF had improved to 45% (Video 48-2) and LV longitudinal strain was improved (Figure 48-3B). At 3-month follow up, the patient is symptom free and back to work, his LV EF is 68% (Video 48-3) and LV longitudinal strain was totally recovered three month later (Figure 48-3C).

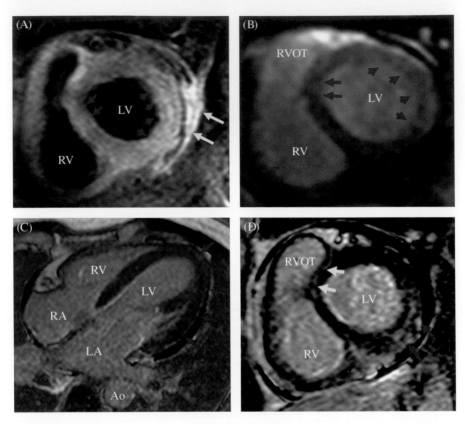

Figure 48-4 Cardiac magnetic resonance T2-weighted short tau inversion recovery (STIR) imaging showed myocardial edema in the intraventricular septum, anterior and lateral wall of left ventricle (red arrow). Pericardial effusion is detected as hyperintense (A). Early T1-weighted (early gadolinium enhancement [EGE]) images showed patch hyperintense in myocardia in the washout phase (B). Late gadolinium enhanced areas were detected in the subepicardial layers of the LV inferolateral wall and in the intraventricular septum of short-axis image (C) and in LV lateral wall of four-chamber image (D).

Discussion

Myocarditis is a disease marked by inflammation and damage of the heart muscle. Although the exact incidence of myocarditis is not known, it is estimated that several thousand patients per year are diagnosed in the United States. Myocarditis is an important cause of cardiac morbidity and mortality, accounting for up to 20% of sudden unexpected deaths in young adults [1]. Fulminant myocarditis is characterized by a distinct viral prodrome, the sudden onset of severe hemodynamic compromise and marked myocardial inflammation. In contrast, patients with acute myocarditis have an indistinct onset of symptoms, less severe hemodynamic embarrassment, and a more variable degree of myocardial inflammation. If patients with fulminant myocarditis are aggressively supported in a timely manner, nearly all can have an excellent recovery.

There are many causes of myocarditis, including viral infections, autoimmune diseases, environmental toxins, and adverse reactions to medications. The prognosis is variable but chronic heart failure is the major long-term complication. Myocarditis and the associated disorder of idiopathic dilated cardiomyopathy are the cause of approximately 45% of heart transplants in the United States [2].

Diagnosis

Because patients with acute myocarditis present in many different ways, often accompanied by unspecific symptoms, correct diagnosis is often challenging [3]. Although endomyocardial biopsy is still regarded as the gold standard for diagnosis [3], non-invasive cardiac magnetic resonance (CMR) is increasingly used for the diagnostic evaluation of patients suspected of having acute myocarditis [4, 5].

Cardiac magnetic resonance uses three types of images to diagnose myocarditis: T2-weighted (T2-W) with fat saturation, early T1-weighted (early gadolinium enhancement [EGE]) images taken 1 min after the injection of gadolinium and delayed enhanced images (LGE) taken 15 min after the injection of gadolinium [6]. These techniques can help determine the extent and hemodynamic significance of effusions [6, 7]. The widely adopted Lake Louise criteria state that two of the following three CMR findings must be present to indicate myocardial inflammation consistent with myocarditis: increased regional or global myocardial signal intensity in T2-weighted images (supporting myocardial edema), increased global myocardial early gadolinium enhancement (EGE) ratio between myocardium and skeletal muscle in gadolinium enhanced T1-weighted images (supporting hyperemia/capillary leakage), and at least one focal lesion with nonischemic distribution in late gadolinium-enhanced (LGE) T1-weighted images (supporting irreversible cell injury/necrosis) [6]. T2-W is indicative of tissue-free water and is increased during an inflammatory or necrotic process. There is a high sensitivity and specificity of T2-W compared to myocardial biopsy [6, 8]. However, differentiation between inflammation and necrosis cannot be achieved only by using T2-W images, as observed in myocarditis or myocardial infarction. Early gadolinium enhancement (EGE) can detect hyperintense myocardial regions of gadolinium uptake and evaluate hyperemia in myocarditis. Early gadolinium enhancement is described as increased distribution into the interstitial space early in the washout phase [6]. This occurs because of cell damage, increased blood flow, and vasodilation in myocarditis [9]. T1-weighted late gadolinium enhancement (LGE) can detect irreversible cell injury, myocyte necrosis, and myocardial fibrosis in the setting of myocarditis [6, 10]. Late gadolinium enhancement is commonly found in the septal wall or in a patchy distribution in the subepicardial layers of the ventricular free wall, but can also be seen in transmural patterns [9]. LGE as an independent diagnostic marker for myocarditis has high specificity but relatively poor sensitivity and diagnostic accuracy for acute myocarditis [6, 9]. CMR can also identify structural abnormalities suggestive of myocarditis, such as global LV dysfunction, increased myocardial wall thickening, and pericardial effusion [11]. Nonspecific pericardial effusion is commonly associated with myocarditis and can be detected with short and long-axis steady-state free precession (SSFP) images or T2-weighted short tau inversion recovery (STIR) imaging. Although pericardial effusion was not included in the Lake Louise criteria, it is valuable supporting evidence of myocarditis [12]. The all of characteristics of CMRI were detected in our patient.

Echocardiography remains one of the primary imaging tools to assess left-ventricular function. In comparison with nonfulminant myocarditis, patients with fulminant myocarditis are more likely to have right-ventricular systolic dysfunction, a normal left ventricular end-diastolic diameter, and increased septal wall thickness [13, 14–18]. As a consequence of the ease with which echocardiography can be performed at the bedside and valuable information obtained, it is recommended as the first-choice imaging modality for these patients. One MRI study [19] indicated global longitudinal and circumferential strain displayed a good accuracy in detecting acute myocarditis (75% and 70%, respectively), suggesting that myocardial deformation analysis can provide incremental diagnostic information in suspected acute myocarditis. In our case, we analyzed the longitudinal strain by the speckle tracking echocardiography, the results demonstrated LV function was global impaired severely excepted apex, and recovered completely 3 month later, which is good quantification recording.

Angiography is recommended for adult patients with risk factors to rule out epicardial coronary artery disease.

Classification

Previously, patients with suspected myocarditis were classified as having fulminant, acute, chronic active or chronic persistent myocarditis on the basis of their clinical course, histological findings, and response to immunosuppressive therapy [20]. In 2000, a classification system was proposed that was based on an analysis of data on 750 patients followed up for more than 7 years. This system incorporated echocardiographic findings, hemodynamic data obtained from right heart catheterization, and the Dallas histologic criteria [13]. Under this new classification system, the distinguishing features of fulminant myocarditis as opposed to nonfulminant myocarditis included histological findings of more severe inflammation, lower mean arterial pressure, higher heart rate, and higher right atrial and pulmonary capillary wedge pressure. Normal left ventricular diastolic dimension and increased thickness of the interventricular septum were also considered characteristic of fulminant myocarditis; the latter feature might possibly result from increased myocardial edema.

In our case, the patient presented with acute pulmonary edema, tachycardia and lower blood pressure and recovered very well. We think this case should be classified as fulminant myocarditis.

Management

Of note, it is notable that there were no specific therapies for fulminant myocarditis. As patients with this disease present with hemodynamic instability and are often in cardiogenic shock, the first-line treatment is supportive care. The majority of these patients require inotropic support, in some cases with an intra-aortic balloon pump, to maintain blood pressure and improve cardiac output. If the patient does not respond to aggressive supportive therapy within a few hours to days, insertion of a ventricular assist device (VAD) should be considered.

Prognosis

If the disease is recognized quickly and appropriate supportive care is initiated early, long-term survival of patients with fulminant myocarditis is excellent.

Key Points

1. Myocarditis could account for up to 10% of acute-onset heart failure cases; viral infections are responsible in the majority of instances.
2. Patients with fulminant myocarditis often present with cardiogenic shock and multiorgan failure; several clinical and laboratory findings enable the practicing physician to differentiate fulminant from nonfulminant myocarditis.
3. Endomyocardial biopsy serves a critical role in the management of fulminant myocarditis and is an essential diagnostic tool to help differentiate myocarditis from giant cell myocarditis and necrotizing eosinophilic myocarditis.
4. Patients with fulminant myocarditis should be managed with aggressive inotropic support with or without placement of an intra-aortic balloon pump; if the patient does not respond rapidly to aggressive supportive therapy, insertion of a ventricular assist device should be considered at an early stage

References

1. Drory, Y., Turetz, Y., Hiss, Y. et al. (1991) Sudden unexpected death in persons less than 40 years of age. *Am J Cardiol* 68:1388–1392
2. Liu, P.P. and Mason, J.W. (2001). Advances in the understanding of myocarditis. *Circulation* 104: 1076–1082.
3. Fabre, A. and Sheppard, M.N. (2006). Sudden adult death syndrome and other nonischaemic causes of sudden cardiac death. *Heart* 92 (3): 316–320.
4. Magnani, J.W., Danik, H.J., Dec, G.W., Jr et al. (2006). Survival in biopsy-proven myocarditis: A long-term retrospective analysis of the histopathologic, clinical, and hemodynamic predictors. *Am Heart J* 151 (2): 463–470.
5. Caforio, A.L., Calabrese, F., Angelini, A. et al. (2007). A prospective study of biopsy-proven myocarditis: prognostic relevance of clinical and aetiopathogenetic features at diagnosis. *Eur Heart J* 28 (11): 1326–1333.
6. Friedrich, M.G., Sechtem, U., Schulz-Menger, J. et al. (2009). Cardiovascular magnetic resonance in myocarditis: a JACC White Paper. *J Am Coll Cardiol* 53: 1475–1487.
7. Friedrich, M.G. and Marcotte, F. (2013). Cardiac magnetic resonance assessment of myocarditis. *Circ Cardiovasc Imaging* 6: 833–839.
8. Gagliardi, M.G., Polletta, B., Di Renzi, P. (1999). MRI for the diagnosis and follow-up of myocarditis. *Circulation* 99: 458–459.
9. Yilmaz, A., Ferreira, V., Klingel, K. et al. (2013). Role of cardiovascular magnetic resonance imaging (CMR) in the diagnosis of acute and chronic myocarditis. *Heart Fail Rev* 18: 747–760.
10. Park, C.H., Choi, E.Y., Greiser, A. et al. (2013). Diagnosis of acute global myocarditis using cardiac MRI with quantitative t1 and t2 mapping: case report and literature review. *Korean J Radiol* 14: 727–732.
11. Rottgen, R., Christiani, R., Freyhardt, P. et al. (2011). Magnetic resonance imaging findings in acute myocarditis and correlation with immunohistological parameters. *Eur Radiol* 21: 1259–1266.
12. Lurz, P., Eitel, I., Klieme, B. et al. (2014). The potential additional diagnostic value of assessing for pericardial effusion on cardiac magnetic resonance imaging in patients with suspected myocarditis. *Eur Heart J Cardiovasc Imaging* 15: 643–650.
13. Felker, G.M., Boehmer, J.P., Hruban, R.H. et al. (2000). Echocardiographic findings in fulminant and acute myocarditis. *J Am Coll Cardiol* 36: 227–232.
14. Pinamonti, B., Alberti, E., Cigalotto, A. et al. (1988). Echocardiographic findings in myocarditis. *Am J Cardiol* 62: 285–291.
15. Mendes, L.A., Dec, G.W., Picard, M.H. et al. (1994). Right ventricular dysfunction: An independent predictor of adverse outcome in patients with myocarditis. *Am Heart J* 128: 301–307. |

16. Lieback, E., Hardouin, I., Meyer, R. (1996). Clinical value of echocardiographic tissue characterization in the diagnosis of myocarditis. *Eur Heart J* 17: 135–142.
17. Carvalho, J.S., Silva, C.M., Shinebourne, E.A. et al. (1996). Prognostic value of posterior wall thickness in childhood dilated cardiomyopathy and myocarditis. *Eur Heart J* 17: 1233–1238.
18. Hiramitsu, S., Morimoto, S., Kato, S. et al. (2001). Transient ventricular wall thickening in acute myocarditis: a serial echocardiographic and histopathologic study. *Jpn Circ J* 65: 863–866.
19. Luetkens, J.A., Schlesinger-Irsch, U., Kuetting, D.L. et al. (2014). Feature-tracking myocardial strain analysis in acute myocarditis: diagnostic value and association with myocardial oedema. *Eur Heart J Cardiovasc Imaging* 15: 643–650.
20. Lieberman, E.B., Hutchins, G.M., Herskowitz, A. et al. (1991). Clinicopathologic description of myocarditis. *J Am Coll Cardiol* 18: 1617–1626.

49 Cardiac Amyloidosis

Jing Ping Sun, Xing Sheng Yang, Bryan P. Yan, and Ka-Tak Wong

The Chinese University of Hong Kong, Hong Kong

History

Case 1 is a 64-year-old male and Case 2 is a 47-year-old female. Both presented with increasing shortness of breath with no significant past history.

Physical Examination

Both patients were normotensive and in sinus rhythm. Cardiovascular examination was unremarkable in both cases. There were no murmurs or signs of heart failure.

Electrocardiogram

Case 1: Diffuse low voltages (presence of QRS voltage amplitude <0.5 mV) in all limb leads with QS pattern in pericardial leads V1-4 (Figure 49-1, top). Case 2: Diffuse low voltages (≤0.5 mV) in all limb leads (Figure 49-1, bottom).

Chest X-ray

Case 1: Bilateral moderate pleural effusion. Case 2: Unremarkable.

Transthoracic Echocardiogram

Case 1: Echocardiogram revealed biatrial enlargement, severe concentric left ventricular (LV) hypertrophy with global hypokinesis (left ventricular eject fraction was 38%), and severe diastolic dysfunction with restrictive filling pattern. There were diffuse echogenetic dots throughout the myocardium (speckled appearance). There was mild right-ventricular hypertrophy with preserved systolic function. There was a small amount of pericardial effusion and moderate pleural effusion. All four cardiac valves and annulus were thickened and echogenetic. There was mild mitral, tricuspid, pulmonary and aortic valvular regurgitation. (See Figures 49-2, 49-3; Videos 49-1, 49-2, and 49-3).

Case 2: There was mild concentric LV hypertrophy with normal size and systolic function and stage 1 diastolic dysfunction. The left atrium was moderately enlarged. The right ventricular free wall was mildly thickened with normal size and systolic function. The mitral and aortic annuluses were mildly thickened with mild regurgitation. There was a small amount of pericardial effusion. (See Figure 49-4; Videos 49-4, 49-5, and 49-6).

Comparative Cardiac Imaging: A Case-based Guide, First Edition.
Edited by Jing Ping Sun, Xing Sheng Yang, and Bryan P. Yan.
© 2018 John Wiley & Sons Ltd. Published 2018 by John Wiley & Sons Ltd.
Companion website: www.wiley.com/sun/comparative_cardiac_imaging

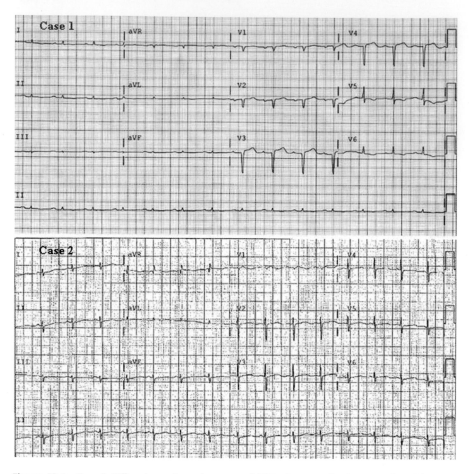

Figure 49-1   Case 1: Diffuse low voltages (presence of QRS voltage amplitude <0.5 mV) in all limb leads with QS pattern in pericardial leads V1-4 (top). Case 2: Diffuse low voltages (≤0.5 mV) in all limb leads (bottom).

Two-D strain imaging showed reduced LV longitudinal and circumferential strain, especially in the septal and anterior walls (Figure 49-5A and B). Basal and apical rotation was decreased and desynchronized resulting in reduced LV twist (Figure 49-5C). Radial strain rate showed decreased early diastolic velocity (Figure 49-5D).

Cardiac Magnetic Resonance Imaging
Case 1: Left ventricle was hypertrophied with global hypokinesis; mild RV hypertrophy with normal systolic function. Late gadolinium enhancement cardiovascular magnetic resonance (CMR) showed diffuse extensive circumferential enhancement involving both the subendocardium and entire myocardium of the LV from basal to apical regions, and RV wall (Figure 49-6). Pulmonary truck and branch pulmonary arteries were not dilated. Pericardium thickness was normal. Mild pericardial effusion and moderate bilateral effusion (more on the right) were detected.

Case 2: Left ventricular hypertrophy with preserved ventricular function. There was no characteristic CMR late gadolinium enhancement for typical cardiac amyloidosis.

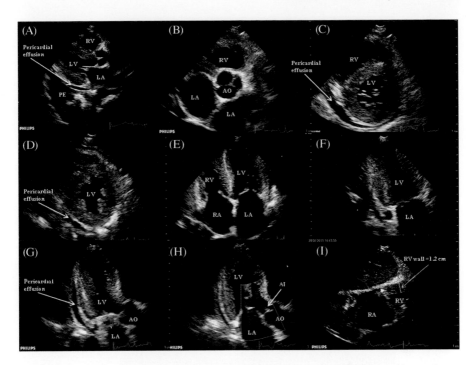

Figure 49-2 Two-D echocardiography images recorded from Case 1: A. The parasternal long-axis view shows left atrial enlargement, severe concentric left-ventricular hypertrophy. There were echogenetic dots diffusing in the myocardium. There is small amount pericardial effusion and moderate pleural effusion (PE). B. The aortic level of parasternal short axis view shows aortic valves and annulus are thickened and both of atriums are enlarge. C. The basal level of parasternal short-axis view shows LV walls and mitral valves are thickened, there is small amount pericardial effusion. D. The middle level of the parasternal short-axis view shows thickened LV walls and pericardial effusion. E. The apical four-chamber view indicates both of atriums enlargement with thickened interatrial septum, and LV hypertrophy. F. An apical two-chamber view shows concentrated LV hypertrophy. G. An apical three-chamber view shows LV hypertrophy and pericardial effusion. H. An apical three-chamber view with color Doppler shows aortic valvular regurgitation. I. The subcustal four-chamber view indicates that the RV free wall is thickened.

Biopsy

Case 1: Cardiac biopsy confirmed the diagnosis of cardiac amyloidosis. Case 2: The diagnosis of amyloidosis was confirmed by kidney biopsy.

Discussion

Amyloidosis is a clinical disorder caused by extracellular deposition of insoluble abnormal fibrils, derived from aggregation of misfolded normally soluble protein [1, 2]. Systemic amyloidosis, in which amyloid deposits are present in the viscera, blood vessel walls, and connective tissues, is usually fatal and is the cause of about 1 per 1000 deaths in developed countries [3]. There are also various localized forms of amyloidosis in which the deposits are confined to specific foci or to a particular organ or tissue. Cardiac amyloidosis is used to describe amyloid depositing in the heart, whether as part of systemic amyloidosis or as a localized phenomenon.

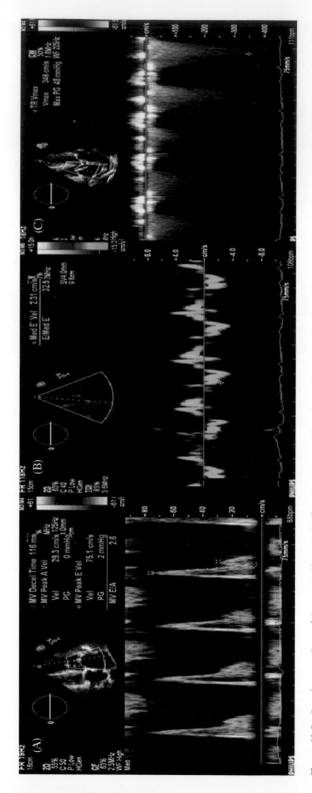

Figure 49-3 Doppler recordings of Case 1: A. The mitral inflow Doppler recording showed E/A >2.5, deceleration time = 116 ms. B. The peak velocity of mitral annulus was 2.3 cm/s, and E/e' was 32.5. C. The peak velocity of tricuspid regurgitation was elevated (346 cm/s).

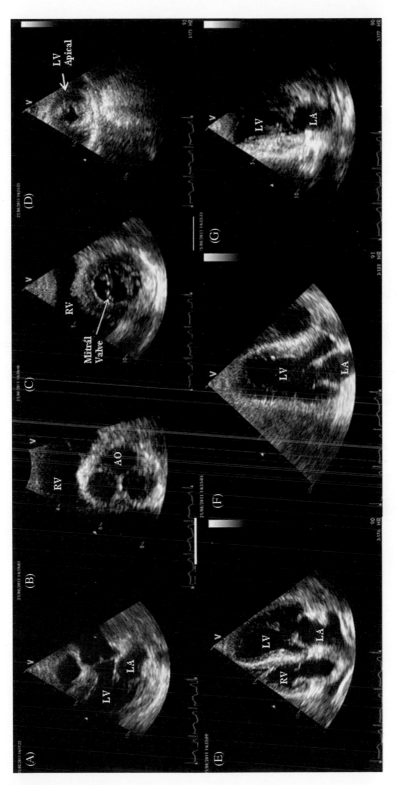

Figure 49-4 Two-D echocardiography images recorded from Case 2: A. The parasternal long axis view shows left atrial enlargement, mild concentric left ventricular hypertrophy. B. The aortic level of parasternal short axis view shows aortic valves and annulus are thickened. C. The basal level of parasternal short axis view shows LV walls and mitral valves are thickened. D. The apical level of parasternal short axis view shows thickened LV walls. E. The apical level of parasternal short axis view indicates left atrial enlargement with thickened inter atrial septum, and concentrate LV hypertrophy. F. Apical three-chamber view shows concentrate LV hypertrophy. G. Apical two-chamber view shows LV hypertrophy.

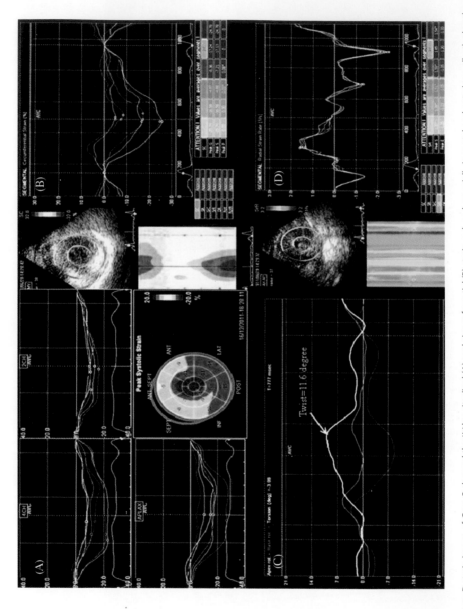

Figure 49-5 A two-D strain image of Case 2 showed the LV longitudinal (A) and circumferential (B) strain reduced especially in septal and anterior walls; the basal and apical rotation were decreased and desynchronized resulting in a decreased LV twist (C); the radial strain rate showed that the velocity of early diastole was decreased in this 43-year-old woman (D).

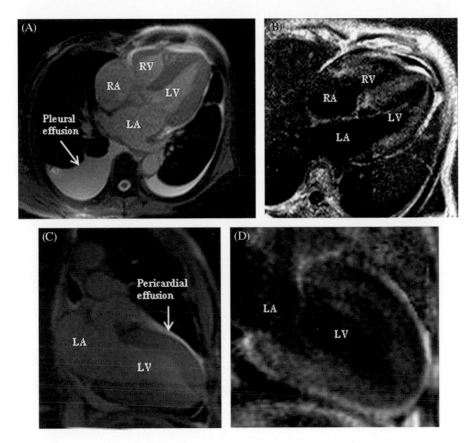

Figure 49-6 A. A four-chamber steady-state free precession image of Case 1 with cardiac amyloido-sis shows diffuse thickening of the myocardium and moderate atrial enlargement. B. A four-chamber view from a postgadolinium delayed enhancement image shows widespread enhancement in the right and left ventricular myocardium involving both the subendocardial and entire myocardium of the LV from basal to apical regions, and RV wall. C. Two-chamber steady-state free precession image of shows diffuse thickening of myocardium and moderate left atrial enlargement. D. Two-chamber long-axis views from postgadolinium delayed enhancement images show widespread enhancement in the left ventricular myocardium.

Types of Amyloidosis

The most frequent types of amyloidosis are the AL (primary) and AA (secondary) types.

AL Amyloidosis AL amyloid is due to deposition of protein derived from immunoglobulin light chain fragments. AL amyloid can occur alone or in association with multiple myeloma or, much less often, Waldenström's macroglobulinemia or non-Hodgkin lymphoma.

AA Amyloidosis AA amyloidosis may complicate chronic diseases in which there is ongoing or recurring inflammation, such as rheumatoid arthritis, spondyloarthropathy, or inflammatory bowel disease; chronic infections; or periodic fever syndromes [4]. The fibrils are composed of fragments of the acute phase reactant serum amyloid A.

Dialysis-related Amyloidosis Dialysis-related amyloidosis is due to deposition of fibrils derived from beta-2 microglobulin, which accumulates in patients with end-stage renal disease who are being maintained for prolonged periods of time by dialysis. This disorder has a predilection for osteoarticular structures.

Heritable Amyloidosis Many mutations lead to heritable types of amyloidosis. An example of this heterogeneous group of disorders is heritable neuropathic and/or cardiomyopathic amyloidosis due to deposition of fibrils derived from transthyretin (also referred to as prealbumin). In addition to the foregoing forms of amyloidosis, certain hereditary types have been reported in which heart may become involved, and in one type it is the organ predominantly affected.

Age-related (Senile) Systemic Amyloidosis Deposition of otherwise normal (wild-type) transthyretin in myocardium and other sites has been referred is referred to as systemic senile amyloidosis (SSA) [5]. Compared with patients with AL amyloidosis, those with the senile systemic disease survive longer (75 versus 11 months) despite having ventricular free wall and septal thickening due to amyloid deposits [6]. Significant renal involvement is rare in the senile systemic disorder; carpal tunnel syndrome may be seen. The disease affects elderly persons, usually in the seventh to ninth decades, and thus seems to be a manifestation of senescence. It is sometimes referred to as senile cardiac amyloidosis.

Organ-specific Amyloid Amyloid deposition can be isolated to a single organ, such as the skin, eye, heart, pancreas, or genitourinary tract, resulting in specific syndromes. Forms of primary localized cutaneous amyloidosis include macular, nodular, and lichen amyloidosis, with the last occurring in some families with multiple endocrine neoplasia type 2 [7–9].

Amyloidosis Restricted to the Heart A distinctive type of amyloidosis has been described in which amyloid is restricted largely to the heart. Deposits either do not appear in other organs or are present in insignificant amounts. This is in contrast to the systemic forms of amyloidosis in which involvement of other organs is extensive.

Less commonly, cardiac amyloidosis may be sufficiently severe to cause cardiac symptoms, and in only rare instances can death from congestive cardiac failure be attributed to cardiac amyloidosis. When the heart is severely involved, amyloid deposits may occur throughout the interstitium of ventricular and atrial myocardium. Subendocardial deposits are especially common in the atria. The wall of the coronary arteries and conduction pathways also may be involved. Discrete nodular deposits of amyloid may be evident on cross sections of the ventricles or under the atrial endocardium. There are multiple subendocardial deposits of glistening, partially translucent amyloid deposits in the atrium. Similar nodules may occur on the epicardial surface or the parietal pericardium. Involvement of the valvular endocardium may also occur.

Microscopically, amyloid occurs in extracellular, eosinophilic, amorphous hyaline deposits. Deposits may form rings completely surrounding and compressing individual myocytes. In systemic amyloidosis of immunoglobulin light chain (AL) and transthyretin (TTR) types, cardiac involvement is frequent and is a major determinant of treatment options and prognosis [10]. Amyloidosis was diagnosed with Congo red staining and demonstration of red-green birefringence under crosspolarized light. In cases of doubt, additional DNA analysis should be performed.

Clinical Manifestation
Cardiac involvement can lead to systolic or diastolic dysfunction and the symptoms of heart failure. Other manifestations that can occur include syncope due to arrhythmia or heart block, and angina or infarction due to accumulation of amyloid in the coronary arteries [11].

Diagnosis
Biopsy
The diagnosis of amyloidosis can be confirmed only by tissue biopsy, although the presence of amyloidosis may be suggested by the history and clinical manifestations (e.g., nephrotic syndrome in a patient with multiple myeloma or long-standing, active rheumatoid arthritis). Biopsies may be directed to dysfunctional organs (e.g. kidney, nerve) or to clinically uninvolved sites such as subcutaneous fat, minor salivary glands, or rectal mucosa.

Echocardiography
Echocardiography can show several features that are suggestive of cardiac amyloidosis, though the classical features are commonly present only in the later stages of disease [12, 13], and there is a wide spectrum of echocardiographic findings. Echocardiography cannot confirm diagnosis in isolation, and the images should be interpreted in the context of the clinical picture and other investigations. The most common echocardiographic feature is thickening of the LV wall, particularly in the absence of hypertension [12, 14, 15]. This feature has poor specificity for amyloidosis because of its occurrence with other conditions, such as hypertensive heart disease, hypertrophic cardiomyopathy, and other infiltrative cardiac diseases (glycogen storage diseases, sarcoidosis, and hemochromatosis). However, the two-D strain image can detect the early systolic function impaired and distinguishes the cardiac amyloidosis from the left ventricular hypertrophy caused by hypertension or hypertrophic cardiomyopathy [16].

The combination of increased LV mass in the absence of high ECG voltages may be more specific for infiltrative diseases, of which amyloid is the most common. High sensitivity (72% to 79%) and specificity (91% to 100%) have been reported for this combination [15, 17]. Increased echogenicity of the myocardium, particularly with a granular or "sparkling" appearance, has been reported in several studies [15, 18–20]. Systolic dysfunction, as measured by low ejection fraction or absence of wall hypertrophy, is uncommon until the more severe stages of disease and can be absent in up to 75% of cases [14, 15, 21, 22]. Diastolic dysfunction is the hallmark, and may be present in all patients, with 21% to 88% of patients showing a restrictive pattern on Doppler mitral inflow assessment [21, 22, 23]. The variable prevalence of diastolic dysfunction may also be related to the severity of disease in the group studied, as the likelihood of a restrictive physiological pattern increases with the severity of disease [21, 23]. Tissue Doppler and two-D strain imaging has shown reduced diastolic velocities in both early and late cardiac amyloid [24], so even early diastolic dysfunction could be identified (when wall thickening is minimal). Other features of cardiac amyloid include thickened valves and a small pericardial effusion; other parameters such as atrial strain and ventricular strain rate imaging show mean differences between amyloid groups with and without heart failure [25] but the considerable overlap in values between groups limits the clinical application of these techniques.

In this study, Case 1 had all of echocardiographic features noted in amyloidosis, including marked LV wall thickening, biatrial enlargement, thickened valve leaflets, and a pericardial effusion; as well as left ventricular systolic dysfunction and diastolic function in restrictive pattern. In case 2, there were all of mild echocardiographic features above and diastolic dysfunction but left ventricular function was reserved. Meanwhile, the results of two-D strain showed the left ventricular longitudinal, circumferential and twist were significantly reduced, even though cardiac MRI did not show late gadolinium enhancement in the myocardium. This case may present that two-D strain imaging might be helpful in diagnose of cardiac amyloidosis early stage.

Cardiovascular Magnetic Resonance

A strength of CMR using the late gadolinium enhancement technique is the ability to "phenotype" various forms of cardiomyopathy with high spatial resolution and reproducibility. In a summary of studies using gadolinium-enhanced CMR, cardiac amyloidosis was associated with qualitative global and subendocardial gadolinium enhancement of the myocardium, subendocardial longitudinal relaxation time (T1) was shorter than in control subjects and was correlated with markers of increased myocardial amyloid load, such as LV mass, wall thickness, interatrial septal thickness, and diastolic function [26]. Gadolinium enhancement could be localized or diffuse, and subendocardial or transmural [27]. The number of enhanced segments correlated with LV end-diastolic volume, end-systolic volume, and left atrial size. There was diffusing transmural gadolinium enhancement in both ventricular myocardia in our Case 1, but it was not detected in Case 2.

Electrocardiography

Systematic study of ECG findings in biopsy-confirmed cardiac amyloidosis is relatively sparse. An ECG voltage is strongly suggests cardiac amyloid. Murtagh et al. [28] from the Mayo Clinic provide the largest report to date of ECG findings in a population of patients with AL amyloidosis and biopsy-proven cardiac involvement. In 127 patients, they found that low ECG voltage (presence of QRS voltage amplitude <0.5 mV in all limb leads or < 1 mV in all precordial leads) was present in 46% of patients, and a pseudo-infarct pattern (i.e., no infarct actually evident on echocardiography) was present in 47% of patients. The pseudo-infarct patterns were anterior (36%), inferior (12%), and lateral (14%). Both low ECG voltage and pseudo-infarct pattern were present in 25% of patients. There was a moderate correlation between the presence of low voltage and pericardial effusion but no correlation between voltage and the ejection fraction. Atrial fibrillation and flutter were the most common arrhythmia.

The present study showed low ECG voltage (presence of QRS voltage amplitude <0.5 mV) in all limb leads and QS pattern in precordial V1-4 leads in Case 1; it showed low ECG voltage of QRS ($\leq$0.5 mV) in all limb leads in Case 2.

Comparison of Diagnosis Techniques

Biopsy: Histological findings in cardiac amyloidosis are characterized by interstitial expansion with amyloid protein [29] and associated endomyocardial fibrosis [30].The gold standard for diagnosis of cardiac amyloidosis is endomyocardial biopsy, although clinically significant amyloid can be missed with small biopsies because of heterogeneous deposition, and incidental wild-type TTR amyloid deposits occurs in elderly patients. A biopsy of another area, such as the abdomen, kidney, or bone marrow, is often done to confirm the diagnosis.

Elecrocadiograph abnormality is a clue to cardiac disease, and is a low-cost noninvasive test. A pattern of low voltage (QRS voltage amplitude ≤0.5 mV in all limb leads or ≤1 mV in all precordial leads) and pseudo infarct pattern are commonly seen in cases with severe amyloid infiltration. Echocardiography is usually considered the technique of choice, with advance two-D strain image can detect the ventricular dysfunction in early stage of cardiac amyloidosis, as seen in our Case 2. The combination of thickening of the LV wall by echocardiography and a pattern of low voltage ECG is very important diagnosis clue of cardiac amyloidosis, particularly in the absence of hypertension. Cardiovascular magnetic resonance late gadolinium enhancement is a more specific and quantitative technique in diagnosis of cardiac amyloidosis. Screening of subclinical early cardiac involvement may become possible. Combined all of information from our cases, the features of echocardiogram and CMR late gadolinium enhancement indicated that the diagnosis of cardiac amyloidosis in Case 1 is in late stage, and Case 2 is in early stage.

Key Points

1. The combination of increased LV mass detected by echocardiography in the absence of high ECG voltages may be more specific for infiltrative diseases, of which amyloid is the most common.
2. CMR late gadolinium enhancement is a more specific and quantitative technique for the diagnosis of cardiac amyloidosis.
3. The gold standard for diagnosis of cardiac amyloidosis is endomyocardial biopsy; a positive result can confirm the diagnosis but a negative result cannot exclude the diagnosis.
4. Two-D strain imaging may be useful in the diagnose of early stages of cardiac amyloidosis.

References

1. Merlini, G. and Westermark, P. (2004). The systemic amyloidoses: clearer understanding of the molecular mechanisms offers hope for more effective therapies. *J Intern Med* 255: 159–178.
2. Selkoe, D.J. (2003). Folding proteins in fatal ways. *Nature* 426(6968): 900–904.
3. Kyle, R.A., Linos, A., Beard, C.M., et al. (1992). Incidence and natural history of primary systemic amyloidosis in Olmsted County, Minnesota, 1950 through 1989. *Blood* 79: 1817–1822.
4. Lachmann, H.J., Goodman, H.J., Gilbertson, J.A., et al. (2007). Natural history and outcome in systemic AA amyloidosis. *N Engl J Med* 356: 2361.
5. Westermark, P., Bergström, J., Solomon, A., et al. (2003). Transthyretin-derived senile systemic amyloidosis: clinicopathologic and structural considerations. *Amyloid* 10 Suppl 1: 48.
6. Ng, B., Connors, L.H., Davidoff, R. et al. (2005). Senile systemic amyloidosis presenting with heart failure: a comparison with light chain-associated amyloidosis. *Arch Intern Med* 165: 1425.

7. Tanaka, A., Arita, K., Lai-Cheong, J.E., et al. (2009). New insight into mechanisms of pruritus from molecular studies on familial primary localized cutaneous amyloidosis. *Br J Dermatol* 161: 1217.

8. Meijer, J.M., Schonland, S.O., Palladini, G. et al. (2008). Sjögren's syndrome and localized nodular cutaneous amyloidosis: coincidence or a distinct clinical entity? *Arthritis Rheum* 58:1992.

9. Baykal, C., Buyukbabani, N., Boztepe, H., et al. (2007). Multiple cutaneous neuromas and macular amyloidosis associated with medullary thyroid carcinoma. *J Am Acad Dermatol* 56: S33.

10. Kyle, R.A., Greipp, P.R. and O'Fallon, W.M. (1986). Primary systemic amyloidosis: multivariate analysis for prognostic factors in 168 cases. *Blood* 68: 220–224.

11. Dubrey, S.W., Hawkins, P.N. and Falk, R.H. (2011). Amyloid diseases of the heart: assessment, diagnosis, and referral. *Heart* 97: 75.

12. Cueto-Garcia, L., Tajik, A.J., Kyle, R.A., et al. (1984). Serial echocardiographic observations in patients with primary systemic amyloidosis: an introduction to the concept of early (asymptomatic) amyloid infiltration of the heart. *Mayo Clin Proc* 59: 589–597.

13. Falk, R.H. (2005). Diagnosis and management of the cardiac amyloidoses. *Circulation* 112: 2047–2060.

14. Nishikawa, H., Nishiyama, S., Nishimura, S. et al. (1988). Echocardiographic findings in nine patients with cardiac amyloidosis: their correlation with necropsy findings. *J Cardiol* 18(1): 121–133.

15. Rahman, J.E., Helou, E.F., Gelzer-Bell, R. et al. (2004). Noninvasive diagnosis of biopsy-proven cardiac amyloidosis. *J Am Coll Cardiol* 43: 410–415.

16. Sun, J.P., Stewart, W.J., Yang, X.S. et al. (2009). Differentiation of Hypertrophic Cardiomyopathy and Cardiac Amyloidosis from Causes of Ventricular Wall Thickening by Two-D Strain Imaging Echocardiography. *Am J Cardiol* 103 (3): 411–415.

17. Carroll, J.D., Gaasch, W.H., McAdam, K.P. (1982). Amyloid cardiomyopathy: characterization by a distinctive voltage/mass relation. *Am J Cardiol* 49: 9–13.

18. Hamer, J.P., Janssen, S., van Rijswijk, M.H. et al. (1992). Amyloid cardiomyopathy in systemic non-hereditary amyloidosis. Clinical, echocardiographic and electrocardiographic findings in 30 patients with AA and 24 patients with AL amyloidosis. *Eur Heart J* 13: 623–627.

19. Bhandari, A.K. and Nanda, N.C. (1983). Myocardial texture characterization by two-dimensional echocardiography. *Am J Cardiol* 51: 817–825.

20. Child, J.S., Levisman, J.A., Abbasi, A.S. et al. (1976). Echocardiographic manifestations of infiltrative cardiomyopathy. A report of seven cases due to amyloid. *Chest* 70: 726–731.

21. Klein, A.L., Hatle, L.K., Taliercio, C.P. et al. (1990). Serial Doppler echocardiographic follow-up of left ventricular diastolic function in cardiac amyloidosis. *J Am Coll Cardiol* 16: 1135–1141.

22. Simons, M. and Isner, J.M. (1992). Assessment of relative sensitivities of noninvasive tests for cardiac amyloidosis in documented cardiac amyloidosis. *Am J Cardiol* 69: 425–427.

23. Klein, A.L., Hatle, L.K., Taliercio, C.P. et al. (1991). Prognostic significance of Doppler measures of diastolic function in cardiac amyloidosis. A Doppler echocardiography study. *Circulation* 83: 808–816.

24. Koyama, J., Ray-Sequin, P.A., Davidoff, R. et al. (2002). Usefulness of pulsed tissue Doppler imaging for evaluating systolic and diastolic left ventricular function in patients with AL (primary) amyloidosis. *Am J Cardiol* 89: 1067–1071.

25. Koyama, J., Ray-Sequin, P.A. and Falk, R.H. (2003). Longitudinal myocardial function assessed by tissue velocity, strain, and strain rate tissue Doppler echocardiography in patients with AL (primary) cardiac amyloidosis. *Circulation* 107: 2446–2452.

26. Maceira, A.M., Joshi, J., Prasad, S.K. et al. (2005). Cardiovascular magnetic resonance in cardiac amyloidosis. *Circulation* 111:186–193.

27. Perugini, E., Rapezzi, C., Piva, T. et al. (2006). Non-invasive evaluation of the myocardial substrate of cardiac amyloidosis by gadolinium cardiac magnetic resonance. *Heart* 92: 343–349.

28. Murtagh, B., Hammill, S.C., Gertz, M.A. et al. (2005). Electrocardiographic findings in primary systemic amyloidosis and biopsy-proven cardiac involvement. *Am J Cardiol* 95: 535–537.

29. Yazaki, M., Tozuda, T., Nakamura, A. et al. (2000). Cardiac amyloid in patients with familial amyloid polyneuropathy consists of wild-type transthyretin. *Biochem Biophys Res Commun* 11: 702–706.

30. Ishikawa, Y., Ishii, T., Masuda, S. et al. (1996). Myocardial ischemia due to vascular systemic amyloidosis: A quantitative analysis of autopsy findings on stenosis of the intramural coronary arteries. *Pathol Int* 46: 189–194.

50 Hypertrophic Cardiomyopathy with Apical Aneurysm

Jing Ping Sun, Xing Sheng Yang, and Ka-Tak Wong

The Chinese University of Hong Kong, Hong Kong

History

A 66-year-old man, presented with shortness of breath on exertion. There is no history of hypertension; family history was unremarkable.

Physical Examination

Heart rate was regular at 89 bpm. Blood pressure was 105/78 mm Hg. There was a systolic murmur III/VI at the fourth left parasternal intercostal space, radiating to the apex. No ankle edema was noted.

Electrocardiogram

This demonstrated a sinus rhythm with a right bundle branch block pattern and old anterior myocardial infarction (V4-6 QS pattern) (Figure 50-1).

Angiogram

The coronary arteries were normal.

Echocardiography

There was significant hypertrophy of the mid-ventricular septum and posterior wall (1.4 and 1.6 cm separately) causing mid-ventricular cavity obliteration. There was no obstruction in the left ventricular outflow tract (mean pressure gradient was 1.7 mmHg). The LV apex was thin with dyskinesia compatible with an aneurysm (Figure 50-2, Videos 50-1, and 50-2). The left atrium was dilated. Mild to moderate mitral and tricuspid regurgitation were present. The peak velocity of tricuspid regurgitation was 3.69 m/s, with an estimated pulmonary artery pressure of 65 mm Hg.

Magnetic Resonance Imaging (MRI)

The apex is thin with dyskinesia compatible with LV aneurysm (Videos 50-3 and 50-4). Asymmetrical LV hypertrophy (septal wall = 1.7 cm, lateral wall = 1.4 cm), most pronounced at mid-ventricular level were noted causing mid-ventricular obstruction. Left ventricular systolic function is moderately impaired with an LVEF of 40%. A mild degree of RV apical hypertrophy was also seen (Figure 50-3). Perfusion at rest and at stress showed subtle stress-induced hypoperfusion at the anteroseptal wall at the basal level

Comparative Cardiac Imaging: A Case-based Guide, First Edition.
Edited by Jing Ping Sun, Xing Sheng Yang, and Bryan P. Yan.
© 2018 John Wiley & Sons Ltd. Published 2018 by John Wiley & Sons Ltd.
Companion website: www.wiley.com/sun/comparative_cardiac_imaging

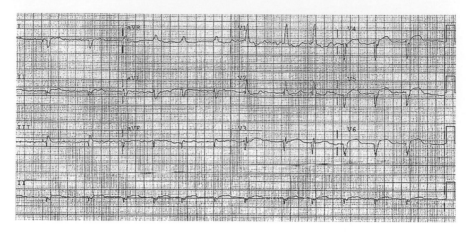

Figure 50-1   Electrcardiogram: Sinus rhythm with a right bundle branch block pattern and old anterior myocardial infarction (V4-6 QS pattern).

and the inferior wall at the mid-ventricular level. Delayed gadolinium enhancement was seen in the LV apex (transmural), anteroseptal / inferoseptal and inferior walls from basal to apical level (mid-layer) (Figure 50-3). Overall, features are compatible with hypertrophy cardiomyopathy with LV apical aneurysm formation and multifocal scarring. The distribution of patchy stress induced myocardial ischemia is more in favor of microvascular disease rather than coronary artery stenosis.

Discussion

Hypertrophic cardiomyopathy (HCM) is a primary disease that affects the muscle of the heart. With HCM, the sarcomeres (contractile elements) in the heart replicate causing heart muscle cells to increase in size, which results in the thickening of the heart muscle. In addition, the normal alignment of muscle cells is disrupted, a phenomenon known as myocardial disarray. Hypertrophic cardiomyopathy is a genetically determined disease with diverse clinical manifestations and pathophysiological substrates. Although several factors have been associated with an unfavorable outcome, the identification of patients at risk for sudden death or progression to heart failure remains a formidable challenge.

Patients with HCM and an LV apical aneurysm are an under-recognized but clinically important subset within the broad HCM disease spectrum. Mid-ventricular obstruction is an uncommon variant of LV obstructive HCM. It may lead to the development of an apical aneurysm, creating two distinct (basal and apical) LV chambers.

Maron et al [1] reported 28 cases of HCM with apical aneurysm. The prevalence of LV apical aneurysms was 2% in the overall HCM population. The clinical course of patients with HCM and those with LV apical aneurysms varies but is largely unfavorable overall. Patients with HCM and large LV apical aneurysms (>4 cm diameter) are more likely to experience adverse disease complications than patients with small aneurysms (≤4 cm diameter) [1]. The mechanisms of sudden death and syncope in HCM are not understood entirely but may be related to lethal ventricular arrhythmias, myocardial ischemia, or the severity of LV outflow tract obstruction [1, 2]. More than 40% of the patients with

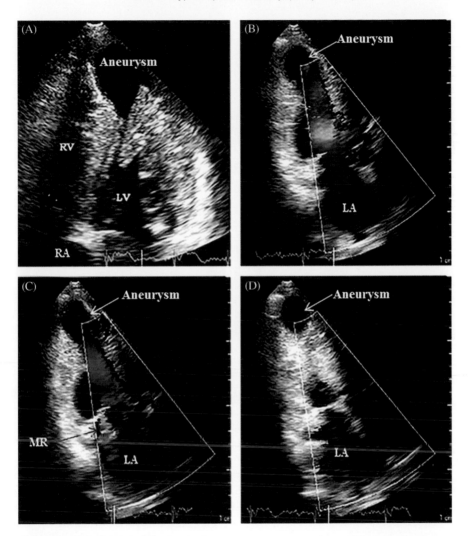

Figure 50-2 Echocardiography: A.An apical four-chamber view showed the apical aneurysm and left ventricle hypertrophy, most pronounced at mid-ventricular, the left ventricular outflow tract was normal. B. The apical three-chamber view at early diastole showed left ventricle hypertrophy, but the apical wall was thin. C.The apical three-chamber view at early systole showed mitral regurgitation and normal blood flow in the left ventricular outflow tract. D. The apical three-chamber view at the end systole showed mid-ventricular hypertrophy causing LV obstruction and apical aneurysm.

an LV apical aneurysm reported by Maron et al. presented with bursts of nonsustained monomorphic VT on Holter ECGs. Nonsustained monomorphic VT has been reported to be a determinant of increased risk for sudden death in HCM [3, 4]. The scarred rim of the aneurysm and associated extensive areas of LV myocardial fibrosis form an arrhythmogenic substrate for the generation of malignant ventricular tachyarrhythmia [5, 6]. The dyskinetic/akinetic apical aneurysm in HCM can also provide a structural basis for intracavitary thrombus formation.

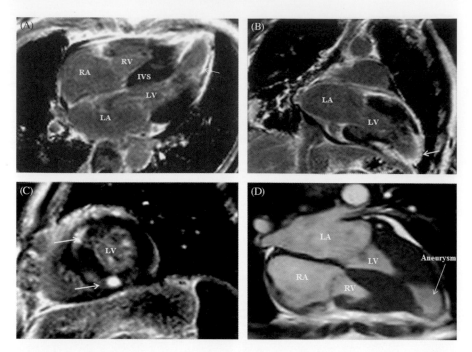

Figure 50-3 The cardiovascular magnetic resonance four-chamber, two-chamber and short axis of mid-ventricular level views showed late gadolinium enhancement involving the interventricular septum, anterior, posterior, and apical wall (A, B, C. white arrows) consistent with fibrosis (D) The cardiovascular magnetic resonance four-chamber view demonstrates LV hypertrophy with mid-ventricular obstruction and an apical aneurysm.
Notes: LA, left atrium; IVS, ventricular septum, LV, left ventricle; RV right ventricle; RA, right ventricle.

The overall rate of HCM-related adverse cardiovascular events such as sudden cardiac death, cardiac arrest, or progressive cardiac failure was 10.5% per year, significantly higher than that reported in the general HCM population [1].

Echocardiography has been used extensively in diagnosis of HCM. However, it is likely to underestimate the true prevalence of apical aneurysms in the overall HCM population as two-dimensional echocardiography is unreliable for detecting small apical aneurysms compared to MRI, which has higher spatial resolution and detection ability [7]. Gadolinium-enhanced CMR has been validated for the detection of irreversible injury in myocardial infarction [8]. Hyperenhancement is considered to occur in areas of expanded extracellular space. Gadolinium bound to DTPA diffuses into the interstitial space between cells but does not cross cell membranes. In fibrosis and extracellular expansion, there is a greater extracellular space for gadolinium-DTPA accumulation, and the distribution kinetics are slower than the normal myocardium [9, 10]. These two effects result in a delayed and persistently higher relative concentration of gadolinium in areas of the heart where extracellular tissue is abnormal. In myocardial infarction, fibrosis always involves the subendocardium because of the nature of the ischemic wave front that starts there. In HCM, gadolinium enhancement is seen in areas of myocardial fibrosis but this may well show different characteristics. First, fibrosis in HCM can occur throughout the myocardial wall, even with subendocardial sparing. In addition, areas of focal myocardial disarray and fine interstitial fibrosis may be seen. Therefore, the distribution and pattern of gadolinium uptake will be different between these two conditions. The different patterns of hyper enhancement seen are likely to be related to the different pathologic processes occurring in different patients, and the different stages of the disease processes at the time of scanning.

Our case is 66-year-old man with symptom of heart failure. The findings of echocardiography and MRI were compatible with the diagnosis of hypertrophic cardiomyopathy with apical aneurysm. Angiogram was normal in our case, thus the apical aneurysm would have been a result of microvascular disease. Microvascular dysfunction is a common feature of hypertrophic cardiomyopathy [11, 12]. Moreover, structural abnormalities of small vessels have been described in patients with hypertrophic cardiomyopathy and are thought to represent a primary abnormality [13]. The failure of myocardial blood flow to increase adequately on demand in patients with hypertrophic cardiomyopathy is clinically relevant in that it predisposes them to myocardial ischemia, which in turn has been implicated in the pathogenesis of syncope, an abnormal blood-pressure response to exercise, left-ventricular systolic dysfunction, and sudden death [14, 15]

A few studies have reported successful surgical therapy in patients with HCM and an LV apical aneurysm [16]. Maron et al. successfully treated 24 of 28 patients with LV apical aneurysm with β-blockers, calcium channel blockers, or both, for relief of heart-failure symptoms and ventricular tachyarrhythmia. Seventeen patients were implanted with cardioverter defibrillator (ICD) to prevent ventricular tachyarrhythmia. No patient underwent invasive septal reduction therapy or surgical treatment [1]. Implantation of ICDs has proven to be highly effective for prevention of sudden cardiac death. However, ICD implantation does not prevent recurrence of arrhythmia nor does it address ongoing heart failure. Furthermore, ICD shock might contribute to rehospitalization and myocardial injury, and backup ventricular pacing may impair LV function [17, 18].

Optimal treatment would prevent further episodes of arrhythmia and normalize LV shape and geometry. A surgical procedure that can correct the underlying structural cardiac abnormality to the maximum extent may not only prevent recurrent arrhythmia but also offer additional improvements in quality of life as well as prolonged survival [19, 20].

Key Points

1. Patients with HCM and an LV apical aneurysm represent a previously under-recognized but clinically important subset within the broad HCM disease spectrum, associated with adverse clinical outcomes, such as sudden death, embolic stroke, and progressive heart failure.
2. Microvascular dysfunction is a common feature of hypertrophic cardiomyopathy. Moreover, structural abnormalities of small vessels have been described in patients with hypertrophic cardiomyopathy and are thought to represent a primary abnormality.
3. Echocardiography has been used extensively in the diagnosis of HCM.
4. Gadolinium-enhanced CMR has been validated for the detection of irreversible myocardial injury; it is superior than echocardiography in diagnosis of myocardial diseases.

References

1. Maron, M.S., Finley, J.J., Bos, J.M. et al. (2008). Prevalence, clinical significance, and natural history of left ventricular apical aneurysms in hypertrophic cardiomyopathy. *Circulation* 118: 1541–1549.
2. Maron, B.J. (2002). Hypertrophic cardiomyopathy: a systematic review. *JAMA* 287: 1308–1320.
3. Adabag, A.S., Casey, S.A., Kuskowski, M.A. et al. (2005). Spectrum and prognostic significance of arrhythmias on ambulatory Holter electrocardiogram in hypertrophic cardiomyopathy. *J Am Coll Cardiol* 45: 697–704.
4. Monserrat, L., Elliott, P.M., Gimeno, J.R. et al. (2003). Non-sustained ventricular tachycardia in hypertrophic cardiomyopathy: An independent marker of sudden death risk in young patients. *J Am Coll Cardiol* 42: 873–879.
5. Paul, M., Schafers, M., Grude, M. et al. (2006). Idiopathic left ventricular aneurysm and sudden cardiac death in young adults. *Europace* 8: 607–612.
6. Ouyang, F., Antz, M., Deger, F.T. et al. (2003). An underrecognized subepicardial reentrant ventricular tachycardia attributable to left ventricular aneurysm in patients with normal coronary arteriograms. *Circulation* 107: 2702–2709.
7. Moon, J.C., McKenna, W.J., McCrohon, J.A. et al. (2003). Toward clinical risk assessment in hypertrophic cardiomyopathy with gadolinium cardiovascular magnetic resonance. *J Am Coll Cardiol* 41: 1561–1567.
8. Kim, R.J., Wu, E., Rafael, A. et al. (2000). The use of contrast-enhanced magnetic resonance imaging to identify reversible myocardial dysfunction. *N Engl J Med* 16: 1445–1453.
9. Kim, R.J., Chen, E.L., Lima, J.A.C. et al. (1996). Myocardial Gd-DTPA kinetics determine MRI contrast enhancement and reflect the extent and severity of myocardial injury after acute reperfused infarction. *Circulation* 94: 3318–3326.
10. Flacke, S.J., Fischer, S.E., and Lorenz, C.H. (2001). Measurement of the gadopentetate dimeglumine partition coefficient in human myocardium in vivonormal distribution and elevation in acute and chronic infarction. *Radiology* 218: 703–710.
11. Camici, P.G., Chiriatti, G., Lorenzoni, R., et al. (1991). Coronary vasodilation is impaired in both hypertrophied and nonhypertrophied myocardium of patients with hypertrophic cardiomyopathy: a study with nitrogen-13 ammonia and positron emission tomography. *J Am Coll Cardiol* 17: 879–886.
12. Krams, R., Kofflard, M.J., Duncker, D.J. et al. (1998). Decreased coronary flow reserve in hypertrophic cardiomyopathy is related to remodeling of the coronary microcirculation. *Circulation* 97: 230–233.
13. Maron, B.J., Wolfson, J.K., Epstein, S.E. et al. (1986). Intramural ("small vessel") coronary artery disease in hypertrophic cardiomyopathy. *J Am Coll Cardiol* 8: 545–557.
14. Dilsizian, V., Bonow, R.O., Epstein, S.E. et al. (1993). Myocardial ischemia detected by thallium scintigraphy is frequently related to cardiac arrest and syncope in young patients with hypertrophic cardiomyopathy. *J Am Coll Cardiol* 22: 796–804.
15. Yoshida, N., Ikeda, H., Wada, T. et al. (1998). Exercise-induced abnormal blood pressure responses are related to subendocardial ischemia in hypertrophic cardiomyopathy. *J Am Coll Cardiol* 32: 1938–1942.
16. Mantica, M., Della Bella, P. and Arena, V. (1997). Hypertrophic cardiomyopathy with apical aneurysm: a case of catheter and surgical therapy of sustained monomorphic ventricular tachycardia. *Heart* 77: 481–483.
17. Moss, A.J., Zareba, W., Hall, W.J. et al. (2002). Prophylactic implantation of a defibrillator in patients with myocardial infarction and reduced ejection fraction. *N Engl J Med* 346: 877–883.
18. Steinberg, J.S., Fischer, A., Wang, P. et al. (2005). The clinical implications of cumulative right ventricular pacing in the Multicenter Automatic Defibrillator Trial II. *J Cardiovasc Electrophysiol* 16: 359–365.
19. Von Oppell, U.O., Milne, D., Okreglicki, A. et al. (2002). Surgery for ventricular tachycardia of left ventricular origin: risk factors for success and long-term outcome. *Eur J Cardiothorac Surg* 22: 762–770.
20. Sartipy, U., Albåge, A., Strååt, E. et al. (2006). Surgery for ventricular tachycardia in patients undergoing left ventricular reconstruction by the Dor procedure. *Ann Thorac Surg* 81: 65–71.

51 Arrythmogenic Right Ventricular Dysplasia

Doris T. Chan, Anna K. Y. Chan, and Jing Ping Sun

The Chinese University of Hong Kong, Hong Kong

History

A 51-year-old man presented to hospital with sudden onset of fast irregular palpitations, with prior similar episodes for a few months which spontaneously subsided. There was no history of dizziness or syncope.

Physical Examination

Cardiovascular examination was unremarkable.

Electrocardiogram

Initial ECG showed frequent premature ventricular complexes (Figure 51-1A). Second ECG after a few minutes showed ventricular tachycardia, with blood pressure 98/57 (Figure 51-1B). Direct- current cardioversion (DCCV) was delivered and the rhythm was reverted instantly back to sinus (Figure 51-1C). T- wave inversions were seen from leads V1 to V3.

Cardiac Catheterization

Cardiac catheterization showed normal coronary arteries.

Transthoracic Echocardiography

Transthoracic echocardiography showed a mildly dilated right ventricle (Figure 51-2A, B, C, D) with hypokinesis of right ventricular free wall (Video 51-1 and Video 51-2). The left ventricular systolic ejection fraction is around 50%.

Cardiac Magnetic Resonance Imaging

Cardiac magnetic resonance imaging showed a dilated right ventricle (Figure 51-3A, B and Video 51-3) with impairment of right ventricular contraction, together with focal aneurysm (Figure 51-3C and Video 51-4) at the right ventricle and fatty infiltration in the myocardium (Figure 51-3D).

Comparative Cardiac Imaging: A Case-based Guide, First Edition.
Edited by Jing Ping Sun, Xing Sheng Yang, and Bryan P. Yan.
© 2018 John Wiley & Sons Ltd. Published 2018 by John Wiley & Sons Ltd.
Companion website: www.wiley.com/sun/comparative_cardiac_imaging

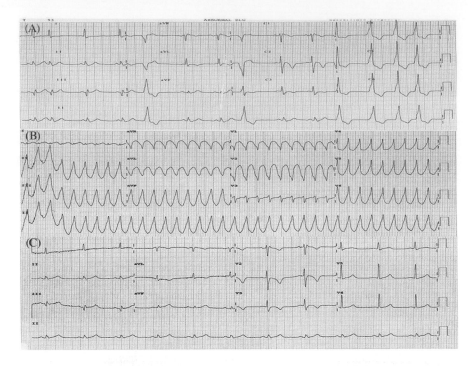

Figure 51-1 The initial ECG showed frequent premature ventricular complexes (A). The second ECG, after a few minutes, showed ventricular tachycardia (B). Direct-current cardioversion (DCCV) was delivered and the rhythm was reverted instantly back to sinus. T-wave inversions were seen from leads V1 to V3 (C).

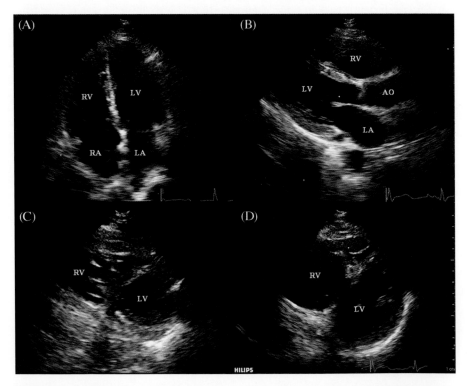

Figure 51-2 Transthoracic echocardiography four-chamber (A), parasternal long (B), short (C) and subcostal four-chamber (D) views showed a mildly dilated right ventricle.

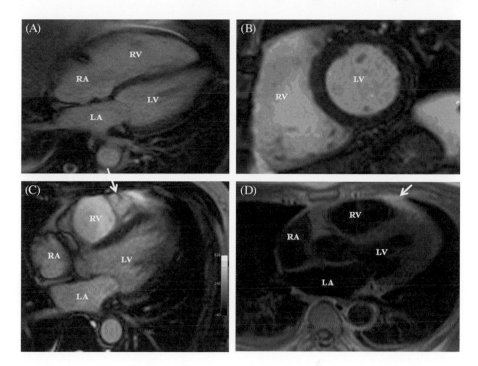

Figure 51-3 Cardiac magnetic resonance imaging four-chamber view showed a dilated right ventricle (A and B) with focal aneurysm (C, arrow) at the right ventricle and fatty infiltration in the myocardium (D, arrow).

Hospital Course

Implantable cardioverter-defibrillator (ICD) was implanted uneventfully after the diagnosis of ARVD was made based on the ECG, echocardiography, and cardiac MRI findings.

Discussion

The prevalence of arrythmogenic right ventricular dysplasia (ARVD) in the general adult population is estimated to be approximately 1 : 1000 [1]. This is likely to be an underestimation of the disease. It accounts for 5% to 10% of unexplained sudden cardiac deaths in individuals aged below 65 years old [2].

Clinical presentations of ARVD are highly variable, ranging from asymptomatic forms to palpitations, syncope, fatigue, or even cardiac arrest especially during exercise. The symptoms are due to ventricular ectopic beats, sustained ventricular tachycardia of left bundle branch block configuration, or right ventricular failure [3].

Arrythmogenic right ventricular dysplasia (ARVD) is a disease of the heart muscle associated with ventricular arrhythmias and sudden death [4]. Macroscopically, it is an inherited disease characterized by structural and functional abnormalities of the right ventricle (RV) caused by the replacement of the myocardium by fatty and fibrous tissue. The RV myocardial scarring initially produces typical regional wall motion abnormalities but later may involve the free wall and become global, producing RV dilatation, sometimes involving areas of the left ventricle as well [5]. Microscopically, it is a genetic disease of dysfunction of desmosomes, which are intracellular adhesion complexes connecting cardiac myocytes. The defect in the intracellular connections between the cardiac myocytes leads to fatty and fibrous tissue infiltration. Arrythmogenic right ventricular dysplasia is typically inherited as an autosomal dominant trait with variable penetrance and incomplete expression [4]. There is an autosomal recessive variant associated with palmoplantar keratosis and wally hair named Naxos disease [6].

Diagnostic Evaluation

Definitive diagnosis of ARVD requires histological confirmation of fibrofatty replacement of right ventricle myocardium at postmortem surgery. This is, however, certainly not feasible in a clinical setting, even by endomyocardial biopsy, because of the segmental nature of the disease and the risks associated including tamponade and perforation. Diagnosis is based on the presence of structural, histological, electrocardiographic and genetic factors based on 1994 Task Force Criteria, which were further revised in 2010. Both the original and revised criteria are divided into minor and major criteria and are classified into six categories [6]:

- Global and / or regional dysfunction and structural alterations.
- Tissue characterization of wall.
- Repolarization abnormalities on ECG.
  - T- wave inversions from V1 to V3.
- Depolarization/ conduction abnormalities on ECG.
  - Epsilon wave (electric potentials after the end of QRS complexes), signifying slowed intraventricular conduction.
- Arrhythmias.
- Family history.

Definite diagnosis requires the presence of two major criteria, one major plus two minor criteria, or four minor criteria from different categories [5].

Diagnostic Tests
Electrocardiogram (ECG)

Echocardiography is the initial diagnostic tool. Principal findings are right ventricular dilatation and hypokinesia. These two characteristics were present in this case. But echocardiography is limited by a lack of spatial resolution in diagnosing the typical fatty and fibrofatty changes of the right ventricular myocardium.

Cardiovascular Magnetic Resonance (CMR)

Cardiovascular magnetic resonance (CMR) imaging is an excellent tool for visualizing the right ventricle. It enables identification of global and regional ventricular dilatation, and systolic and diastolic phase dysfunction. It also better recognizes the replacement of myocardial fatty and fibrofatty tissue. Typical features that can be identified in CMR include presence of high-signal intensity areas indicating substitution of myocardium by fat, fibrofatty tissue, which leads to diffuse thinning of the right ventricular myocardium, right ventricle and right ventricular outflow tract, dilatation of right ventricle and right ventricular outflow tract, regional contraction abnormalities, and global systolic and diastolic dysfunction. According the MRI characteristics (fibro fatty replaced right ventricular apical wall and ventricular aneurysm) combined with ventricular tachycardia by ECG, the diagnosis of ARVD should be reasonable in this case. The recognition of mild and localized forms of ARVD remains a clinical challenge. Arrythmogenic right ventricular dysplasia is difficult to detect in patients with minimal right ventricular abnormalities using echocardiography, ultrafast computed tomography (CT) scanning, radionuclide angiography, or contrast-enhanced angiography. Cardiovascular magnetic resonance is a promising technique for showing the anatomy and function of the right ventricle, as well as for characterizing the composition of the right ventricle's wall, especially with regard to adipose tissue. Several studies have reported on the use of MR imaging to detect the characteristic high signal intensity of fat in the right ventricular myocardium on T1-weighted images [4, 7]. However, the diagnostic sensitivity and specificity of MRI remain to be defined because the quality of images detected is observer-dependent. Signal intensity suggesting the presence of fat in the right ventricle may be related to a latent form of the disease or to the dissociation of myocardial tissue by fat. Therefore, only the combination of MRI signs, including the size, function, and fat content in the free wall, is necessary to support the diagnosis.

Endomyocardial Biopsy
In some cases, endomyocardial biopsy may be necessary to confirm the diagnosis.

Prognosis and Management
Arrythmogenic right ventricular dysplasia is a progressive disease. The disease course is unpredictable, as illustrated by the highly variable clinical presentations ranging from incidental findings at autopsy in older adults who have had no symptoms at all, to the cause of sudden cardiac death in younger patients. Multiple studies have demonstrated a favorable long-term prognosis in properly treated patients [8].

Arrythmogenic right ventricular dysplasia patients should be restricted from competitive and high-intensity sports or recreational activities. Implantable cardioverter-defibrillators (ICD) are recommended as secondary prevention of sudden cardiac death (SCD) for patients with ARVD who have experienced sustained ventricular tachycardia or ventricular fibrillation. They work by providing antitachycardia pacing and defibrillation shocks when arrhythmias occur. Radiofrequency ablation (RFA) and antiarrhythmic drugs, including sotalol and amiodarone, are not definitive treatment. They are for patients who are not candidates for ICD, or to act as adjunct therapy for patients with ICD still experiencing frequent shocks due to ventricular arrhythmias.

Key Points
1. Arrhythmogenic right ventricular dysplasia (ARVD) is an inherited disease typically as autosomal dominant trait, characterized by structural and functional abnormalities of the right ventricle caused by the replacement of the myocardium by fibrofatty tissue, leading to ventricular arrhythmias and sudden cardiac death.
2. Clinical manifestations range from asymptomatic to sudden cardiac death.

3. The Task Force Criteria (newly revised in 2010) are the diagnostic criteria for ARVD based on the presence of structural, histological, electrocardiographic, and genetic factors.

4. Restrictions from competitive sports, radiofrequency ablation and antiarrhythmic drugs are useful to manage ARVD patients but none of them is definitive treatment. Patients with high risk of sudden cardiac death should receive an implantable cardioverter- defibrillator (ICD) as secondary prevention.

References

1. Gemayel, C., Pelliccia, A. and Thompson, P.D. (2001). Arrhythmogenic right ventricular cardio-myopathy. *J Am Coll Cardiol* 38: 1773–1781.

2. Tabib, A., Loire, R., Chalabreysse, L. et al. (2003). Circumstances of death and gross and micro-scopic observations in a series of 200 cases of sudden death associated with arrythmogenic right ventricular cardiomyopathy and/or dysplasia. *Circulation* 108: 3000–3005.

3. Anderson, E.L. (2006). Arrhythmogenic right ventricular dysplasia. *Am Fam Physician* 73: 1391–1398.

4. Auffermann, W., Wichter, T., Breithardt, G. et al. (1993). Arrhythmogenic right ventricular disease: MR imaging vs angiography. *Am J Roentgenol* 161: 549–555.

5. Hamid, M.S., Norman, M., Quraishi, A. et al. (2002). Prospective evaluation of relatives for familial arrhythmogenic right ventricular cardiomyopathy/dysplasia reveals a need to broaden diagnostic criteria. *J Am Coll Cardiol* 40: 1445.

6. European Heart Rhythm Association, Heart Rhythm Society, Zipes, D.P. et al. (2006). ACC/AHA/ESC 2006 guidelines for management of patients with ventricular arrhythmias and the prevention of sudden cardiac death: a report of the American College of Cardiology/American Heart Association Task Force and the European Society of Cardiology Committee for Practice Guidelines (Writing Committee to Develop Guidelines for Management of Patients With Ventricular Arrhythmias and the Prevention of Sudden Cardiac Death). *J Am Coll Cardiol* 48: e247.

7. Globits, S., Kreiner, G., Frank, H. et al. (1997). Significance of morphological abnormalities detected by MRI in patients undergoing successful ablation of right ventricular outflow tract tachycardia. *Circulation* 96: 2633–2640.

8. Anderson, E.L. (2006). Arrhythmogenic right ventricular dysplasia. *Am Fam Physician 15*; 73 (8): 1391–1398.

52 Danon Disease

Ligang Fang[1] and Jing Ping Sun[2]

[1] Affiliated Hospital of Peking Union Medical College, Beijing, China
[2] The Chinese University of Hong Kong, Hong Kong

History

A 14-year-old male was admitted with intermittent palpitation and syncope with loss of consciousness for a few seconds. He had mental retardation. His grandmother died of heart disease at the age of 40 years, and an aunt has "heart disease."

Physical Examination

Blood pressure 110/70 mmHg, regular heart rate 72 bpm. There was no heart murmur.

Biochemical Tests

NT-proBNP 1012 pg/mL, creatine kinase 2167 U/L, creatine kinase MB quantitative 4.0 µg / L, troponin I 0.04 g /L. Creatine kinase-MM isoenzyme in a CK isoenzyme electrophoresis assay was abnormal. The concentrations of serum hepatic enzymes, including ALT (248 U/L, normal: 5–40 U/L), AST (237 U/L, normal: 5–37 U/L), LDH (990 U/L, normal: 97–270 U/L), and CK (1707 U/L, normal: 18–198 U/L), were elevated.

Cardiac tropoin I was negative. The thyroid function was normal.

Molecular Genetics and cDNA Analysis

Molecular genetics and cDNA analysis: Indicated a novel mutation in exon 2 of the Lamp-2 gene (257_258 delCC).

X-Ray

The chest X-ray was normal.

Electrocardiogram

An electrocardiogram showed Wolff–Parkinson–White syndrome with very high voltage of the left ventricle (SV1 + RV5 = 13.2 mV) and inverted T-wave (Figure 52-1).

Endomyocardial Biopsy

Found myocardia hypertrophy, disorganized, and large vacuoles were seen within the myocardial fibers. The interstitial hyperplasia is not obvious and Congo red staining was negative. Light microscope examinations revealed an autophagosome-like vesicle. Electron microscopic examination revealed some autophagic vacuoles containing

Comparative Cardiac Imaging: A Case-based Guide, First Edition.
Edited by Jing Ping Sun, Xing Sheng Yang, and Bryan P. Yan.
© 2018 John Wiley & Sons Ltd. Published 2018 by John Wiley & Sons Ltd.
Companion website: www.wiley.com/sun/comparative_cardiac_imaging

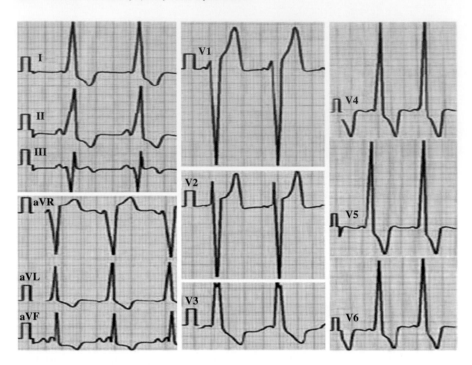

Figure 52-1   An electrocardiogram showed Wolff–Parkinson–White syndrome with very high voltage of the left ventricle (SV1 + RV5 = 13.2 mV) and inverted T-wave.

glycogen particles (Figure 52-2). These findings are in line with vacuolar myopathy due to lysosome deficiency.

Echocardiography

Left Ventricular Hypertrophy The thickness of ventricular septum was 14 mm. The lateral wall was 15 mm. The diameter of the left ventricle was 41 mm; the left ventricular ejection fraction was normal (68%) (Figure 52-3, Video 52-1–4). Left ventricular diastolic function was abnormal in stage 1.

Cardiac Magnetic Resonance Imaging (MRI)

The MRI short axis view showed severe LV hypertrophy (Figure 52-4A, during diastole; B, during systole). Gadolinium-DTPA delayed-enhancement magnetic resonance imaging identified abnormal enhancement at the left ventricular apex (arrows) (Figure 52-4C).

Discussion

In this 14-year-old Asian male with no evidence of skeletal muscle weakness but with intermittent palpitation, syncope, retardation, the echocardiogram demonstrated left ventricular hypertrophy, while electrocardiogram showed Wolff–Parkinson–White syndrome with very high voltage of the left ventricle (SV1 + RV5 = 13.2 mV) and inverted T-wave. Magnetic resonance imaging showed severe LV hypertrophy and abnormal

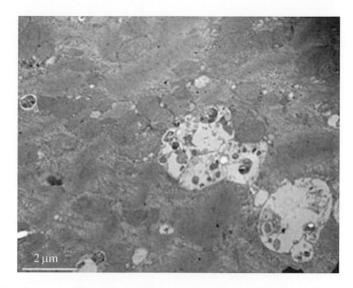

Figure 52-2   Electron microscopic examination revealed some autophagic vacuoles containing glycogen particles.

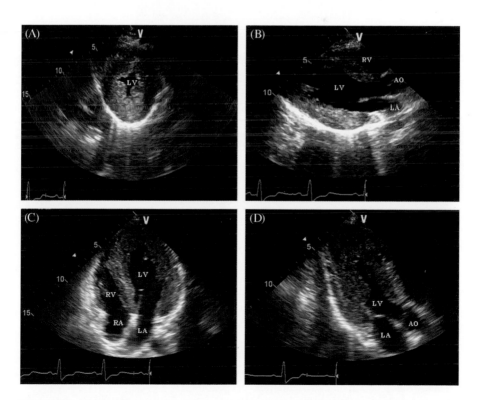

Figure 52-3   The transthoracic echocardiography parasternal short (A) and long-axis (B), apical four-chamber (C) and three-chamber (D) views showed severe LV concentric hypertrophy.

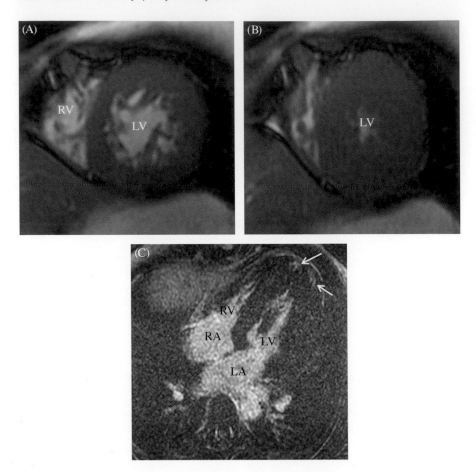

Figure 52-4 Cardiac magnetic resonance imaging (MRI): The MRI short-axis view showed severe LV hypertrophy (A, during diastole; B, during systole). Gadolinium-DTPA delayed-enhancement magnetic resonance imaging identified abnormal enhancement at the left ventricular apex (arrows) (C).

enhancement in the LV apex myocardium. The concentrations of serum hepatic enzymes were elevated. Endomyocardial biopsy confirmed the vacuolar cardiomyopathy. All of these characteristics are consistent with Danon disease. The disease was first described by Danon in 1981 [1].

The Danon disease patients were younger. Significantly elevated serum hepatic enzymes and CK and WPW syndrome on ECG were more common. Maron et al. [2] reported that six of seven Danon disease patients were boys with a median age of 14 years, and six patients had WPW syndrome and deeply inverted T-waves at diagnosis. Their patients also had markedly elevated serum hepatic enzymes and CK concentrations, consistent with our case.

Another important finding of this case was the 2 bp deletion (257_258 delCC) in exon 3, leading to frameshift mutation of lysosome-associated membrane protein 2 and a premature stop codon on cDNA analysis.

Maron et al. [2] reported that each of the seven Danon disease patients experienced serious adverse clinical consequences by 14–24 years of age (mean: 21 years). Four patients died of acute or progressive heart failure, and one patient underwent heart transplantation; all seven patients had received implantable cardioverter defibrillators (ICDs), which ultimately failed to terminate lethal ventricular tachyarrhythmias in five. Physicians should therefore consider early intervention with heart transplantation [3, 4] once left ventricular dysfunction occurs, despite the possibility of extracardiac organ involvement of this disease [3, 5].

It is important to distinguish hypertrophic cardiomyopathy (HCM) from Danon disease. Some patterns of myocardial late-gadolinium enhancement on CMR have been reported more frequently in particular cardiomyopathies, for example, midmyocardial posterolateral scarring in the LV (Fabry disease, glycogen storage disease) [6] and diffuse myocardial pattern in cardiac amyloidosis [7]. However, these patterns are not specific and must be interpreted in light of the clinical presentation.

Improved cardiac imaging and advances in our understanding of a genetic basis for HCM have dramatically increased our ability to diagnose and manage patients with this condition. In the future, integration of structural and functional information with detailed molecular analysis will provide the basis for new therapeutic interventions that improve quality of life and protect patients and families from disease-related complications.

Key Points

1. Danon disease is a congenital metabolic syndrome with an early age of onset of muscle weakness and heart disease (onset in childhood or adolescence).
2. Some learning problems or mental retardation can be present.
3. The heart disease (cardiomyopathy) can be severe. It usually progresses to heart failure, commonly complicated by atrial fibrillation and embolic strokes, with severe neurological disability, leading to death unless heart transplant is performed.
4. Problems with the electrical conduction in the heart can occur. Some patients had Wolff–Parkinson–White syndrome.
5. Danon disease is rare and unfamiliar to most physicians. It can be mistaken for other forms of heart disease and / or muscular dystrophies.

References

1. Danon, M.J., Oh, S.J., DiMauro, S. et al. (1981). Lysosomal glycogen storage disease with normal acid maltase. *Neurology* 31 (1): 51–57.
2. Maron, B.J., Roberts, W.C., Arad, M. et al. (2009). Clinical outcome and phenotypic expression in LAMP2 cardiomyopathy. *JAMA* 301:1253–1259.
3. Sugie, K., Yamamoto, A., Murayama, K. et al. (2002). Clinicopathological features of genetically confirmed Danon disease. *Neurology* 58: 1773–1778.
4. Echaniz-Laguna, A., Mohr, M., Epailly, E. et al. (2006). Novel Lamp-2 gene mutation and successful treatment with heart transplantation in a large family with Danon disease. *Muscle Nerve* 33: 393–397.
5. Charron, P., Villard, E., Sébillon, P. et al. (2004). Danon's disease as a cause of hypertrophic cardiomyopathy: A systematic survey. *Heart* 90: 842–846.
6. Mahrholdt, H., Wagner, A., Judd, R.M. et al. (2005). Delayed enhancement cardiovascular magnetic resonance assessment of non-ischaemic cardiomyopathies. *Eur Heart J* 26:1461–1474.
7. Austin, B.A., Tang, W.H., Rodriguez, E.R. et al (2009). Delayed hyper-enhancement magnetic resonance imaging provides incremental diagnostic and prognostic utility in suspected cardiac amyloidosis. *J Am Coll Cardiol Cardiovasc Imaging* 2: 1369–1377.

53 Acute Eosinophilic Myocarditis

Xianda Ni[1] and Jing Ping Sun[2]

[1] The First Affiliated Hospital of Wenzhou Medical University, Wenzhou, China
[2] The Chinese University of Hong Kong, Hong Kong

History

A 43-year-old man was admitted to our hospital with fever, chills, and a persistent headache accompanied by dizziness, nausea, vomiting. He had a history of hypertension for 4 years and gout for 5 years.

Patient had cervical resistance and positive Klinefelter syndrome.

Laboratory Tests

White blood neutrophils, eosinophil cell count, cardiac troponins and C- reactive protein were abnormal. Cerebrospinal fluid examination: showed that leukocytosis, Pan's test (+), the level of protein was increased, while the level of glucose and chloride were decreased. Bone marrow results showed: hyperplasia, myeloid hyperplasia, increased eosinophils, giant hyperplasia. All myocardial enzymes, troponin and C- reactive protein were significantly elevated.

Electrocardiogram (ECG)

The first ECG at admission was normal. The second ECG at 1 week later (when the patient felt severe chest pain) showed ST-segment elevation and T-wave change in all leads.

Coronary Angiography

Coronary angiography revealed a normal coronary artery.

Transthoracic Echocardiography (TTE)

The first TTE was normal. But one week later after cardiac arrest, TTE revealed thickness of left ventricular walls and the right ventricular free wall was significantly increased, and the myocardium was apparently echogenic with a normal ejection fraction (Figure 53-1, Videos 53-1 and 53-2), left ventricular diastolic function was impaired (E/E' = 22), there was moderate mitral regurgitation, moderate to severe tricuspid regurgitation, and mild pulmonary hypertension. The characteristics of echocardiography suggested an infiltrative myocardial disease.

Comparative Cardiac Imaging: A Case-based Guide, First Edition.
Edited by Jing Ping Sun, Xing Sheng Yang, and Bryan P. Yan.
© 2018 John Wiley & Sons Ltd. Published 2018 by John Wiley & Sons Ltd.
Companion website: www.wiley.com/sun/comparative_cardiac_imaging

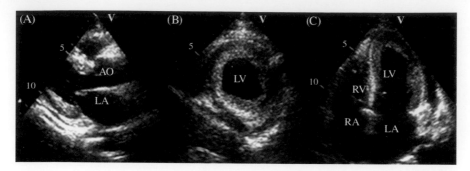

Figure 53-1   Parasternal long-axis (A), short-axis (B) and apical four-chamber (C) views revealed thickness of left ventricular walls and right ventricular free wall was significantly increased, and the myocardium was apparently echogenic.

Computed Tomography (CT)

A CT scan of the chest revealed the pleural effusion in both sides, enlarged cardiac shadow with pericardial effusion.

Magnetic Resonance Imaging (MRI)

At admission, MRI revealed multiple lesions scattered in the brain. The possibility of tuberculous meningitis was considered.

One week later, MRI scans showed an abnormal delayed enhancement signal within the myocardium and pericardial effusion (Figure 53-2).

Endomyocardial Biopsy

The myocardial endoplasmic reticulum stroma showed myocardial disarranged with eosinophilic infiltrationin the myocardial interstitial focal area, which was in line with eosinophils endocarditis and myocarditis (Figure 53-3).

Hospital Course

Tests confirmed tuberculous meningitis. The antituberculous meningitis therapy began. One week later, during examinations, cardiac arrest occurred suddenly. The patient fortunately recovered after cardiopulmonary resuscitation. The diagnosis of eosinophilic myocarditis was confirmed by echocardiography, MRI, and endomyocardial biopsy. The patient received prednisone combined with antituberculous therapy. A week later, the patient's symptoms had improved, and the count of eosinophils significantly decreased. After 3 months, repeat echocardiography showed thickened myocardium of left and right ventricle was significantly improved, atrioventricular valve regurgitation was significantly reduced, pericardial effusion disappeared; the left ventricular systolic function estimated by 2-D (Videos 53-3 and 53-4) and longitudinal strain of speckle tracking imaging was significantly improved compared with the results obtained during acute myocarditis (Figure 53-4A and B). The diastolic function also recovered (E/E' from 22 return to 8). Magnetic resonance imaging showed that the lesions in the myocardium had apparently improved.

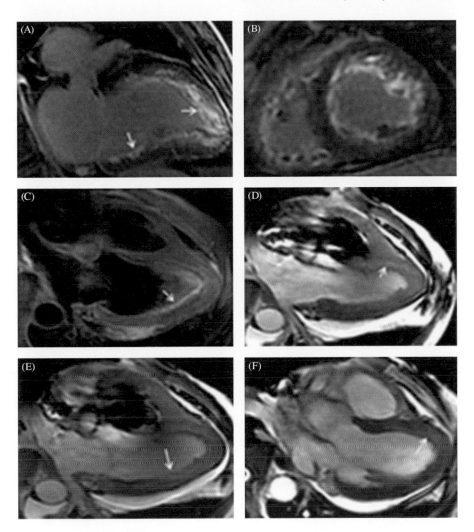

Figure 53-2 Magmatic resonance imaging showed abnormal delayed enhancement signal within the myocardium (A, B, C) and pericardial effusion (C, D, E, F).

Discussion

The process of this patient most likely occurred as a result of a hypersensitivity reaction. The eosinophilic myocarditis is typically associated with Drugs [1, 2]. Patients with eosinophilic myocarditis may present with various signs and symptoms including fever, chills, malaise, weight loss, acute coronary syndrome-like features, heart failure, tachy- or brady-type arrhythmias, and sudden death [3, 4]. To date, there are no universally accepted guidelines for the diagnosis of eosinophilic myocarditis. Essential diagnostic features include eosinophilia > 500/µL, cardiac symptoms, elevated cardiac enzymes, electrocardiogram (ECG) changes, and cardiac dysfunction on echocardiography, especially in the setting of unremarkable coronary angiography. Definitive diagnosis requires an endomyocardial biopsy [5]. In the present case, the initial disease was tuberculous

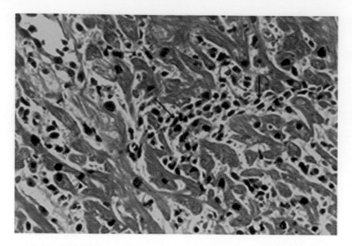

Figure 53-3 Endomyocardial biopsy. Microscopically, myocardial disarray and eosinophilic infiltrate (arrows) can be seen in the myocardial interstitial focal area, which was in line with eosinophils endocarditis and myocarditis.

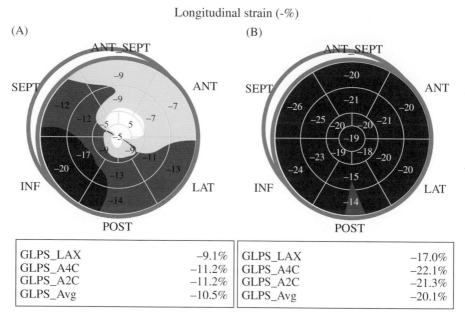

Figure 53-4 The left ventricular systolic function estimated by the longitudinal strain of speckle tracking was significantly reduced during acute myocarditis (A), and completely recovered after therapy (B).

meningitis, and antituberculous meningitis drugs were involved. One week after antituberculous therapy, the patient felt severe chest pain. All results of laboratory examinations fulfilled the criteria for a diagnosis of eosinophilic myocarditis, which was confirmed by endomyocardial biopsy. The etiology of eosinophilic myocarditis in this patient might be the antituberculous drugs, but it is hard to exclude the tuberculosis itself. Steroids are the cornerstone of treatment in eosinophilic myocarditis [6, 7]. Our patient took steroid therapy, which was followed by a dramatic response within weeks, documented via serial echocardiograms, MRI and biomarker measurements of the course of cardiac dysfunction and recovery.

This case also clearly highlights the persistently important role of echocardiography in the evaluation of patients with myocarditis, despite the very prominent role of MRI in this field. It remains indisputable that MRI's late enhancement images and edema sequences (as direct evidence of myocardial infiltration and inflammation) provide an excellent tool for the diagnosis of myocarditis [8], particularly if the echocardiogram is inconclusive. But the role of MRI in the evaluation of cardiac function is limited to the accurate measurement of left and right ventricular volumes and ejection fractions. In contrast, transthoracic echocardiography using tissue-Doppler and speckle tracking echocardiography enabled excellent functional evaluation at the initial examination and during follow-up in our patient. In our patient, the results of initial and follow-up MRI examination were consistent with the echocardiographic findings. It is important to note that echocardiography, in comparison with MRI, is relatively inexpensive and broadly available. Tissue-Doppler readings can be obtained in nearly all patients even if 2-D quality is imperfect; and experience renders the measurements highly reproducible [9]. In patients with myocarditis, echocardiography clearly cannot replace MRI in general. However, in patients with obvious abnormalities in the initial echocardiogram, comprehensive echocardiography includes tissue-Doppler and speckle tracking echocardiographic measurement can be used for the serial evaluation of LV structure and function during follow-up.

Conclusion

Eosinophilic myocarditis remains a rare and likely underdiagnosed subtype of myocarditis. The main characteristics of this disease include myocardial injury in the setting of noncontributory coronary artery disease. Endomyocardial biopsy remains the definitive gold standard for the diagnosis of noninfectious myocarditis [10]. Non-invasive cardiac imaging is important tool for earlier diagnosis of eosinophilic myocarditis in patients with peripheral eosinophilia. The early diagnose and therapies are the key to prevent the irreversible myocardial injury in patients with myocarditis. Large prospective studies in validating therapies of eosinophilic myocarditis are needed.

Key Points

1. Acute eosinophilic myocarditis is a rare cause of acute heart failure.
2. Acute eosinophilic myocarditis has an excellent response to steroids.
3. Two-D and tissue-Doppler echocardiographic measurements are useful as simple, broadly available bedside tools for the evaluation and follow up of patients with myocarditis.

References

1. Ginsberg, F. and Parrillo, J.E. (2005). Eosinophilic myocarditis. *Heart Fail Clin* 1 (3): 419–429.
2. Sabatine, M.S., Poh, K.K., Mega, J.L. et al. (2007). Case records of the Massachusetts General Hospital. Case 36-2007. A 31-year-old woman with rash, fever, and hypotension. *N Engl J Med* 357 (21): 2167–2178.

3. Al Ali, A.M., Straatman, L.P., Allard, M.F. et al. (2006). Eosinophilic myocarditis: case series and review of literature. *Can J Cardiol* 22 (14): 1233–1237.

4. Bleakley, C. and McEneaney, D. (2010). Eosinophilic myocarditis presenting as acute myocardial infarction. *J Cardiovasc Med* 12: 761–764.

5. Talierco, C.P., Olney, B.A. and Lie, J.T. (1985) Myocarditis related to drug hypersensitivity. *Mayo Clin Proc* 60: 463–468.

6. Caforio, A., Pankuweit, S., Arbustini, E. et al. (2013). Current state of knowledge on aetiology, diagnosis, management, and therapy of myocarditis: a position statement of the European Society of Cardiology Working Group on Myocardial and Pericardial Diseases. *Eur Heart J* 34 (33): 2636–2648.

7. Amini, R. and Nielsen, C. (2010). Eosinophilic myocarditis mimicking acute coronary syndrome secondary to idiopathic hypereosinophilic syndrome: a case report. *J Med Case Reports* 4: 40.

8. Friedrich, M.G., Sechtem, U., Schulz-Menger, J. et al. (2009). Cardiovascular magnetic resonance in myocarditis: A JACC white paper. *J Am Coll Cardiol* 53 (17): 1475–1487.

9. Nagueh, S.F., Appleton, C.P., Gillebert, T.C. et al. (2009) Recommendations for the evaluation of left ventricular diastolic function by echocardiography. *J Am Soc Echocardiogr* 22 (2): 107–133.

10. Caforio, A., Pankuweit, S., Arbustini, E. et al. (2013). Current state of knowledge on aetiology, diagnosis, management, and therapy of myocarditis: a position statement of the European Society of Cardiology Working Group on Myocardial and Pericardial Diseases. *Eur Heart J* 34 (33): 2636–2648.

54 Noncompaction Cardiomyopathy with Apical Aneurysm

Xianda Ni[1], Xing Sheng Yang[2], and Jing Ping Sun[2]

[1] The First Affiliated Hospital of Wenzhou Medical University, Wenzhou, China
[2] The Chinese University of Hong Kong, Hong Kong

History

A 39-year-old asymptomatic woman was found having an apical aneurysm by echocardiography.

Physical Examination

There were no abnormal signs.

Angiogram and Ventriculography

Ventriculography noted numerous trabeculations and recesses with honeycomb-like appearance during diastole and systole (Figure 54-1), which is consistent with evidence of extensive left ventricular noncompaction. The coronary arteries were normal.

Transthoracic Echocardiography

The echocardiography examination revealed a thickened left ventricular lateral wall with apical aneurysm and normal LV systolic function. There were excessively prominent trabeculations with sinusoids of blood flow in apical posterior area and an apical aneurysm (Figure 54-2, Video 54-1, and Video 54-2).

Magnetic Resonance Imaging

The left ventricular short-axis view of magnetic resonance imaging (MRI) showed the thickness of the trabeculations is more than twice of the underlying ventricular wall (Figure 54-3A). Magnetic resonance imaging revealed delayed enhancement of LV apical aneurysm, indicating fibrosis (Figure 54-3B).

Computed Tomography

Computed tomography on the axial plane showed an apical aneurysm (Figure 54-3C). A CT three-dimensional reconstruction image showed apical aneurysm (Figure 54-3D).

All of above cardiac imaging studies were consistent with LV noncompaction cardiomyopathy complicated with apical aneurysm formation in this case.

Comparative Cardiac Imaging: A Case-based Guide, First Edition.
Edited by Jing Ping Sun, Xing Sheng Yang, and Bryan P. Yan.
© 2018 John Wiley & Sons Ltd. Published 2018 by John Wiley & Sons Ltd.
Companion website: www.wiley.com/sun/comparative_cardiac_imaging

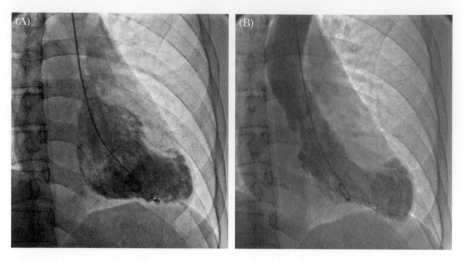

Figure 54-1 Ventriculography found numerous trabeculations and recesses with honeycomb-like appearance during diastole (A) and systole (B).

Discussion

Isolated left ventricular noncompaction (LVNC) is a congenital cardiomyopathy caused by a defect in endomyocardial morphogenesis [1]. Recently, the American Heart Association classified LVNC as a primary genetic cardiomyopathy [2]. In contrast, the European Society of Cardiology considers LVNC to be an "unclassified cardiomyopathy" [3]. Multiple diagnostic criteria for LVNC have been proposed on the basis of echocardiography and cardiac MRI findings. The echocardiographic criteria suggested by Jenni et al. [4] have become widely accepted. They are as follows: (i) thickened myocardium with a two-layered structure consisting of a thin compacted epicardial layer [C] and a much thicker, noncompacted endocardial layer [N] or trabecular meshwork with deep endocardial spaces (N/C ratio > 2.0 at end-systole); (ii) predominant location of the pathology in the midlateral, midinferior, and apical areas; (iii) color Doppler evidence of deep intertrabecular recesses filled with blood from the LV cavity; and (iv) absence of coexisting cardiac abnormalities (in isolated LV isolated noncompaction).

Cardiac magnetic resonance imaging is increasingly recognized as an alternative modality for the noninvasive assessment of patients with noncompaction cardiomyopathy. Compared with traditional echocardiography, cardiac magnetic resonance imaging has less operator dependence, superior spatial resolution, higher contrast between blood and myocardium, which can provide better delineation of the abnormal trabeculations in noncompaction cardiomyopathy patients.

Contrast-enhanced CT is capable of showing the abnormal architecture of the left ventricular wall in noncompaction. Computed tomography also enables quantitative and qualitative assessment of global and regional ventricular function. Additionally, CT can be used to evaluate the coronary arteries to exclude anomalies or coronary artery disease, which is usually not feasible with CMRI or echocardiography.

The clinical manifestations of LVNC vary widely. Patients may be asymptomatic or have symptoms of heart failure, arrhythmias, or thromboembolism, ventricular tachyarrhythmia, and sudden death [5].

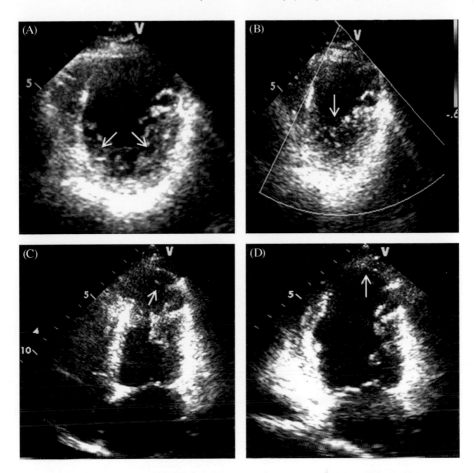

Figure 54-2 Transthoracic echocardiogram. A. Parasternal short-axis view shows excessively prominent trabeculations with sinusoids (arrows). B. Parasternal short-axis view with color Doppler showed excessively prominent trabeculations with blood filling in the sinusoids (arrows). C. An apical four-chamber view indicated a thickened lateral wall with prominent trabeculations and the apical aneurysm at the end of systole (arrow). D. Apical two-chamber view indicated the apical aneurysm at the end of diastole (arrow).

There were only a few cases about coexisting left ventricular aneurysm [6, 7]. The mechanism by which the left ventricular aneurysm developed is uncertain, but microcirculation abnormality may play a role in its pathophysiology. Subendocardial perfusion defects have been demonstrated by magnetic resonance imaging [8–10]. Impaired microperfusion is present not only in the noncompacted segment but also in the compacted segment in autopsy cases [4]. Impaired microcirculation may also account for the contractile dysfunction. Junga et al. [8] suggested that altered perfusion and coronary flow reserve in noncompaction cardiomyopathy may be related to failure of the coronary microcirculation to grow with the increasing ventricular mass, compression of the intramural coronary bed by the hypertrophied myocardium, or both processes.

Our patient had no symptoms before. The diagnosis of noncompaction cardiomyopathy with apical aneurysm was made based on echocardiography, CMRI and CT imaging.

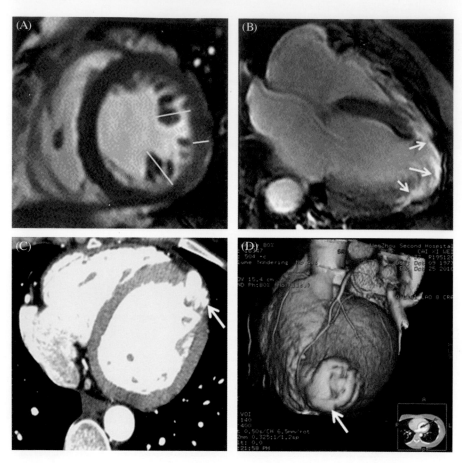

Figure 54-3 A. Magnetic resonance imaging (MRI) showed acquisition with ECG gating, in cine Fiesta sequence (SSFP). At end diastole in the short-axis view, the increase in subendocardial LV trabeculation in the medial, anterior, and inferior segments was noted. The maximum myocardial ratio of noncompacted (N/C) to compacted thickness was 3 (mean ratio = 2.4). B. Magnetic resonance imaging image acquisition with ECG-gating. Delayed enhancement at end-diastole in a four-chamber view showed the present of delayed myocardial enhancement (arrows), compatible with myocardial necrosis/fibrosis. C. Computed tomography an axial plane showed the apical aneurysm (arrow). D. Computed tomography three-dimensional reconstruction image showed the apical aneurysm (arrow).

The coronary arteries were normal in our patient, which suggested that his apical aneurysm was caused by impaired microcirculation.

Limited data are available regarding treatment of this condition, so it is recommended that clinical complications be managed according to the current guidelines for each clinical complication. The prevalence of systemic embolic events in patients with non-compaction cardiomyopathy varied in reports. Based on the high rate of embolic events reported in long-term follow-up data, Oechslin et al. [5] recommended anticoagulant therapy for these patients, independent of ventricular systolic function. However, Oechslin and Jenni [11] recently recommended anticoagulation therapy for patients with impaired systolic function (LV ejection fraction < 40%) because deep intertrabecular recesses and slow blood flow might increase the risk of thrombus formation. Patients with LVNC who have end-stage heart failure are candidates for cardiac transplantation; successful cardiac transplantation in those patients has been reported [12].

Key Points

1. Isolated left ventricular noncompaction is a congenital cardiomyopathy caused by a defect in endomyocardial morphogenesis.
2. Careful evaluation of LVNC patients for coexisting heart abnormalities such as aneurysms is essential for making the best clinical decisions for their management.

References

1. Chin, T.K., Perloff, J.K., Williams, R.G. et al. (1990). Isolated noncompaction of left ventricular myocardium. A study of eight cases. *Circulation* 82: 507–513.
2. Maron, B.J., Towbin, J.A., Thiene, G. et al. (2006). American Heart Association; Council on Clinical Cardiology, Heart Failure and Transplantation Committee; Quality of Care and Outcomes Research and Functional Genomics and Translational Biology Interdisciplinary Working Groups; Council on Epidemiology and Prevention. Contemporary definitions and classification of the cardiomyopathies: an American Heart Association Scientific Statement from the Council on Clinical Cardiology, Heart Failure and Transplantation Committee; Quality of Care and Outcomes Research and Functional Genomics and Translational Biology Interdisciplinary Working Groups; and Council on Epidemiology and Prevention. *Circulation* 113: 1807–1816.
3. Elliott, P., Andersson, B., Arbustini, E. et al. (2008). Classification of the cardiomyopathies: A position statement from the European Society Of Cardiology Working Group on Myocardial and Pericardial Diseases. *Eur Heart J* 29: 270–276.
4. Jenni, R., Oechslin, E., Schneider, J. et al. (2001). Echocardiographic and pathoanatomical characteristics of isolated left ventricular non compaction: a step towards classification as a distinct cardiomyopathy. *Heart* 86: 666–671.
5. Oechslin, E.N., Attenhofer Jost, C.H., Rojas, J.R. et al. (2000). Long-term follow up of 34 adults with isolated left ventricular noncompaction: a distinct cardiomyopathy with poor prognosis. *J Am Coll Cardiol* 36: 493–500.
6. Sato, Y., Matsumoto, N., Yoda, S. et al. (2006). Left ventricular aneurysm associated with isolated noncompaction of the ventricular myocardium. *Heart Vessels* 21 (3): 192–194.
7. Ionescu, C.N. and Turcot, D. (2011). Left ventricular noncompaction and aneurysm revealed by left ventriculography. *Catheter Cardiovasc Interv* 80 (1): 109–111.
8. Junga, G., Kneifel, S., von Smekal, A. et al. (1999). Myocardial ischemia in children with isolated ventricular noncompaction. *Eur Heart J* 20: 910–916.
9. Ichida, F., Hamamichi, Y., Miyawaki, T. (1999). Clinical features of isolated noncompaction of the ventricular myocardium: long-term clinical course, hemodynamic properties, and genetic background. *J Am Coll Cardiol* 34: 233–240.
10. Soler, R., Rodriguez, E., Monserrat, L. et al. (2002). MRI of subendocardial perfusion deficits in isolated left ventricular noncompaction. *J Comput Assist Tomogr* 26: 373–375.
11. Oechslin, E. and Jenni, R. (2011). Left ventricular non-compaction revisited: A distinct phenotype with genetic heterogeneity? *Eur Heart J* 32: 1446–1456.
12. Roberts, W.C., Karia, S.J., Ko, J.M. (2011). Examination of isolated ventricular noncompaction (hypertrabeculation) as a distinct entity in adults. *Am J Cardiol* 108 (5): 747–752.

Part V
Diversification

Part V
Diversification

55 A Fistula between Aortic Pseudoaneurysm and Right Atrium

Ligang Fang[1] and Jing Ping Sun[2]

[1] Affiliated Hospital of Peking Union Medical College, Beijing, China
[2] The Chinese University of Hong Kong, Hong Kong

History

A 19-year-old female presented with a 1-month history of high fever, weight loss and dyspnea. Initial transthoracic echocardiography (TTE) revealed a large amount of pericardial effusion with normal cardiac structure and function. Thoracic computed tomography(CT)showed mediastinal lymphadenopathy and discrete infiltrations in the right lung with right-side pleural effusion. She underwent diagnostic pericardial drainage, which aspirated exudative hemoserous fluid. Interferon-γ release assay for tuberculosis was 2044 SFC (normal < 24), which confirmed the diagnosis of tuberculosis. Antituberculosis therapy was started and her symptoms resolved after 2 weeks. However, progressive dyspnea relapsed after 1 month.

Transthoracic Echocardiography

Repeat echocardiogram showed a large pseudoaneurysm arising from the ascending aorta (Ao) (Figure 55-1, left), which communicated with the right atrium (Figure 55-1, middle and right).

Computed Tomography Angiogram

Computed tomography examination confirmed the pseudoaneurysm between the ascending aorta and right atrium (Figure 55-2).

Treatment

Urgent surgery was recommended to prevent rupture of the pseudoaneurysm but the patient declined surgery.

Discussion

A tuberculous aneurysm of the aorta is exceedingly rare. Before 1950, most of the reported cases were from autopsies [1, 2, 3]; in later years, antemortem diagnosis and successful treatment became more common with the availability of better diagnostic facilities and enhanced awareness [4, 5, 6].

Comparative Cardiac Imaging: A Case-based Guide, First Edition.
Edited by Jing Ping Sun, Xing Sheng Yang, and Bryan P. Yan.
© 2018 John Wiley & Sons Ltd. Published 2018 by John Wiley & Sons Ltd.
Companion website: www.wiley.com/sun/comparative_cardiac_imaging

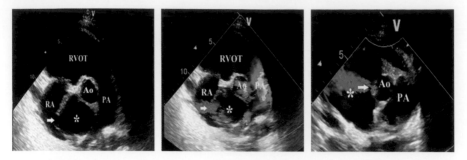

Figure 55-1 Transthoracic echocardiography. A large pseudoaneurysm was seen arising from the right side of the ascending aorta (AO) in parasternal short axis view (left). There was a blood flow communication between pseudoaneurysm and RA as well as aorta (arrows at middle and right). *Notes*: AO, aorta; *, pseudoaneurysm; RVOT, right ventricular outflow tract; RA, right atrium; PA, pulmonary artery.

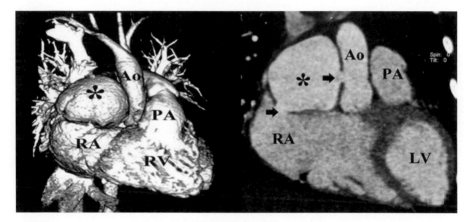

Figure 55-2 Computed tomography angiogram confirmed the pseudoaneurysm was arising from ascending aorta and communicated with right atrium (arrows). *Notes*: AO, aorta; *, pseudoaneurysm; RA, right atrium; PA, pulmonary artery; RV, right ventricle; LV, left ventricle.

Tubercle bacilli may reach the aortic wall in one of four ways: (i) the bacilli may implant directly on the internal surface of the vessel wall in patients suffering from miliary tuberculosis; (ii) the bacilli may be carried to the adventitia or media by the vasa vasorum; (iii) infection may reach the vessel wall by the lymphatics of the vasa vasorum; (iv) the outside of the vessel wall may be affected by direct extension from a neighboring tuberculous lymph node, abscess, or bone. This has been reported as the most common cause (75%) in literature [4]. In our case, the patient had tuberculosis pericarditis and mediastinal lymphadenopathy; the aortic pseudoaneurysm could have been caused by mediastinal lymphadenopathy. The arterial system may be affected by miliary tuberculosis of the intima, tubercular polyps attached to the intima, tuberculosis involving several layers of the arterial wall, aneurysm formation, or even by hypersensitivity reaction to the tubercular antigens [4, 5, 6]. Tubercular aneurysms are mostly pseudoaneurysm and are rarely true or dissecting [5].

Clinically, tuberculosis of the aorta manifests only after the onset of its major complications [2, 7]. One should have a high index of suspicion, and an aneurysm should be suspected in patients with active tuberculosis if they deteriorate suddenly or if a mass lesion is present [5]. The patient may present initially with persistent pain related to the location of the aneurysm. Other symptoms include fever, weight loss, hoarseness, dysphasia, palpable para-aortic mass (especially if pulsatile and expanding), hemoptysis, and hypovolemic shock or other evidence of massive bleeding, particularly into the lungs, gastrointestinal tract, peritoneal cavity, retroperitoneum, or even pericardial space.

The auscultatory presence of a continuous systolo-diastolic murmur should raise suspicion for fistulization. Fistulizing paeudoaneurysm of aorta (PSA) should be differentiated from ruptured sinus of Valsalva aneurysm [8]. Echocardiography, computed tomography, aortography, right heart catheterization and magnetic resonance angiography can differentiate and confirm the diagnosis. During pulmonary artery catheter placement, high oxygen saturation in the right atrium and the pulmonary artery are useful clues for the diagnosis of aortoatrial fistulization. In this case, cardiac CT illustrated the exact relationship between the paeudoaneurysm of aorta and the right atrium, the size and location of the aneurysmal sac, the adjacent structures and the shunts between the paeudoaneurysm and the right atrium, as well as communication with the ascending aorta. It was the most useful diagnostic tool in planning the surgical strategy and approach.

The management of tuberculous aortitis is both surgical and medical. There is no evidence that either of these alone will cure the disease [4, 6, 7]. All the survivors in literature have received both [6]. Antitubercular treatment must be instituted the moment tuberculosis is suspected [4].

Key Points

1. Pseudoaneurysm in the ascending aorta has been described as an uncommon and serious complication of trauma, inflammation, and aortic surgery. It may also occur as a result of atherosclerotic disease.
2. Aortic pseudoaneurysm is often fatal and results in death from rupture.
3. Despite the use of modern medicine therapy and imaging techniques, this disastrous complication still occurs and reinforces the need for early suspicion, diagnosis, surgical resection, and antitubercular therapy, along with close postoperative follow-up to prevent recurrence.

References

1. Allins, A.D., Wagner, W.H., Cossman, D.V. et al. (1999). Tuberculous infection of the descending thoracic and abdominal aorta: case report and literature review. *Ann Vasc Surg* 13: 439–444.
2. Wetteland, P. and Scott, D. (1956). Tuberculous aortic perforations; review of the literature and report of a case of false aneurysm with rupture into a bronchus. *Tubercle* 37, 177–182.
3. Stiefel, J.W. (1958). Rupture of a tuberculous aneurysm of the aorta; review of the literature and report of a case. *AMA Arch Pathol* 65: 506–512.
4. Long, R., Guzman, R., Greenberg, H. (1999). Tuberculous mycotic aneurysm of the aorta: review of published medical and surgical experience. *Chest* 115: 522–531.
5. Chowdhary, S.K., Bhan, A., Talwar, S. et al. (2001). Tubercular pseudoaneurysms of aorta. *Ann Thorac Surg* 72: 1239–1244.

6. Golzarian, J., Cheng, J., Giron, F. et al. (1999). Tuberculosis pseudoaneurysm of the descending thoracic aorta: successful surgical treatment by surgical excision and primary repair. *Tex Heart Inst J* 26: 232–235.

7. Volini, F.I., Olfield, R.C. Jr., Thompson, J.R. et al. (1962). Tuberculosis of the aorta. *JAMA* 181, 78–83.

8. Missault, L., Callens, B. and Taeymans, Y. (1995). Echocardiography of sinus of Valsalva aneurysm with rupture into the right atrium. *Int J Cardiol* 47: 269–272.

56 Dual Aortic and Mitral Valve Aneurysms in a Patient with Infective Endocarditis

Weihua Wu[1], Lan Ma[1], Xing Sheng Yang[2], Bryan P. Yan[2], and Jing Ping Sun[2]

[1] Jiaotong University, Shanghai, China
[2] The Chinese University of Hong Kong, Hong Kong

History

A 47-year-old man was admitted with acute shortness of breath, after experiencing 2 weeks of fever and malaise.

Physical Examination

On examination, the patient was hemodynamically stable. On auscultation, both systolic and diastolic murmurs were detected.

Laboratory

Three out of three sets of blood culture were positive for *Streptococcus sanguinis*.

Transthoracic Echocardiography

On admission, echocardiography was performed and showed a bicuspid aortic valve, a large aneurysm arising from the anterior leaflet of the bicuspid valve with severe aortic insufficiency (Figure 56-1A–F; Videos 56-1, 56-2, and 56-3); a second large aneurysm was found in the anterior leaflet of the mitral valve with severe mitral valve regurgitation (Figure 56-2 and Videos 56-4 and 56-5). The left ventricle was dilated. Several small instances of vegetation were seen on both the aortic and mitral-valve leaflets. Transesophageal echocardiography identified perforation of the aneurysms as part of the cause of aortic and mitral regurgitation.

Hospital Course

After the patient had recieved a course of intravenous antibiotic treatment and blood cultures tested negative, he underwent successful surgical operation including aortic valve replacement and mitral valve repaired. Operative findings (Figure 56-2) concurred with echocardiography described above.

Comparative Cardiac Imaging: A Case-based Guide, First Edition.
Edited by Jing Ping Sun, Xing Sheng Yang, and Bryan P. Yan.
© 2018 John Wiley & Sons Ltd. Published 2018 by John Wiley & Sons Ltd.
Companion website: www.wiley.com/sun/comparative_cardiac_imaging

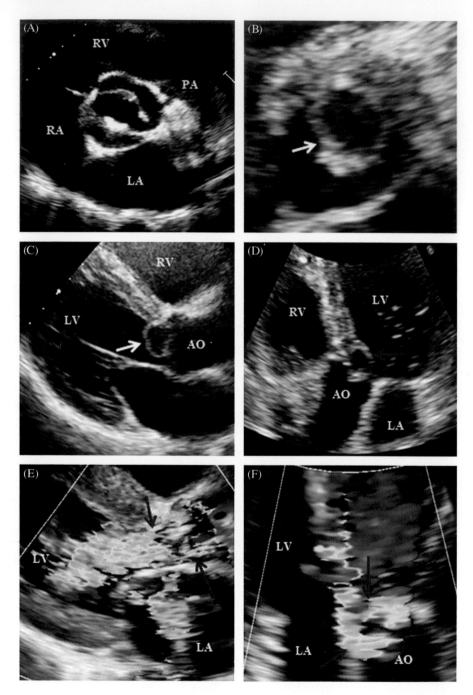

Figure 56-1   Echocardiography: A. Parasternal short-axis view showed bicuspid aortic valve. B. Parasternal short-axis view showed anterior aortic valve aneurysm. C. Parasternal long-axis view showed an aneurysm of bicuspid aortic anterior valve (arrow). D. Apical five-chamber view showed an aneurysm of the bicuspid aortic anterior valve (arrow). E and F. Color Doppler echocardiography demonstrated aortic insufficiency was partially from the perforation of the aneurysm.

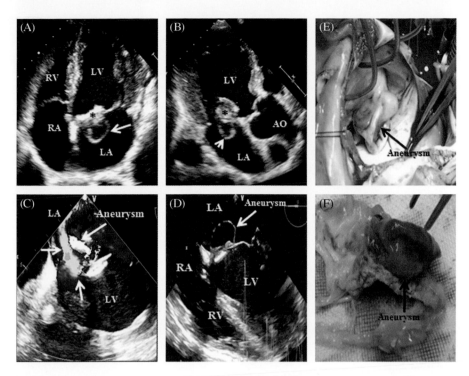

Figure 56-2 Echocardiography: A. An apical four-chamber showed anterior mitral valve with vegetation (*) and aneurysm (arrow). B. An apical three-chamber showed anterior mitral valve with vegetation (*) and aneurysm (arrow). C. A transesophageal color Doppler showed blood flow flowing through an aneurysm perforation into the left atrium (arrow). D. A transesophageal echocardiography four-chamber view showed an aneurysm (arrow) of mitral anterior valve toward the left atrium. E. Surgery field showed the mitral valve aneurysm. F. The gross picture of mitral valve aneurysm.

Pathology Examination

Histology examination of the mitral and aortic leaflets showed fibrous tissue hyperplasia with myxoid degeneration.

Discussion

Mitral valve aneurysm is a rare condition with reported incidence of 0.29% on 4500 TEE examinations [1]. On transthoracic echocardiography, it looks like a saccular bulge of the mitral leaflet protruding toward the left atrium with systolic expansion and diastolic collapse. The diastolic expansion may occur with aortic regurgitation or after the rupture of the mitral valve aneurysm [2]. The anterior mitral valve aneurysm is more commonly observed than the posterior mitral valve [3].

The development of mitral valve aneurysm is likely due to the infected aortic regurgitant jets striking the ventricular surface of the anterior mitral leaflet, causing physical trauma and possible occult mitral leaflet infection. This is manifested by valvulitis and the formation of saclike outpouchings due to formation of scar tissue and granulation tissue on microscopic examination. However, the posterior mitral valve occurs as a result of weakness of the mitral valve secondary to myxomatous degeneration and latent infective endocarditis [3]. Vilacosta et al. studied the natural course of these aneurysms with serial echocardiography and concluded that they undergo progressive expansion and subsequent rupture or perforation [1].

Vegetation or thrombus formation may occur within the aneurysm leading to thromboembolism and spread of infection [2]. The extension of infection to the mitral–aortic intervalvular fibrosis results in abscess or aneurysm formation [4]. The most probable cause of valve aneurysm is infectious endocarditis.

Our case met two of the major and three minor Duke criteria for the diagnosis of definite infective endocarditis: positive blood culture, echocardiography findings, new valvular insufficiency, fever, and predisposing bicuspid aortic valve.

Aortic valve aneurysm is very rare, with limited cases reported in the literature [5]. The bicuspid aortic valve and anterior mitral valve aneurysms occurred simultaneously in our case, with infective endocarditis. To the best of our knowledge, this is the first reported case of combined aortic and mitral valvular aneurysms in one patient.

Key Points

1. Aortic and mitral valve aneurysm is a very rare complication of infective endocarditis.
2. Early accurate diagnosis and treatment is the key for successful surgery therapy.

References

1. Vilacosta, I., San Roman, J.A., Sarria, C. et al. (1999). Clinical, anatomic, and echocardiographic characteristics of aneurysms of the mitral valve. *Am J Cardiol* 84: 110–113.
2. Guler, A., Karabay, C.Y., Gursoy, O.M. et al. (2014). Clinical and echocardiographic evaluation of mitral valve aneurysms: a retrospective, single center study. *Int J Cardiovasc Imag* 30: 535–541.
3. Hotchi, J., Hoshiga, M., Okabe, T. et al. (2011). Impressive echocardiographic images of a mitral valve aneurysm. *Circulation* 123: e400–e402.
4. Reid, C.L., Chandraratna, A.N., Harrison, E. et al. (1983). Mitral valve aneurysm: clinical features, echocardiographic-pathologic correlations. *J Am Col Cardiol* 2: 460–464.
5. de Juan, J., Moya, J.L. and Zamorano, J.L. (2014). Perforated aortic valve aneurysm due to infective endocarditis. *Rev Esp Cardiol* (Engl. edn) 67 (3): 222.

57 Intracardiac Thrombus in Behçet's Disease

Ligang Fang[1], Jing Ping Sun[2], and Yining Wang[1]

[1] Affiliated Hospital of Peking Union Medical College, Beijing, China
[2] The Chinese University of Hong Kong, Hong Kong

History

A 37-year-old male presented with intermittent fever, oral ulcers, and lower extremity erythema for 2 months.

Physical Examination

Temperature was 36.9 °C. Heart rate was 84 bpm. Breathing rate was 19 times/min. Blood pressure was 96/62 mmHg. An oral aphthous ulcer was noticed. There was no jugular vein engorgement. No heart murmur was heard.

Laboratory

Laboratory examination of blood showed hemoglobin 9.8 g/L, white blood cell 6.9×10^9/L, neutral classification of 53.8%, platelet 408 * 10^9/L. Erythrocyte sedimentation rate >140 mm/h. Activated partial thromboplastin time (APTT) for 28.5 s; prothrombin time: 13.5 s; prothrombin activity: 74.6%; thrombin time: 19.5 s. Immune index: ANA, anti dsDNA, anti ENA, lupus anticoagulant, anti beta 2 glycoprotein 1, anticardiolipin antibody (aCL), ANCA and rheumatoid factor were normal or negative. Blood gas analysis: PH7.438, 98.7 mmHg, PO2, pCO2 42.2 mmHg, high sensitive C reactive protein (hs-CRP) >10 mg/L (normal value 0~3), complement CH50 was 58.2 U/ml (25~55); complement C3 and C4 normal, antituberculosis antibody (–), purified protein derivative of ruberculin (PPD) (+ +), sputum smear, –D (–) 1-3 beta glucan antigen detection test (G test) (–), procalcitonin (PCT) (3–), blood culture (–). Human leukocyte antigen B5 (–). Bone marrow smear: some of the neutrophil granules were thick and numerous. Pathergy reaction was positive. Electrocardiogram: Sinus rhythm was normal.

Echocardiography

Apical 4- and 2-chamber views showed: The cardiac chambers were normal in size and function. The arrow point to an ellipse mass (2×1.4 cm) with a stalk attached to middle segment of right ventricle free wall, the mass center was low echo density with clear boundary (Figure 57-1A and B, Videos 57-1 and 57-2).There was mild to moderate tricuspid

Comparative Cardiac Imaging: A Case-based Guide, First Edition.
Edited by Jing Ping Sun, Xing Sheng Yang, and Bryan P. Yan.
Companion website: www.wiley.com/sun/comparative_cardiac_imaging

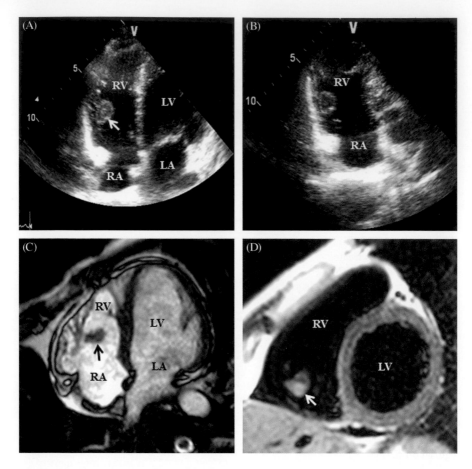

Figure 57-1 A and B. Apical four- and two-chamber echocardiography views. The cardiac chambers were normal in size and function. There was an elliptical mass (2 × 1.4 cm) with a stalk attached to the middle segment of the right ventricle free wall. The mass had a low echo density and a clear boundary. Figure C and D. Magnetic resonance imaging showed a 2 × 1.4 cm mass with a narrow base attached to the trabecular of the right ventricle.

regurgitation. The pulmonary artery systolic pressure was 28 mmHg estimated by the velocity of the tricuspid.

Chest CT Scan
Pulmonary angiography showed multiple pulmonary embolisms in the left and right lungs. Multiple patchy shadows were seen in the left lingual lobe and inferior field of both pulmonaries, which suggested as pulmonary infarction.

Magnetic Resonance Imaging (MRI)
Magnetic resonance imaging (MRI) showed a 2 × 1.4 cm mass with a narrow base attached to the trabecular of the right ventricle. The shape and position of the mass changed during the cardiac cycle (Figure 57-1C and D).

Hospital Course

The diagnosis of cardiac thrombus was considered and the patient was given anticoagulant therapy. After 4 weeks of treatment, the mass was 1.4 × 0.9 cm measured by echocardiography. The mass was 1.5 × 1.1 cm measured by magnetic resonance imaging. In order to further clarify the etiology and treatment, an operation was performed. Surgical inspection found an oval mass (about 2 × 1 cm) attached to the myocardial trabeculae of the right ventricle near the apical anterior septum. The mass and part of the trabecular were resected.

Pathology

Histology The organized thrombus contained an acute and chronic severe inflammatory cell infiltrate composed of a mixture of granulocytes and mononuclear inflammatory cells, which was consistent with the diagnosis of Behçet's disease.

The patient was admitted to hospital due to fever and genital ulcers 2 months after operation, and was treated with prednisone and cyclophosphamide. His symptoms were resolved one week after treatment.

Discussion

Behçet's disease (BD) is a chronic inflammatory multisystem disorder of unknown etiology. In addition to the triple symptom complex originally described by Hulusi Behçet, which encompassed oral ulcerations, genital ulcerations, and uveitis [1], the disease may also involve other organs, including the skin, joints, vessels, gastrointestinal tract, heart, lungs, and central nervous system (CNS). The diagnosis is made on the basis of the criteria proposed by the International Study Group (ISG) for BD in 1990 [2]. Cardiac complications (in up to 6% of BD patients) include pericarditis, endocarditis with valvular regurgitation, myocardial lesions (myocardial infarction, myocarditis, and endomyocardial fibrosis), and intracardiac thrombosis [3]. The innate and adaptive immune systems both play an important role in the disease pathogenesis [4], but the pathophysiology of the thrombotic predisposition among these patients is still mainly unknown. Several mechanisms have been proposed, such as endothelial lesions, increased levels of prothrombotic factors, and immune complex deposition in the blood vessels [5].

It is important to exclude other diagnoses, such as endocarditis, cardiac tumor and thrombus, in order to assume the presence of intracardiac lesions caused by BD. Although transthoracic echocardiography is an excellent imaging modality to screen and evaluate intracardiac lesions, in some cases it lacks sensitivity for identifying and characterizing the thrombi when compared to cardiac MRI [6]. Chest CT and MRI could be helpful in the assessment of associated thoracic manifestations of BD including thrombus of the systemic veins and pulmonary arteries [7]. In our case, the CT scan found multiple pulmonary embolisms.

Treatment of intracardiac thrombus is unclear. Some patients have been treated surgically with the removal of the thrombus. In our case, the cardiac mass was resected by surgery. The histological finding of cardiac mass was consistent with the cardiac lesion of Behçet's disease. The patient's symptoms were controlled by medical therapy. In the small number of cases published in the literature, patients treated with medical therapy tend to do better than those treated surgically [8]. Most patients have been treated with colchicine and steroids. Some have also been treated with cyclophosphamide and have shown a good response. Anticoagulation in patients with cardiac thrombus is controversial because these have a low chance of thromboembolism and a high risk of bleeding in the presence of pulmonary artery aneurysm, which can be life threatening. Often, resolution of the thrombus has been seen with just immunosuppression with or without an antiplatelet agent [9].

Key Points

1. Behçet's disease (BD) is a chronic inflammatory multisystem disorder of unknown etiology.
2. Clinical acumen is essential to diagnose these patients in time and institute life-saving immunosuppression as soon as possible.
3. The treatment of Behçet's disease with intracardiac thrombosis is mainly medical treatment, including anticoagulant, hormonal, and immunosuppressive therapy.

References

1. Behert, H. (1937). Über rezidivierende aphthöse, durch ein virus verursachte geschwüre ammund, am auge und an den genitalian. *Dermatol Wochenschr* 105: 1152–1157.
2. [No authors listed]. (1990). International Study Group for Behçet's Disease Criteria for diagnosis of Behçet's disease. *Lancet* 335: 1078–1080.
3. Aksu, T. and Tufekcioglu, O. (2015). Intracardiac thrombus in Behçet's disease: Four new cases and a comprehensive literature review. *Rheumatol Int* 35: 1269–1279.
4. Direskeneli, H. (2006). Autoimmunity vs autoinflammation in Behçet's disease: Do we oversimplify a complex disorder? *Rheumatology (Oxford)* 45: 1461–1465.
5. Jagadeesh, L.Y., Wajed, J., Sangle, S.R. et al. (2014). Cardiac complications of Behçet's disease. *Clin Rheumatol* 33:1185–1187.
6. Mollet, N.R., Dymarkowski, S., Volders, W. et al. (2002). Visualization of ventricular thrombi with contrast-enhanced magnetic resonance imaging in patients with ischemic heart disease. *Circulation* 106: 2873–2876.
7. Ben Ghorbel, I., Ibn Elhadj, Z., Khanfir, M. et al. (2004). Intracardiac thrombus in Behçet's disease. A report of three cases. *J Mal Vasc* 29: 159–161.
8. Zhu, Y.-L, Wu, Q.-J, Guo, L.-L. et al. (2012). The clinical characteristics and outcome of intracardiac thrombus and aortic valvular involvement in Behçet's disease: an analysis of 20 cases. *Clin Exper Rheumatol* 30 (suppl. 72), S40–S45.
9. Mogulkoc, N., Burgess, M.I., and Bishop, P.W. (2000). Intracardiac thrombus in Behçet's disease: A systematic review. *Chest* 118 (2): 479–487.

58 Cardiac Hydatid Disease

Ligang Fang¹, Jing Ping Sun², and Yining Wang¹

¹ Affiliated Hospital of Peking Union Medical College, Beijing, China
² The Chinese University of Hong Kong, Hong Kong

History

A 37-year-old male presented with headache and chest pain for 6 months. The patient grew up in rural areas of Tibet and had a history of cattle and sheep exposure. He was used to drinking raw milk and ate uncooked meat.

Physical Examination

Blood pressure was 145/89 mmHg. Heart rate was roughly 66 bpm. No heart murmur was heard.

Transthoracic Echocardiography

Transthoracic echocardiography showed a low echo-density cyst (16×20 mm) with a clear border in the left ventricular lateral wall (Figure 58-1, Video 58-1). There was mild to moderate mitral valvular regurgitation. The left ventricular ejection fraction was 66%.

Cardiac Magnetic Resonance Imaging

A low-density area with visible enhancement edge was in the middle of the left ventricular lateral wall (Figure 58-1A, B).

Thoracic and Abdominal Plain and Enhanced Computed Tomography (CT) Scan

There was a left-ventricular mass (Figure 58-2C, D), renal infarction, spleen infarction, and mesenteric artery, renal artery, and splenic artery embolization. Skull enhancement CT showed a large amount of cerebral hemorrhage in the left occipital lobe, rupturing into the ventriculus sinister cerebri.

According to the history and findings of echocardiography, MRI and CT, a diagnosis of cardiac hydatid associated with multiple organ embolism was made. The patient refused to receive operation.

Comparative Cardiac Imaging: A Case-based Guide, First Edition.
Edited by Jing Ping Sun, Xing Sheng Yang, and Bryan P. Yan.
© 2018 John Wiley & Sons Ltd. Published 2018 by John Wiley & Sons Ltd.
Companion website: www.wiley.com/sun/comparative_cardiac_imaging

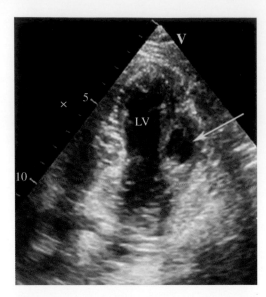

Figure 58-1 Echocardiography. A low echo density cyst with clear border (arrow) in left ventricular lateral wall was seen in an apical four-chamber view.

Discussion

The first description of cardiac hydatidosis was made in 1846 by Griensinger. Marten and de Crespigny were pioneers of surgical treatment of cardiac hydatidosis in 1921 [1]. The hexacanth embryos of the hydatid released from the ova into the human intestine enter the portal or lymphatic circulation. A few of these embryos may escape from the vascular beds of the liver and lungs and travel to the myocardium via the coronary circulation. When this occurs, the left ventricle is the most frequently involved site (60%), followed by the right ventricle (15%), the interventricular septum (9%), the left atrium (8%), the right atrium (4%), and the interatrial septum (2%) [2–5]. Primary pericardial cysts are extremely rare, and they generally develop secondary to intrapericardial rupture of a myocardial cyst or to spillage of cysts' contents during surgical removal [2, 6, 7].

Various symptoms and signs (from a simple dyspnea to anaphylactic reaction and sudden death) have been described depending on cyst location. Cardiac hydatidosis may lead to arrhythmia due to direct invasion or compression of the conducting system, which is usually seen in septal cysts. It can also mimic valvular lesions or intracardiac masses. If the parasite invades the papillary muscles or obstructs the ventricular outflow tract to produce valve dysfunction, so murmurs could be detected. Myocardial ischemia and congestive heart failure may result due to compression of the coronary arteries [8]. Cyst rupture is a serious complication and may cause death by anaphylactic shock or cardiac tamponade or acute pericarditis if the cyst is below the epicardium [9]. Acute or chronic cerebral occlusion, pulmonary embolism or acute arterial occlusion by embolism of small cyst pieces are nonfatal complications of cyst rupture [10]. The left ventricular mass, renal infarction, spleen infarction, mesenteric artery, renal artery, splenic artery embolization were detected by CT scan in our case. The patient suffered multiple organ failures caused by the multiple emboli from hydatidosis.

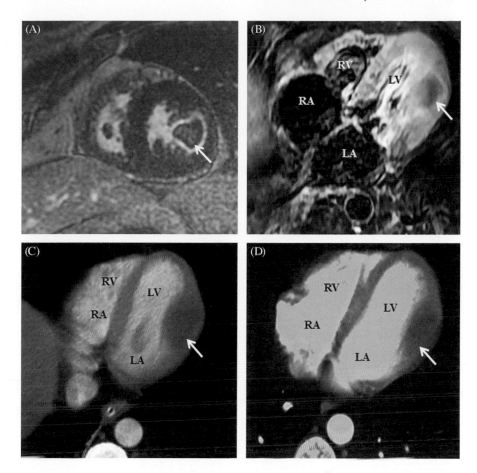

Figure 58-2   Cardiac magnetic resonance ECG gated SE sequence images. A. A low density area with visible enhancement edge was in the middle of left ventricular lateral wall (arrow). B. A left-ventricle apical four-chamber view showed a low-density area with a visible enhancement edge (arrow). A cardiac enhanced CT scan showed (C and D) there is a low-density area in left ventricular lateral wall.

Suspicion is essential in the diagnosis of cardiac hydatid cysts, especially in endemic geographic areas. Although the electrocardiogram and chest radiograph can be abnormal, they are usually not diagnostic [2]. Echocardiography is an efficient, easy-to-perform, and highly sensitive noninvasive technique, which should be the first choice for diagnostic method to detect and localize cardiac hydatid cysts. Computed tomography and magnetic resonance imaging are additional useful diagnostic methods [7]. Computed tomography body scan is very useful for detecting multiple organs involved, as in our case.

The treatment of choice even for asymptomatic cardiac hydatid cysts is surgical excision, which yields complete recovery and excellent prognosis [11]. Supplemental medical therapy with mebendazole or albendazole is recommended to reduce the risk of recurrence, especially in the event of intracardiac rupture. In order to exclude the possibility of recurrence due to inadvertent spillage or a small cyst not noticed at the time of the operation, serologic and echocardiographic monitoring is recommended during the first 5 postoperative years [12].

Key Points
1. Cardiac hydatid cysts may present with a variety of signs and symptoms.
2. Physician should be aware the possibility of hydatid disease especially in endemic zones.
3. Due to the high risk of associated complications, surgical excision combined with antiparasite medical therapy seems to be the first-line treatment even in asymptomatic patients.

References

1. Tellez, G., Nojek, C., Juffe, A., et al. (1976). Cardiac echinococcosis: Report of three cases and review of the literature. *Ann Thorac Surg* 21: 425–430.
2. Salih, O.K., Celik, S.K., Topcuoglu, M.S. et al. (1998). Surgical treatment of hydatid cysts of the heart: A report of three cases and a review of the literature. *Can J Surg* 41: 321–327.
3. Abid, A., Ben Omrane, S., Kaouel, K. et al. (2003). Intracavitary cardiac hydatid cyst. *Cardiovasc Surg* 11: 521–525.
4. Ozer, N., Aytemir, K., Kuru, G. et al. (2001). Hydatid cyst of the heart as a rare cause of embolization: report of 5 cases and review of published reports. *J Am Soc Echocardiogr* 14: 299–302.
5. Kaplan, M., Demirtas, M., Cimen, S. et al. (2001). Cardiac hydatid cysts with intracavitary expansion. *Ann Thorac Surg* 71: 1587–1590.
6. Narin, N., Mese, T., Unal, N. et al. (1996). Pericardial hydatid cyst with a fatal course. *Acta Paediatr Jpn* 38: 61–62.
7. Birincioglu, C.L., Bardakci, H., Kucuker, S.A. et al. (1999). A clinical dilemma: Cardiac and pericardiac echinococcosis. *Ann Thorac Surg* 68: 1290–1294.
8. Rezaian, G.R. and Aslani, A. (2008). Endocardial hydatid cyst: A rare presentation of echinococcal infection. *Eur J Echocar-diogr* 9 (2): 342–343.
9. Kaplan, M., Demirates, M., Cimen, S. et al. (2001). Cardiac hydatid cysts with intracavitary expansion. *Ann Thorac Surg* 71: 1587–1590.
10. Kelle, S., Köhler, U., Thouet, T. et al. (2009). Cardiac involvementof *Echinococcus granulosus* evaluated by multi-contrast CMR imaging. *Int J Cardiol* 131 (2): e59–e60.
11. Miralles, A., Bracamonte, L., Pavie, A. et al. (1994). Cardiac echinococcosis. Surgical treatment and results. *J Thorac Cardiovasc Surg* 107: 184–190.
12. Kutay, V., Ekim, H. and Yakut, C. (2003). Infected myocardial hydatid cyst imitating left ventricular aneurysm. *Cardiovasc Surg* 11: 239–241.

59 Diagnosis of Constrictive Pericarditis with Multimodality Imaging

Alex Pui-Wai Lee and Jing Ping Sun

The Chinese University of Hong Kong, Hong Kong

History

A 48-year-old gentleman presented with a 6-month history of abdominal and lower limbs swelling.

Physical Examination

Cardiovascular examination revealed severe ascites, peripheral edema, and elevated jugular venous pressure with rapid x and y descent (Video 59-1).

Laboratory Investigation and Hospital Course

Laboratory blood tests showed a decreased serum albumin of 22 g/L. A 99mTc-albumin scan revealed protein extravasation in the transverse colon. Protein-losing enteropathy was suspected but extensive gastrointestinal investigations, including endoscopy and biopsies, were diagnostically unrevealing. The patient was subsequently referred to cardiology for evaluation.

Echocardiography

The left ventricle (LV) was normal in size with a preserved ejection fraction of 65%. There was a brisk, diastolic bounce of the interventricular septum (Video 59-2). The inferior vena cava was dilated with absent collapse during inspiration (Figure 59-1A). A preserved mitral annular velocity was detected on tissue Doppler imaging (Figure 59-1B). Pulsed wave Doppler examination of the transvalvular flow demonstrated reciprocal respiratory variation in left and right ventricular (RV) filling (Figure 59-1C).

Cardiac Computed Tomography (CCT)

The thickness of the pericardium was increased (maximum thickness 6.1 mm) without pericardial calcification (Figure 59-2).

The diagnosis of idiopathic constrictive pericarditis was established. Pericardectomy was performed and the patient's symptoms completely resolved after surgery. The interventricular septal paradoxical motion returned to normal after operation (Video 59-3).

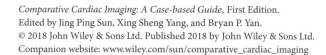

Comparative Cardiac Imaging: A Case-based Guide, First Edition.
Edited by Jing Ping Sun, Xing Sheng Yang, and Bryan P. Yan.
© 2018 John Wiley & Sons Ltd. Published 2018 by John Wiley & Sons Ltd.
Companion website: www.wiley.com/sun/comparative_cardiac_imaging

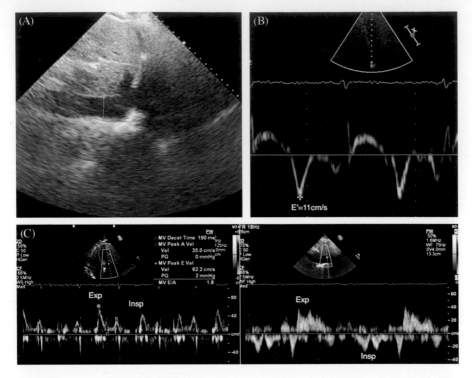

Figure 59-1 Echocardiographic features of constrictive pericarditis. The inferior vena cava is severely dilated with absent collapse during inspiration, consistent with high right atrial pressure (A). Tissue Doppler imaging shows a preserved early diastolic mitral annular velocity (B). Doppler echocardiography demonstrates reciprocal respiratory changes of LV and RV filling, with a respiratory variation of >25% in the mitral inflow E velocity after inspiration (Insp) and increased diastolic flow reversal with expiration (Exp) in the hepatic vein. This reflects disassociation between the intrathoracic and intracardiac pressures (C).

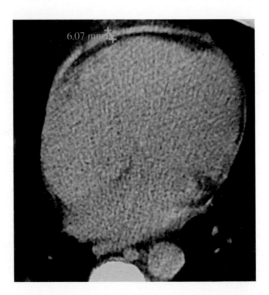

Figure 59-2 A cardiac computed tomography (CCT) scan depicts increased pericardial thickness without calcification.

Discussion

Constrictive pericarditis is the result of chronic inflammation and scarring of the pericardial sac. This results anatomically in thickening, fibrosis, and calcification of the pericardium. Physiologically, an inflamed pericardium hinders transmission of the respiratory changes of intrathoracic pressure to the pericardial and intracardiac cavities (disassociation between intrathoracic and intracardiac pressures). Moreover, diastolic filling of the LV and of the RV rely on each other as a result of the fixed total cardiac volume that is constrained within a stiff pericardium (exaggerated ventricular interdependence).

Echocardiography is an essential diagnostic modality in patients with suspected pericardial constriction. The M-mode and 2D echocardiography features of constrictive pericarditis include a thickened pericardium, septal bounce, rapid diastolic flattening of the LV posterior wall, respiratory variation in ventricular size, and a plethoric inferior vena cava. Trasnesophageal echocardiography may be helpful in measuring pericardial thickness with a reportedly good correlation with cardiac CT [1].

The hemodynamic hallmark of constrictive pericarditis is an exaggerated change in transvalvular flow during respiration. Optimally, a respiratory variation of 25% or more in the mitral inflow E velocity and increased diastolic flow reversal with expiration in the hepatic vein have to be demonstrated to establish the diagnosis of constriction [2]. However, in patients with markedly increased atrial pressure, the respiratory variation in mitral inflow may be less prominent [3]. The early diastolic mitral annulus velocity (E′) recorded with tissue Doppler imaging is a valuable Doppler variable for establishing the diagnosis of pericardial constriction (typically >8 cm/s) and for differentiating it from myocardial restriction [4]. Constrictive pericarditis should be considered in all patients who have symptoms of heart failure, with a normal LV ejection fraction and an E′ >8 cm/s. Speckle strain echocardiography can be used to demonstrate a reduced circumferential strain in the presence of preserved longitudinal early diastolic velocities, as well as significantly reduced left ventricular twist and torsion [5].

Cardiac CT is very sensitive for the detection of pericardial thickening and/or calcification. When there is clinical and/or echocardiographic evidence of impaired filling, pericardial thickening (>4 mm, diffuse or localized) is highly suggestive of constrictive pericarditis [6]. The absence of thickening, however, does not rule out constriction, as 20% of patients with surgically proven constrictive pericarditis have normal pericardial thickness [7]. Cardiac CT is also useful for detailed descriptions of the location and extent of thickening and calcification, which will aid the surgeon in risk assessment and surgical planning for pericardectomy.

A cardiac magnetic resonance (CMR) myocardial tagging sequence can be used to show adhesion and immobility of the pericardial-myocardial interface [8]. It is a valuable imaging tool—in both the morphologic and the functional assessments—for evaluating pericardial abnormalities. It also has good spatial resolution, high inherent soft-tissue contrast, a wide field of view, and multiplanar imaging capabilities; these characteristics of MRI are useful in the evaluation of pericardium, particularly for tissue characterization, assessment of inflammation, and evaluation for other potential cardiac abnormalities. Although accurate measurement of pericardial thickness using CMR is clinically feasible, calcification may not be as well visualized as on CCT [9].

Key Points

1. Echocardiography revealed a respiratory variation of >25% in the mitral inflow E velocity; increased diastolic flow reversal with expiration in the hepatic vein; symptoms of heart failure, with a normal LV ejection fraction and an E' >8 cm/s.
2. Cardiac CT is very sensitive for the detection of pericardial thickening and/or calcification.
3. Cardiac magnetic resonance (CMR) is a valuable imaging tool in both the morphologic and the functional assessments for evaluating pericardial abnormalities. Calcification may not be as well visualized as on CCT.

References

1. Ling, L.H., Oh, J.K., Tei, C. et al. (1997). Pericardial thickness measured with transesophageal echocardiography: feasibility and potential clinical usefulness. *J Am Coll Cardiol* 29: 1317–1323.
2. Oh, J.K., Hatle, L.K., Seward, J.B. et al. (1994). Diagnostic role of Doppler echocardiography in constrictive pericarditis. *J Am Coll Cardiol* 23: 154–162.
3. Oh, J.K., Tajik, A.J., Appleton, C.P. et al. (1997). Preload reduction to unmask the characteristic Doppler features of constrictive pericarditis. A new observation. *Circulation* 95: 796–799.
4. Rajagopalan, N., Garcia, M.J., Rodriguez, L. et al. (2001). Comparison of new Doppler echocardiographic methods to differentiate constrictive pericardial heart disease and restrictive cardiomyopathy. *Am J Cardiol* 87: 86–94.
5. Sengupta, P.P., Krishnamoorthy, V.K., Abhayaratna, W.P. et al. (2008). Disparate patterns of left ventricular mechanics differentiate constrictive pericarditis from restrictive cardiomyopathy. *JACC Cardiovasc Imaging* 1: 29–38.
6. Isner, J.M., Carter, B.L., Bankoff, M.S. et al. (1982). Computed tomography in the diagnosis of pericardial heart disease. *Ann Intern Med* 97: 473–479.
7. Talreja, D.R., Edwards, W.D., Danielson, G.K. et al. (2003). Constrictive pericarditis in 26 patients with histologically normal pericardial thickness. *Circulation* 108: 1852–1857.
8. Yared, K., Baggish, A.L., Picard, M.H. et al. (2010). Multimodality imaging of pericardial diseases. *JACC Cardiovasc Imaging* 3: 650–660.
9. Masui, T., Finck, S., Higgins, C.B. (1992). Constrictive pericarditis and restrictive cardiomyopathy: Evaluation with MR imaging. *Radiology* 182: 369–373.

60 Inverted Left-Atrial Appendage

Haiping Zhang¹ and Jing Ping Sun²

¹ The Second Affiliated Hospital of Wenzhou Medical University, Wenzhou, China
² The Chinese University of Hong Kong, Hong Kong

History

A 2-month-old boy was confirmed to have ventricular and atrial septal defect, coarctation of descending aorta, and patent ductus arteriosus by preoperative echocardiogram.

With the aid of cardiopulmonary bypass, the ventricular and atrial septal defects were closed using pericardium, the patent ductus arteriosus was ligated, the coarctation portion of aorta excised with anastomosis reconstituted with distal part of the descending aorta. The child suffered from respiratory distress on the second postoperative day.

Transthoracic Echocardiography

An abnormal homogenous mass in the left atrial cavity was detected. The mass was attached to the left atrial lateral wall and prolapsed toward the mitral annulus during diastole, causing left ventricular inflow obstruction (Figure 60-1 and Videos 60-1, 60-2, and 60-3).

The patient underwent a second operation without cardiopulmonary bypass. During the operation, the left atrial mass (1.2 × 1.3 cm²) was found appearance purplish, representing an inverted left atrial appendage. Reversion of the atrial appendage was done without complication. Postoperative echocardiography revealed no abnormal mass in the left atrial cavity and the patient recovered very well.

Discussion

Inverted left atrial appendage is a rare complication of cardiac surgery. The reversal atrial appendage presents as a left atrial mass postoperatively mimicked as a blood clot or vegetation. The differential diagnosis is very important. Unnecessary investigations and treatment may be employed if this entity is not recognized. Once the diagnosis is defined early, the treatment is simple. We report an infant with inverted left atrial appendage following repair of congenital heart disease. This report aimed to improve the awareness of sonographers toward this rare cause of left atrial mass. New left atrial mass found after cardiac surgery on echocardiography may be attributed to blood clot, vegetation or, rarely, an inverted left atrial appendage. Although vegetation is less likely in a patient immediately after surgery, blood clot is a possibility. A new mass in the left atrium after surgery, and the absence of the long tubular pyramidal left atrial appendage

Comparative Cardiac Imaging: A Case-based Guide, First Edition.
Edited by Jing Ping Sun, Xing Sheng Yang, and Bryan P. Yan.
© 2018 John Wiley & Sons Ltd. Published 2018 by John Wiley & Sons Ltd.
Companion website: www.wiley.com/sun/comparative_cardiac_imaging

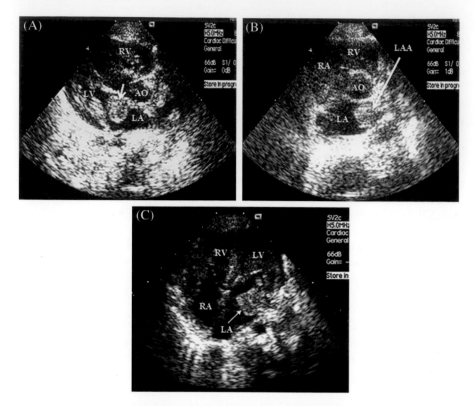

Figure 60-1   A. Parasternal long-axis view demonstrating a homogenous and mobile mass with a hingelike motion in the left atrium swinging into left ventricle. B. Modified parasternal short-axis view showed a mass extending from the left atrial appendage into the left atrium. C. The apical four-chamber view showed a mass from the atrial lateral wall prolapsing into left ventricle through the mitral valve.

shadow in its normal anatomic location by echocardiography made an inverted left atrial appendage a more possible suspect. Moreover, the mass was freely mobile and had a smooth tongue-like appearance, which favored this diagnosis.

Inverted left atrial appendage can be caused by the excessive negative pressure created by a left ventricular event or during evacuation of air intraoperatively [1]. There is a published case with inverted appendage caused by massive pericardial effusion, suggesting that left-atrium appendage inversion can probably be caused by significantly elevated intrapericardial pressure due to massive effusion [2]. Surgery remains the gold standard in diagnosing this lesion [3–5]. Inverted left atrial appendage can cause severe and occasionally life threatening complications, so we believe intraoperative transesophageal echocardiography is essential to diagnose this pathology and to avoid restorative operation. However, if intraoperative transesophageal echocardiography is not performed and the lesion is discovered late, the differential diagnosis should be made between infective vegetation and thrombus. Therapy may vary for each of these conditions and may include anticoagulation, antibiotics, or operation. Cardiac magnetic resonance imaging had been used to diagnose the lesion by observing the mass coming out from the left atrial appendage and having the same characteristics as the left atrial wall, but it may not be helpful in all cases [1–3]. Being aware of this lesion and recognizing its features on echocardiography is the key to diagnose it. The following echocardiographic characteristics are useful in the diagnosis of this lesion: (i) an homogenous mass arising from the anterolateral wall, in between the pulmonary vein and the mitral valve, which is an unusual position for blood clot or vegetation; (ii) absence of a left-atrial appendage in the short-axis view; (iii) The mass has a broad base and is highly mobile; and (iv) a new postsurgical mass [3].

The natural history of this lesion has yet to be well understood. Treatment of this rare lesion is debatable. Some authors suggest to revert the inversion surgically, while others adopt a more conservative approach and spontaneously reversion has been reported [4]. No approach has thus far proved to be superior to the others. When the condition is treated surgically, it is also uncertain whether the left atrial appendage should be merely reverted, ligated, or even be resected [3–7]. In view of the potential risks of embolic stroke, appendage necrosis, and hemodynamic disturbance, surgery might be necessary [8, 9]. This procedure was simple, quick and had minimal complications. In our case, the reversion of left appendage was done by operation.

Key Points

1. Inverted left atrial appendage is a rare phenomenon but should be considered if there is a newly developed cardiac mass after cardiac surgery.
2. Echocardiography is an excellent imaging modality that will provide adequate information for the diagnosis of this lesion. However, other imaging modalities such as cardiac magnetic resonance is helpful.
3. Awareness of this lesion is the key for diagnosis.

References

1. Fujiwara, K., Naito, Y., Noguchi, Y. et al (1999). Inverted left atrial appendage. An unusual complication in cardiac surgery. *Ann Thorac Surg* 67: 1492–1494.
2. Gecmen, C., Candan, O., Guler, A. et al. (2011). Unusual left atrial mass: Inverted left atrial appendage caused by massive pericardial effusion. *Echocardiography* 28: E134–E136.
3. Leong, M.C., Latiff, H.A. and Hew, C.C. (2013). Inverted left atrial appendage masquerading as a cardiac mass. *Echocardiography* 30: E33–E35.
4. Allen, B.S., Ilbawi, M., Hartz, R.S. et al. (1997). Inverted left atrial appendage: An unrecognized cause of left atrial mass. *J Thorac Cardiovasc Surg* 114: 278–280.
5. Cohen, A.J., Tamir, A., Yanai, O., et al. (1999). Inverted left atrial appendage presenting as a left atrial mass after cardiac surgery. *Ann Thorac Surg* 67: 1489–1491.
6. Vincentelli A, Juthier F, Lettourneau T, et al. (2005). An inverted left atrial appendage mimicking an intraatrial thrombus after ross operation. *J Heart Valve Dis* 14: 780–782.
7. Srichai, M.B., Griffin, B., Banbury, M. et al. (2005). Inverted left atrial appendage ligation mimicking thrombus. *Circulation* 111: e178–e179.
8. Corno, A.F. (1998). Inverted left atrial appendage. *J Thorac Cardiovasc Surg* 115: 1223–1224.
9. Danford, D.A., Cheatham, J.P., Van Gundy, J.C. et al. (1994). Inversion of the left atrial appendage: Clinical and echocardiographic correlates. *Am Heart J* 127: 719–721.

61 Inferior Vena Stent Fracture and Multiple Heart Injuries caused by Migration

Ligang Fang[1], Yining Wang[1], and Jing Ping Sun[2]

[1] Affiliated Hospital of Peking Union Medical College, Beijing, China
[2] The Chinese University of Hong Kong, Hong Kong

History

A 42-year-old man with a history of inferior vena stent placement for Budd–Chiari syndrome 3 years earlier presented with shortness of breath, abdominal distension, and cough for 16 days. The patient underwent pericardiocentesis 14 days ago for large amount of pericardial effusion, which was bloody.

Physical Examinations

The patient's jugular vein was remarkably distended. There was a continuous murmur in the tricuspid valve area.

Echocardiography

One strut of the stent was seen in the right atrium from apical four-chamber and parasternal short-axis views (Figure 61-1A and B; Videos 61-1 and 61-2). A fistula, with continuous flow between the noncoronary sinus and the right atrium, was detected by color Doppler (Figure 61-1C; Video 61-3), and a left-to-right shunt was found in the middle of the atrial septum (Figure 61-1D). The findings above suggested that there is a right-atrial-to-aortic fistula and the atrial septal had a perforation.

Computed Tomogaphy

Cardiac computed tomography (CT) scans revealed the presence of the stent in the right atrium (Figure 61-2A) and metal opacities in the left pulmonary artery (Figure 61-2B) and in the right hepatic vein (Figure 61-2C).

Hospital Course

An emergency operation was performed. Intraoperative inspection demonstrated that there was a laceration of the parietal pericardium close to the junction of the right atrium and the inferior vena cava, an 8 mm defect in the central part (oval fossa) of the atrial septum, and a 10 mm laceration in the noncoronary sinus. The patient recovered well after the operation.

Comparative Cardiac Imaging: A Case-based Guide, First Edition.
Edited by Jing Ping Sun, Xing Sheng Yang, and Bryan P. Yan.
© 2018 John Wiley & Sons Ltd. Published 2018 by John Wiley & Sons Ltd.
Companion website: www.wiley.com/sun/comparative_cardiac_imaging

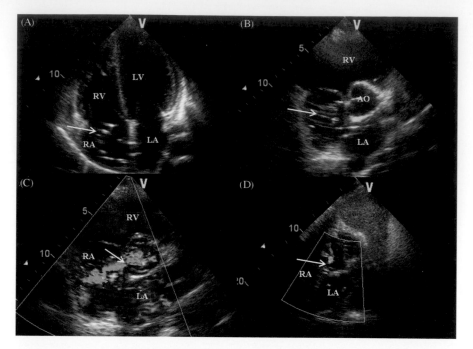

Figure 61-1 One strut of the stent was seen in the right atrium from apical four-chamber and parasternal short axis (A and B). A fistula, with continuous flow between the noncoronary sinus and the right atrium, was detected by color and continuous wave Doppler (C, arrow) and a left-to-right shunt was found in the middle of the atrial septum (D, arrow).

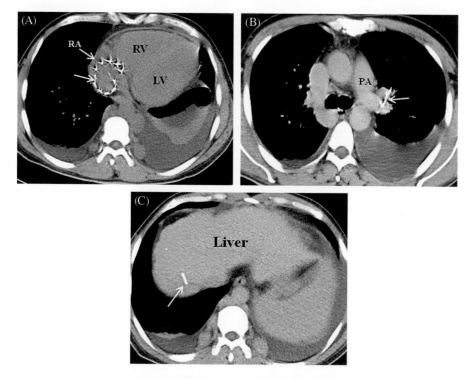

Figure 61-2 Cardiac computed tomography scans revealed the presence of the stent in the right atrium (A) and metal opacities in the left pulmonary artery and in the right hepatic vein (B and C).

Discussion

The Food and Drug Administration (FDA) has received more than 900 reports of adverse events with inferior vena cava (IVC) filters, leading the agency to remind clinicians that the devices should be removed as soon as it is safely possible [1]. Only a few reports have shown that the inferior vena cava stent could migrate into the right atrium [2]. A condition leading to multiple perforations, as in our case, has not been reported.

Some studies suggest that strenuous physical activity and increased intra-abdominal pressure can lead to the fracture and migration of IVC filters [3, 4]. Fracture and migration of a suprarenal IVC filter in a pregnant patient has also been reported [3]. Apart from morbid obesity, our patient did not have any other recognizable precipitating factors. A review of the literature shows that very few cases of fractured IVC filter migrate to the heart, and even fewer cases cause cardiac tamponade [5, 6]. The cause of cardiac tamponade is the perforation of the superior vena cava or the atrium, and in one case report it was due to the perforation of the right ventricle. The patient described above was unique in that the fractured IVC filter was lodged in the right ventricle and caused cardiac tamponade.

In our case, there was a laceration of the parietal pericardium close to the junction of the right atrium and the inferior vena cava, an 8 mm defect in the central part (oval fossa) of the atrial septum, and a 10 mm laceration in the noncoronary sinus. In such a case, a bedside echocardiogram is a good initial modality to find the strut and a fistula between the noncoronary sinus and the right atrium also rules out cardiac tamponade, which leads to prompt open-heart surgery.

Sudden decompensation and death can result from migration of a fractured IVC filter or stent to the heart or lungs [7, 8]. This rare side effect of IVC filters or stent needs to be promptly identified, as the consequences can be fatal.

Key Points

1. Inferior vena cava (IVC) filters or stent can fracture and migrate to the heart, causing tamponade and death.
2. The fracture and migration of IVC filters or stent should be suspected in patients presenting with sudden, unexplained cardiopulmonary symptoms.
3. Echocardiography is a good initial modality to diagnose this situation. Computed tomography can detect the extracardiac injuries.

References

1. Food and Drug Administration (2010). Removing retrievable inferior vena cava filters: Initial communication. August 9.
2. Goelitz, B.W. and Darcy, M. (2007). Longitudinal stent fracture and migration of a stent fragment complicating treatment of hepatic vein stenosis after orthotopic liver transplantation. *Semin Intervent Radiol* 24 (3): 333–336.
3. Ganguli, S., Tham, J.C., Komlos, F. et al. (2006). Fracture and migration of a suprarenal inferior vena cava filter in a pregnant patient. *J Vasc Interv Radiol* 17: 1707–1711.
4. Saeed, I., Garcia, M., McNicholas, K. (2006). Right ventricular migration of a recovery IVC filter's fractured wire with subsequent pericardial tamponade. *Cardiovasc Intervent Radiol* 29: 685– 686.
5. Vergara, G.R., Wallace, W.F., Bennett, K.R. (2007). Spontaneous migration of an inferior vena cava filter resulting in cardiac tamponade and percutaneous filter retrieval. *Catheter Cardiovasc Interv* 69: 300–302.

6. Hussain, S.M., McLafferty, R.B., Schmittling, Z.C. et al. (2005). Superior vena cava perforation and cardiac tamponade after filter placement in the superior vena cava – a case report. *Vasc Endovascular Surg* 39: 367–370.

7. Rossi, P., Arata, F.M., Bonaiuti, P. et al. (1999). Fatal outcome in atrial migration of the Tempofilter. *Cardiovasc Intervent Radiol* 22: 227–231.

8. Kuo, W.T., Loh, C.T. and Sze, D.Y. (2007). Emergency retrieval of a G2 filter after complete migration into the right ventricle. *J Vasc Interv Radiol* 18: 1177–1182.

62 Anterior Mitral Valve Aneurysm: A Rare Complication of Aortic Valve Endocarditis

Jinchuan Yan[1], Fen Zhang[1], Yi Liang[1], and Jing Ping Sun[2]

[1] Affiliated Hospital of Zhenjiang Medical College, Zhenjiang, China
[2] The Chinese University of Hong Kong, Hong Kong

History

A 64-year-old Chinese male presented with a more than 4-week history of worsening shortness of breath and cough. He did not have any antibacterial therapy. The patient had a history of untreated hypertension for more than 10 years.

Examination

At the time of presentation, the patient was extremely weak, with orthopnea and dyspnea. He was afebrile with a normal heart rate of 75 BNP. Blood pressure was 110/40 mm Hg.

Apex impulse was displaced inferolaterally and sustained. Auscultation at the right second interspace revealed a grade 3/6, holodiastolic murmur and a grade 2/6 short, systolic murmur; at the apex a grade 1-2 holosystolic murmur was heard, which radiated into the axilla.

Laboratory

Hemoglobin was 13.0 g/percent and the white blood cell count was 25700/mcL with 93.1% polymorphonuclears. Nutritionally variant streptococci grow in blood culture.

Chest X-ray

The chest radiograph shows both of lower lobes opacities with a predominantly peripheral distribution, consistent with pneumonia.

Transthoracic Echocardiography

The echocardiography was performed on admission and revealed the anterior mitral valve leaflet with an aneurysm bulging toward the left atrium (LA), the aortic noncoronary cusp was ruptured at the bottom and there was a prolapse into the left ventricular outflow tract. The aortic valve regurgitation was clearly seen from the rupture location by color Doppler. The mild mitral regurgitation toward the postlateral wall of left atrium and a color flow filling into anterior mitral valve aneurysm were seen from the apical long-axis view during early diastole (Figure 62-1, Videos 62-1, 62-2, 62-3, and 62-4).

Comparative Cardiac Imaging: A Case-based Guide, First Edition.
Edited by Jing Ping Sun, Xing Sheng Yang, and Bryan P. Yan.
© 2018 John Wiley & Sons Ltd. Published 2018 by John Wiley & Sons Ltd.
Companion website: www.wiley.com/sun/comparative_cardiac_imaging

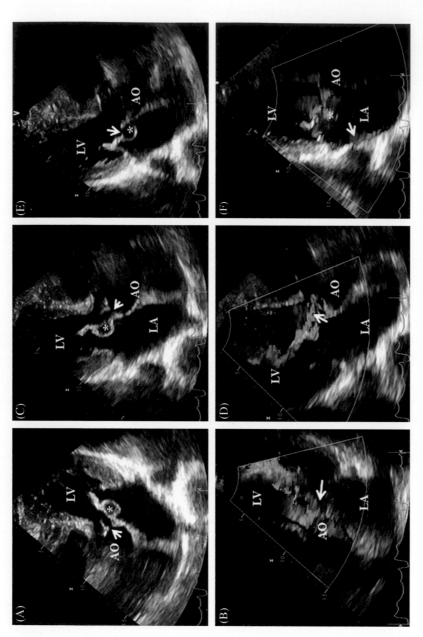

Figure 62-1 Two-dimensional echocardiogram apical long-axis view obtained during early diastole showed a hollow aneurysm [*] of the anterior mitral valve leaflet, which was bulging toward the left atrium (LA)(A), and the aortic noncoronary cusp was ruptured at the bottom (A, arrow). An apical long-axis view with color Doppler obtained at early diastole showed aortic regurgitation was from the rupture location (B, arrow). Apical long axis view without (C) and with color Doppler (D) obtained at mid-diastole showed the anterior mitral leaflet aneurysm (*) and ruptured aortic valve with aortic regurgitation (arrow). An apical long-axis view without (E) and with color Doppler obtained at systole showed a color flow filling in the anterior mitral valve aneurysm (F. *) and a mild mitral regurgitation toward to posterior wall of left atrium (arrow).

Notes: LV, left ventricle; AO, aorta.

Hospital Course

After blood was withdrawn for bacteria culture, antibacteriatherapy began but there was gastrointestinal bleeding on the second day, and the clinical conditions worsened rapidly. Plasma protamine Vice coagulation tests (3p test) were positive. Disseminated intravascular coagulation (DIC) was diagnosed. Multiple organ function failure subsequently occurred, and unfortunately the patient died.

Discussion

Our patient developed endocarditis due to bacteremia secondary to pneumonia. The patient did not receive suitable therapy, so he died due to DIC and multiple organ failure.

Infective endocarditis (IE) due to *Abiotrophia* and *Granulicatella* species, previously referred to as nutritionally variant streptococci (NVS), occurs rarely and is often associated with negative blood cultures. Rates of treatment failure, infection relapse, and mortality are higher than those of endocarditis caused by other viridians streptococci.

Mitral-valve aneurysm (MVA) is a rare condition with a reported incidence of 0.29% on 4500 transoesophageal echocardiogram (TEE) examinations [1]. On TTE it looks like a saccular bulge of the mitral leaflet protruding toward the left atrium with systolic expansion and diastolic collapse. The diastolic expansion may occur with aortic regurgitation or after rupture of the mitral valve aneurysm [2]. Anterior mitral valve aneurysm is more commonly observed than the posterior MVA [3]. In our case, anterior mitral valve aneurysm was a localized saccular bulge of the mitral valve leaflet toward the left atrium demonstrated by transthoracic echocardiography, which persisted throughout the cardiac cycle.

The development of MVA is likely due to the infected aortic regurgitant jets striking the ventricular surface of the anterior mitral leaflet, causing physical trauma and possibly occult mitral leaflet infection. This is manifested by valvulitis and the formation of sac-like outpouchings due to the formation of scar tissue and granulation tissue on microscopic examination. The extension of infection to the mitral–aortic intervalvular fibrosa results in abscess or aneurysm formation [4]. However, the posterior MVA occurs as a result of the weakness of the mitral valve secondary to myxomatous degeneration and latent infective endocarditis [3]. Vilacosta et al. studied the natural course of these aneurysms with serial echocardiographic follow-up and concluded that they undergo progressive expansion and subsequent rupture or perforation [1]. The vegetation or thrombus formation may occur within the aneurysm leading to thromboembolism and spread of infection [2].

Because mitral valve aneurysms rarely occurs in the absence of endocarditis or in patients with pure aortic regurgitation, an infectious etiology is at least partly responsible for leaflet degeneration. The compromised leaflets may then be more susceptible to aneurismal dilatation from a regurgitant jet. Aneurysms of the mitral valve have been reported in patients without a history of endocarditis but these rare cases usually occur in association with connective tissue disorders [5]. In the absence of a valve disease, the mitral valve aneurysm in association with the infected aortic valve indicate that the aneurysm in our case was caused by aortic valve endocarditis.

Mitral-valve aneurysms can be confused with several abnormalities including myxomatous degeneration of the mitral valve, mitral-valve prolapse, flail mitral leaflets, papillofibroelastomas or myxomas involving the mitral valve, and nonendothelialized cysts of the mitral valve [6].

Transthoracic echocardiography may occasionally identify subtle valvular abnormalities but TEE yields a more definitive identification [7]. Color flow Doppler distinguishes the aneurysm from these other abnormalities by demonstrating direct communication between the aneurysm and the left ventricle [8].

Early detection and prompt intervention are important to prevent the complications of valvular aneurysms, which include rupture, embolism, endocarditis and poor outcomes, such as our case.

Echocardiographic follow-up of these lesions has demonstrated progressive expansion and subsequent rupture with development of acute mitral regurgitation. Therefore, in patients with mitral valve aneurysms, repair or replacement of the valve during aortic valve replacement should be performed.

Key Points

1. Mitral valve aneurysms are uncommon, but potentially serious, complications of aortic valve endocarditis.
2. A transoesophageal echocardiogram is an excellent method for diagnosing as well as following the clinical course of mitral aneurysms and may contribute significantly to management decisions.
3. Surgical repair of these aneurysms prevents subsequent rupture and acute mitral regurgitation.

References

1. Vilacosta, I., San Roman, J.A., Sarria, C. et al. (1999). Clinical, anatomic, and echocardiographic characteristics of aneurysms of the mitral valve. *Am J Cardiol* 84: 110–113.
2. Guler, A., Karabay, C.Y., Gursoy, O.M. et al. (2014). Clinical and echocardiographic evaluation of mitral valve aneurysms: a retrospective, single center study. *Int J Cardiovasc Imaging* 30: 535–541.
3. Hotchi, J., Hoshiga, M., Okabe, T. et al. (2011). Impressive echocardiographic images of a mitral valve aneurysm. *Circulation* 123: e400–e402.
4. Reid, C.L., Chandraratna, A.N., Harrison, E. et al. (1983). Mitral valve aneurysm: clinical features, echocardiographic-pathologic correlations. *J Am College Cardiol* 2: 460–464.
5. Rachko, M.R., Safi, A.M., Yeshou, D. et al. (2001). Anterior mitral valve aneurysm: A subaortic complication of aortic valve endocarditis. *Heart Dis* 3: 145–147.
6. Changlani, M., Lieb, D., Kaczkowski, D. et al. (1993). The role of color flow Doppler in the echocardiographic diagnosis of mitral valve aneurysm. *J Am Soc Echocardiogr* 6: 610–612.
7. Mollod, M., Felner, K.J. and Felner, J.M. (1997). Mitral and tricuspid valve aneurysms evaluated by transesophageal echocardiography. *Am J Cardiol* 79: 1269–1272.
8. Vilacosta, I., San Roman, J.A., Sarria, C. et al. (1999). Clinical, anatomic and echocardiographic characteristics of aneurysms of the mitral valve. *Am J Cardiol* 84 (1): 110–113.

Index

Comparative Cardiac Imaging: A Case-based Guide, First Edition.
Edited by Jing Ping Sun, Xing Sheng Yang, and Bryan P. Yan.
© 2018 John Wiley & Sons Ltd. Published 2018 by John Wiley & Sons Ltd.
Companion website: www.wiley.com/sun/comparative_cardiac_imaging